Position, Consensus, Official and Support Statements

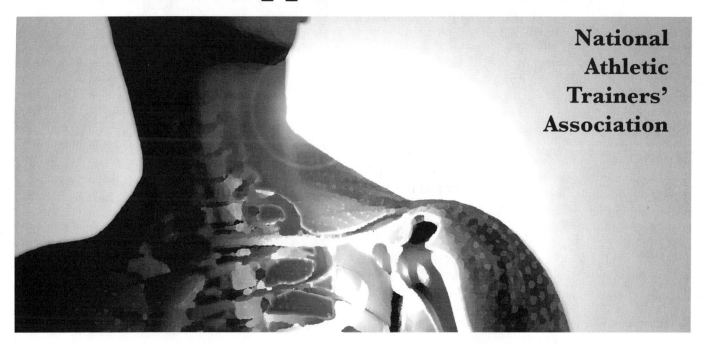

National Athletic Trainers' Association

Our sincere thanks to Douglas Casa, PhD, ATC, FACSM, FNATA and Susan Rozzi, PhD, ATC for their assistance with this project and to Chad Starkey, PhD, ATC, LAT, FNATA for providing the inspiration for this textbook.

Editorial Content Coordinator: **Rachael Oats**
Cover and Book Designer: **Jordan Bostic**
Print Production: **Brian Hawkins**

Contents

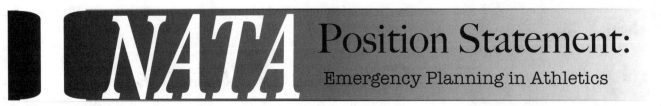

NATA Position Statement:
Emergency Planning in Athletics

In This Section:

The National Athletic Trainers' Association believes emergency planning is essential to handling unpredictable limb- and life-threatening situations that occur in athletics. This position statement discusses the need for emergency planning and details the components of a thorough emergency action plan.

National Athletic Trainers' Association Position Statement: Emergency Planning in Athletics

J. C. Andersen*; Ronald W. Courson†; Douglas M. Kleiner‡; Todd A. McLoda§

*Armstrong Atlantic State University, Savannah, GA; †University of Georgia, Athens, GA; ‡University of Florida, Health Science Center/Jacksonville, Jacksonville, FL; §Illinois State University, Normal, IL

J. C. Andersen, PhD, ATC, PT, SCS, contributed to conception and design; acquisition and analysis and interpretation of the data; and drafting, critical revision, and final approval of the article. Ronald W. Courson, ATC, PT, NREMT-I, CSCS, Douglas M. Kleiner, PhD, ATC, CSCS, NREMT, FACSM, and Todd A. McLoda, PhD, ATC, contributed to acquisition and analysis and interpretation of the data and drafting, critical revision, and final approval of the article.

Address correspondence to National Athletic Trainers' Association, Communications Department, 2952 Stemmons Freeway, Dallas, TX 75247.

Objectives: To educate athletic trainers and others about the need for emergency planning, to provide guidelines in the development of emergency plans, and to advocate documentation of emergency planning.

Background: Most injuries sustained during athletics or other physical activity are relatively minor. However, potentially limb-threatening or life-threatening emergencies in athletics and physical activity are unpredictable and occur without warning. Proper management of these injuries is critical and should be carried out by trained health services personnel to minimize risk to the injured participant. The organization or institution and its personnel can be placed at risk by the lack of an emergency plan, which may be the foundation of a legal claim.

Recommendations: The National Athletic Trainers' Association recommends that each organization or institution that sponsors athletic activities or events develop and implement a written emergency plan. Emergency plans should be developed by organizational or institutional personnel in consultation with the local emergency medical services. Components of the emergency plan include identification of the personnel involved, specification of the equipment needed to respond to the emergency, and establishment of a communication system to summon emergency care. Additional components of the emergency plan are identification of the mode of emergency transport, specification of the venue or activity location, and incorporation of emergency service personnel into the development and implementation process. Emergency plans should be reviewed and rehearsed annually, with written documentation of any modifications. The plan should identify responsibility for documentation of actions taken during the emergency, evaluation of the emergency response, institutional personnel training, and equipment maintenance. Further, training of the involved personnel should include automatic external defibrillation, cardiopulmonary resuscitation, first aid, and prevention of disease transmission.

Key Words: policies and procedures, athletics, planning, catastrophic

---

Although most injuries that occur in athletics are relatively minor, limb-threatening or life-threatening injuries are unpredictable and can occur without warning.[1] Because of the relatively low incidence rate of catastrophic injuries, athletic program personnel may develop a false sense of security over time in the absence of such injuries.[1-4] However, these injuries can occur during any physical activity and at any level of participation. Of additional concern is the heightened public awareness associated with the nature and management of such injuries. Medicolegal interests can lead to questions about the qualifications of the personnel involved, the preparedness of the organization for handling these situations, and the actions taken by program personnel.[5]

Proper emergency management of limb- or life-threatening injuries is critical and should be handled by trained medical and allied health personnel.[1-4] Preparation for response to emergencies includes education and training, maintenance of emergency equipment and supplies, appropriate use of personnel, and the formation and implementation of an emergency plan. The emergency plan should be thought of as a blueprint for handling emergencies. A sound emergency plan is easily understood and establishes accountability for the management of emergencies. Furthermore, failure to have an emergency plan can be considered negligence.[5]

POSITION STATEMENT

Based on an extensive survey of the literature and expert review, the following is the position of the National Athletic Trainers' Association (NATA):

1. Each institution or organization that sponsors athletic activities must have a written emergency plan. The emergency plan should be comprehensive and practical, yet flexible enough to adapt to any emergency situation.

2. Emergency plans must be written documents and should be distributed to certified athletic trainers, team and at-

tending physicians, athletic training students, institutional and organizational safety personnel, institutional and organizational administrators, and coaches. The emergency plan should be developed in consultation with local emergency medical services personnel.

3. An emergency plan for athletics identifies the personnel involved in carrying out the emergency plan and outlines the qualifications of those executing the plan. Sports medicine professionals, officials, and coaches should be trained in automatic external defibrillation, cardiopulmonary resuscitation, first aid, and prevention of disease transmission.

4. The emergency plan should specify the equipment needed to carry out the tasks required in the event of an emergency. In addition, the emergency plan should outline the location of the emergency equipment. Further, the equipment available should be appropriate to the level of training of the personnel involved.

5. Establishment of a clear mechanism for communication to appropriate emergency care service providers and identification of the mode of transportation for the injured participant are critical elements of an emergency plan.

6. The emergency plan should be specific to the activity venue. That is, each activity site should have a defined emergency plan that is derived from the overall institutional or organizational policies on emergency planning.

7. Emergency plans should incorporate the emergency care facilities to which the injured individual will be taken. Emergency receiving facilities should be notified in advance of scheduled events and contests. Personnel from the emergency receiving facilities should be included in the development of the emergency plan for the institution or organization.

8. The emergency plan specifies the necessary documentation supporting the implementation and evaluation of the emergency plan. This documentation should identify responsibility for documenting actions taken during the emergency, evaluation of the emergency response, and institutional personnel training.

9. The emergency plan should be reviewed and rehearsed annually, although more frequent review and rehearsal may be necessary. The results of these reviews and rehearsals should be documented and should indicate whether the emergency plan was modified, with further documentation reflecting how the plan was changed.

10. All personnel involved with the organization and sponsorship of athletic activities share a professional responsibility to provide for the emergency care of an injured person, including the development and implementation of an emergency plan.

11. All personnel involved with the organization and sponsorship of athletic activities share a legal duty to develop, implement, and evaluate an emergency plan for all sponsored athletic activities.

12. The emergency plan should be reviewed by the administration and legal counsel of the sponsoring organization or institution.

BACKGROUND FOR THIS POSITION STAND

Need for Emergency Plans

Emergencies, accidents, and natural disasters are rarely predictable; however, when they do occur, rapid, controlled response will likely make the difference between an effective and an ineffective emergency response. Response can be hindered by the chaotic actions and increased emotions of those who make attempts to help persons who are injured or in danger. One method of control for these unpredictable events is an emergency plan that, if well designed and rehearsed, can provide responders with an organized approach to their reaction. The development of the emergency plan takes care and time to ensure that all necessary contingencies have been included. Lessons learned from major emergencies are also important to consider when developing or revising an emergency plan.

Emergency plans are applicable to agencies of the government, such as law enforcement, fire and rescue, and federal emergency management teams. Furthermore, the use of emergency plans is directly applicable to sport and fitness activities due to the inherent possibility of "an untoward event" that requires access to emergency medical services.[6] Of course, when developing an emergency plan for athletics, there is one notable difference from those used by local, state, and federal emergency management personnel. With few exceptions, typically only one athlete, fan, or sideline participant is at risk at one time due to bleeding, internal injury, cardiac arrest, shock, or traumatic head or spine injury. However, emergency planning in athletics should account for an untoward event involving a game official, fan, or sideline participant as well as the participating athlete. Although triage in athletic emergency situations may be rare, this does not minimize the risks involved and the need for carefully prepared emergency care plans. The need for emergency plans in athletics can be divided into 2 major categories: professional and legal.

Professional Need. The first category for consideration in determining the need for emergency plans in athletics is organizational and professional responsibility. Certain governing bodies associated with athletic competition have stated that institutions and organizations must provide for access to emergency medical services if an emergency should occur during any aspect of athletic activity, including in-season and off-season activities.[6] The National Collegiate Athletic Association (NCAA) has recommended that all member institutions develop an emergency plan for their athletic programs.[7] The National Federation of State High School Associations has recommended the same at the secondary school level.[8] The NCAA states, "Each scheduled practice or contest of an institution-sponsored intercollegiate athletics event, as well as out-of-season practices and skills sessions, should include an emergency plan."[6] The *1999–2000 NCAA Sports Medicine Handbook* further outlines the key components of the emergency plan.[6]

Although the *1999–2000 NCAA Sports Medicine Handbook* is a useful guide, a recent survey of NCAA member institutions revealed that at least 10% of the institutions do not maintain any form of an emergency plan.[7] In addition, more than one third of the institutions do not maintain emergency plans for the off-season strength and conditioning activities of the sports.

Personnel coverage at NCAA institutions was also found to be an issue. Nearly all schools provided personnel qualified to administer emergency care for high-risk contact sports, but fewer than two thirds of institutions provided adequate personnel to sports such as cross-country and track.[9] In a memorandum dated March 25, 1999, and sent to key personnel at all schools, the president of the NCAA reiterated the recommendations in the *1999–2000 NCAA Sports Medicine Handbook* to maintain emergency plans for all sport activities, including skill instruction, conditioning, and the nontraditional practice seasons.[8]

A need for emergency preparedness is further recognized by several national organizations concerned with the delivery of health care services to fitness and sport participants, including the NATA Education Council,[10] NATA Board of Certification, Inc,[11] American College of Sports Medicine, International Health Racquet and Sports Club Association, American College of Cardiology, and Young Men's Christian Association.[12] The NATA-approved athletic training educational competencies for athletic trainers include several references to emergency action plans.[10] The knowledge of the key components of an emergency plan, the ability to recognize and appraise emergency plans, and the ability to develop emergency plans are all considered required tasks of the athletic trainer.[11] These responsibilities justify the need for the athletic trainer to be involved in the development and application of emergency plans as a partial fulfillment of his or her professional obligations.

In addition to the equipment and personnel involved in emergency response, the emergency plan must include consideration for the sport activity and rules of competition, the weather conditions, and the level of competition.[13] The variation in these factors makes venue-specific planning necessary because of the numerous contingencies that may occur. For example, many youth sport activities include both new participants of various sizes who may not know the rules of the activity and those who have participated for years. Also, outdoor sport activities include the possibility of lightning strikes, excessive heat and humidity, and excessive cold, among other environmental concerns that may not be factors during indoor activities. Organizations in areas of the country in which snow may accumulate must consider provisions for ensuring that accessibility by emergency vehicles is not hampered. In addition, the availability of safety equipment that is necessary for participation may be an issue for those in underserved areas. The burden of considering all the possible contingencies in light of the various situations must rest on the professionals, who are best trained to recognize the need for emergency plans and who can develop and implement the venue-specific plans.

Legal Need. Also of significance is the legal basis for the development and application of an emergency plan. It is well known that organizational medical personnel, including certified athletic trainers, have a legal duty as reasonable and prudent professionals to ensure high-quality care of the participants. Of further legal precedence is the accepted standard of care by which allied health professionals are measured.[14] This standard of care provides necessary accountability for the actions of both the practitioners and the governing body that oversees those practitioners. The emergency plan has been categorized as a written document that defines the standard of care required during an emergency situation.[15] Herbert[16] emphasized that well-formulated, adequately written, and periodically rehearsed emergency response protocols are absolutely required by sports medicine programs. Herbert[16] further stated that the absence of an emergency plan frequently is the basis for claim and suit based on negligence.

One key indicator for the need for an emergency action plan is the concept of foreseeability. The organization administrators and the members of the sports medicine team must question whether a particular emergency situation has a reasonable possibility of occurring during the sport activity in question.[14,15,17] For example, if it is reasonably possible that a catastrophic event such as a head injury, spine injury, or other severe trauma may occur during practice, conditioning, or competition in a sport, a previously prepared emergency plan must be in place. The medical and allied health care personnel must constantly be on guard for potential injuries, and although the occurrence of limb-threatening or life-threatening emergencies is not common, the potential exists. Therefore, prepared emergency responders must have planned in advance for the action to be taken in the event of such an emergency.

Several legal claims and suits have indicated or alluded to the need for emergency plans. In *Gathers v Loyola Marymount University*,[18] the state court settlement included a statement that care was delayed for the injured athlete, and the plaintiffs further alleged that the defendants acted negligently and carelessly in not providing appropriate emergency response. These observations strongly support the need to have clear emergency plans in place, rehearsed, and carried out. In several additional cases,[19–21] the courts have stated that proper care was delayed, and it can be reasoned that these delays could have been avoided with the application of a well-prepared emergency plan.

Perhaps the most significant case bearing on the need for emergency planning is *Kleinknecht v Gettysburg College,* which came before the appellate court in 1993.[5,17] In a portion of the decision, the court stated that the college owed a duty to the athletes who are recruited to be athletes at the institution. Further, as a part of that duty, the college must provide "prompt and adequate emergency services while engaged in the school-sponsored intercollegiate athletic activity for which the athlete had been recruited."[17] The same court further ruled that reasonable measures must be ensured and in place to provide prompt treatment of emergency situations. One can conclude from these rulings that planning is critical to ensure prompt and proper emergency medical care, further validating the need for an emergency plan.[5]

Based on the review of the legal and professional literature, there is no doubt regarding the need for organizations at all levels that sponsor athletic activities to maintain an up-to-date, thorough, and regularly rehearsed emergency plan. Furthermore, members of the sports medicine team have both legal and professional obligations to perform this duty to protect the interests of both the participating athletes and the organization or institution. At best, failure to do so will inevitably result in inefficient athlete care, whereas at worst, gross negligence and potential life-threatening ramifications for the injured athlete or organizational personnel are likely.

Components of Emergency Plans

Organizations that sponsor athletic activities have a duty to develop an emergency plan that can be implemented immediately and to provide appropriate standards of health care to all sports participants.[5,14,15,17] Athletic injuries may occur at any time and during any activity. The sports medicine team must be prepared through the formulation of an emergency plan, proper coverage of events, maintenance of appropriate emergency equipment and supplies, use of appropriate emergency medical personnel, and continuing education in the area of emergency medicine. Some potential emergencies may be averted through careful preparticipation physical

_____University Sports Medicine Football Emergency Protocol

1. Call 911 or other emergency number consistent with organizational policies
2. Instruct emergency medical services (EMS) personnel to "report to _____ and meet _____ at _____ as we have an injured student-athlete in need of emergency medical treatment."
   University Football Practice Complex: _____ Street entrance (gate across street from _____) *cross street:* _____ Street
   University Stadium: Gate _____ entrance off _____ Road
3. Provide necessary information to EMS personnel:
   - name, address, telephone number of caller
   - number of victims; condition of victims
   - first-aid treatment initiated
   - specific directions as needed to locate scene
   - other information as requested by dispatcher
4. Provide appropriate emergency care until arrival of EMS personnel: on arrival of EMS personnel, provide pertinent information (method of injury, vital signs, treatment rendered, medical history) and assist with emergency care as needed

Note:

- sports medicine staff member should accompany student-athlete to hospital
- notify other sports medicine staff immediately
- parents should be contacted by sports medicine staff
- inform coach(es) and administration
- obtain medical history and insurance information
- appropriate injury reports should be completed

Emergency Telephone Numbers
_____ Hospital   _____ - _____
_____ Emergency Department   _____ - _____
University Health Center   _____ - _____
Campus Police   _____ - _____

Emergency Signals

Physician: arm extended overhead with clenched first
Paramedics: point to location in end zone by home locker room and wave onto field
Spine board: arms held horizontally
Stretcher: supinated hands in front of body or waist level
Splints: hand to lower leg or thigh

---

screenings, adequate medical coverage, safe practice and training techniques, and other safety measures.[1,22] However, accidents and injuries are inherent with sports participation, and proper preparation on the part of the sports medicine team will enable each emergency situation to be managed appropriately.

The goal of the sports medicine team is the delivery of the highest possible quality health care to the athlete. Management of the emergency situation that occurs during athletic activities may involve certified athletic trainers and students, emergency medical personnel, physicians, and coaches working together. Just as with an athletic team, the sports medicine team must work together as an efficient unit to accomplish its goals.[22] In an emergency situation, the team concept becomes even more critical, because time is crucial and seconds may mean the difference among life, death, and permanent disability. The sharing of information, training, and skills among the various emergency medical care providers helps reach the goal.[22,23]

Implementation. Once the importance of the emergency plan is realized and the plan has been developed, the plan must be implemented. Implementation of the emergency plan requires 3 basic steps.[23]

First, the plan must be committed to writing (Table) to provide a clear response mechanism and to allow for continuity among emergency team members.[14,16] This can be accomplished by using a flow sheet or an organizational chart. It is also important to have a separate plan or to modify the plan for different athletic venues and for practices and games. Emergency team members, such as the team physician, who are present at games may not necessarily be present at practices. Moreover, the location and type of equipment and communication devices may differ among sports, venues, and activity levels.

The second step is education.[23] It is important to educate all the members of the emergency team regarding the emergency plan. All personnel should be familiar with the emergency medical services system that will provide coverage to their venues and include their input in the emergency plan. Each team member, as well as institution or organization administrators, should have a written copy of the emergency plan that provides documentation of his or her roles and responsibilities in emergency situations. A copy of the emergency plan specific to each venue should be posted prominently by the available telephone.

Third, the emergency plan and procedures have to be rehearsed.[16] This provides team members a chance to maintain their emergency skills at a high level of competency. It also provides an opportunity for athletic trainers and emergency medical personnel to communicate regarding specific policies and procedures in their particular region of practice.[22] This rehearsal can be accomplished through an annual in-service meeting, preferably before the highest-risk sports season (eg, football, ice hockey, lacrosse). Reviews should be undertaken as needed throughout the sports season, because emergency medical procedures and personnel may change.

Personnel. In an athletic environment, the first person who responds to an emergency situation may vary widely[22,24]; it may be a coach or a game official, a certified athletic trainer, an emergency medical technician, or a physician. This variation in the first responder makes it imperative that an emergency plan be in place and rehearsed. With a plan in place and rehearsed, these differently trained individuals will be able to work together as an effective team when responding to emergency situations.

The plan should also outline who is responsible for summoning help and clearing the uninjured from the area.

In addition, all personnel associated with practices, competitions, skills instruction, and strength and conditioning activities should have training in automatic external defibrillation and current certification in cardiopulmonary resuscitation, first aid, and the prevention of disease transmission.[5,7]

Equipment. All necessary supplemental equipment should be at the site and quickly accessible.[13,25] Equipment should be in good operating condition, and personnel must be trained in advance to use it properly. Improvements in technology and emergency training require personnel to become familiar with the use of automatic external defibrillators, oxygen, and advanced airways.

It is imperative that health professionals and organizational administrators recognize that recent guidelines published by the American Heart Association call for the availability and use of automatic external defibrillators and that defibrillation is considered a component of basic life support.[26] In addition, these guidelines emphasize use of the bag-valve mask in emergency resuscitation and the use of emergency oxygen and advanced airways in emergency care. Personnel should consider receiving appropriate training for these devices and should limit use to devices for which they have been trained.

To ensure that emergency equipment is in working order, all equipment should be checked on a regular basis. Also, the use of equipment should be regularly rehearsed by emergency personnel, and the emergency equipment that is available should be appropriate for the level of training of the emergency medical providers and the venue.

Communication. Access to a working telephone or other telecommunications device, whether fixed or mobile, should be ensured.[5,17,21] The communications system should be checked before each practice or competition to ensure proper working order. A back-up communication plan should be in effect in case the primary communication system fails. A listing of appropriate emergency numbers should be either posted by the communication system or readily available, as well as the street address of the venue and specific directions (cross streets, landmarks, and so on) (Table).

Transportation. The emergency plan should encompass transportation of the sick and injured. Emphasis should be placed on having an ambulance on site at high-risk events.[15] Emergency medical services response time should also be factored in when determining on-site ambulance coverage. Consideration should be given to the level of transportation service that is available (eg, basic life support, advanced life support) and the equipment and training level of the personnel who staff the ambulance.[23]

In the event that an ambulance is on site, a location should be designated with rapid access to the site and a cleared route for entering and exiting the venue.[19] In the emergency evaluation, the primary survey assists the emergency care provider in identifying emergencies that require critical intervention

and in determining transport decisions. In an emergency situation, the athlete should be transported by ambulance to the most appropriate receiving facility, where the necessary staff and equipment can deliver appropriate care.[23]

In addition, a plan must be available to ensure that the activity areas are supervised if the emergency care provider leaves the site to transport the athlete.

Venue Location. The emergency plan should be venue specific, based on the site of the practice or competition and the activity involved (Table). The plan for each venue should encompass accessibility to emergency personnel, communication system, equipment, and transportation.

At home sites, the host medical providers should orient the visiting medical personnel regarding the site, emergency personnel, equipment available, and procedures associated with the emergency plan.

At away or neutral sites, the coach or athletic trainer should identify, before the event, the availability of communication with emergency medical services and should verify service and reception, particularly in rural areas. In addition, the name and location of the nearest emergency care facility and the availability of an ambulance at the event site should be ascertained.

Emergency Care Facilities. The emergency plan should incorporate access to an emergency medical facility. In selection of the appropriate facility, consideration should be given to the location with respect to the athletic venue. Consideration should also include the level of service available at the emergency facility.

The designated emergency facility and emergency medical services should be notified in advance of athletic events. Furthermore, it is recommended that the emergency plan be reviewed with both medical facility administrators and in-service medical staff regarding pertinent issues involved in athlete care, such as proper removal of athletic equipment in the facility when appropriate.[22,23,27]

Documentation. A written emergency plan should be reviewed and approved by sports medicine team members and institutions involved. If multiple facilities or sites are to be used, each will require a separate plan. Additional documentation should encompass the following[15,16]:

1. Delineation of the person and/or group responsible for documenting the events of the emergency situation
2. Follow-up documentation on evaluation of response to emergency situation
3. Documentation of regular rehearsal of the emergency plan
4. Documentation of personnel training
5. Documentation of emergency equipment maintenance

It is prudent to invest organizational and institutional ownership in the emergency plan by involving administrators and sport coaches as well as sports medicine personnel in the planning and documentation process. The emergency plan should be reviewed at least annually with all involved personnel. Any revisions or modifications should be reviewed and approved by the personnel involved at all levels of the sponsoring organization or institution and of the responding emergency medical services.

SUMMARY

The purpose of this statement is to present the position of the NATA on emergency planning in athletics. Specifically,

9

professional and legal requirements mandate that organizations or institutions sponsoring athletic activities have a written emergency plan. A well-thought-out emergency plan consists of a number of factors, including, but not necessarily limited to, personnel, equipment, communication, transportation, and documentation. Finally, all sports medicine professionals, coaches, and organizational administrators share professional and legal duties to develop, implement, and evaluate emergency plans for sponsored athletic activities.

ACKNOWLEDGMENTS

This position statement was reviewed for the National Athletic Trainers' Association by the Pronouncements Committee and by John Cottone, EdD, ATC; Francis X. Feld, MEd, MS, CRNA, ATC, NREMT-P; and Richard Ray, EdD, ATC.

REFERENCES

1. Arnheim DD, Prentice WE. *Principles of Athletic Training*. 9th ed. Madison, WI: WCB/McGraw-Hill Inc; 1997.
2. Dolan MG. Emergency care: planning for the worst. *Athl Ther Today*. 1998;3(1):12–13.
3. Kleiner DM, Glickman SE. Considerations for the athletic trainer in planning medical coverage for short distance road races. *J Athl Train*. 1994; 29:145–151.
4. Nowlan WP, Davis GA, McDonald B. Preparing for sudden emergencies. *Athl Ther Today*. 1996;1(1):45–47.
5. Shea JF. Duties of care owed to university athletes in light of Kleinecht. *J Coll Univ Law*. 1995;21:591–614.
6. Halpin T, Dick RW. *1999–2000 NCAA Sports Medicine Handbook*. Indianapolis, IN: National Collegiate Athletic Association; 1999.
7. Brown GT. NCAA group raising awareness on medical coverage. *NCAA News*. 1999; March 15:6–7.
8. Shultz SJ, Zinder SM, Valovich TC. *Sports Medicine Handbook*. Indianapolis, IN: National Federation of State High School Associations; 2001.
9. Dempsey CW. *Memorandum to all National Collegiate Athletic Association Institutions: Emergency Care and Coverage at NCAA Institutions*. Indianapolis, IN: National Collegiate Athletics Association; March 25, 1999.
10. National Athletic Trainers' Association Education Council. *Athletic Training Educational Competencies*. 3rd ed. Dallas, TX: National Athletic Trainers' Association; 1999.
11. National Athletic Trainers' Association Board of Certification. *Role Delineation Study of the Entry-Level Athletic Trainer Certification Examination*. 3rd ed. Philadelphia, PA: FA Davis; 1995.
12. Herbert DL. Do you need a written emergency response plan? *Sports Med Stand Malpract Rep*. 1999;11:S17–S24.
13. Rubin A. Emergency equipment: what to keep on the sidelines. *Physician Sportsmed*. 1993;21(9):47–54.
14. Appenzeller H. *Managing Sports and Risk Management Strategies*. Durham, NC: Carolina Academic Press; 1993:99–110.
15. Rankin JM, Ingersoll C. *Athletic Training Management: Concepts and Applications*. St Louis, MO: Mosby-Year Book Inc; 1995:175–183.
16. Herbert DL. *Legal Aspects of Sports Medicine*. Canton, OH: Professional Reports Corp; 1990:160–167.
17. *Kleinknecht v Gettysburg College*, 989 F2d 1360 (3rd Cir 1993).
18. *Gathers v Loyola Marymount University*. Case No. C759027, Los Angeles Super Court (settled 1992).
19. *Mogabgab v Orleans Parish School Board*, 239 So2d 456 (Court of Appeals, Los Angeles, 970).
20. *Hanson v Kynast*, 494 NE2d 1091 (Oh 1986).
21. *Montgomery v City of Detroit*, 448 NW2d 822 (Mich App 1989).
22. Kleiner DM. Emergency management of athletic trauma: roles and responsibilities. *Emerg Med Serv*. 1998;10:33–36.
23. Courson RW, Duncan K. *The Emergency Plan in Athletic Training Emergency Care*. Boston, MA: Jones & Bartlett Publishers; 2000:
24. National Athletic Trainers' Association. Establishing communication with EMTs. *NATA News*. June 1994:4–9.
25. Waeckerle JF. Planning for emergencies. *Physician Sportsmed*. 1991; 19(2):35, 38.
26. American Heart Association. Guidelines 2000 for cardiopulmonary resuscitation and emergency cardiovascular care: international consensus on science. *Curr Emerg Cardiovasc Care*. 2000;11:3–15.
27. Kleiner DM, Almquist JL, Bailes J, et al. *Prehospital Care of the Spine-Injured Athlete: A Document from the Inter-Association Task Force for Appropriate Care of the Spine-Injured Athlete*. Dallas, TX: National Athletic Trainers' Association; 2001.

Emergency Planning Review Questions:

1. Detail the recommended components of an emergency action plan and explain how these components may vary based on sports level (high school, college, professional) and location (soccer field, basketball court, aquatic center).

2. The position statement recommends that emergency action plans are reviewed and rehearsed annually. Explain why this recommendation is important and propose possible negative consequences that might occur if an athletic training site's emergency action plan has not been reviewed or rehearsed in more than three years.

3. Review the emergency action plan at your athletic training site. Note the recommendations in this position statement that your plan is currently meeting and areas where your plan is falling short. Explain changes you can make to adopt more or all of the recommendations in this statement.

NATA Position Statement:
Exertional Heat Illnesses

In This Section: Heat illness is associated with physical activity and is a very important issue to athletic trainers. Athletes participating in outdoor sports in humid climates are especially at risk for exertional heat illness. This position statement defines the various heat illnesses and gives recommendations for the prevention, recognition and treatment of these conditions.

National Athletic Trainers' Association Position Statement: Exertional Heat Illnesses

Helen M. Binkley*; Joseph Beckett†; Douglas J. Casa‡;
Douglas M. Kleiner§; Paul E. Plummer‖

*Mesa State College, Grand Junction, CO; †University of Charleston, Charleston, WV; ‡University of Connecticut, Storrs, CT; §University of Florida, Jacksonville, FL; ‖Indiana State University, Terre Haute, IN

*Helen M. Binkley, PhD, ATC, CSCS*D, NSCA-CPT (Chair), contributed to conception and design; acquisition of the data; and drafting, critical revision, and final approval of the article. Joseph Beckett, EdD, ATC, contributed to acquisition of the data and drafting, critical revision, and final approval of the article. Douglas J. Casa, PhD, ATC, FACSM, contributed to conception and design; acquisition of the data; and drafting, critical revision, and final approval of the article. Douglas M. Kleiner, PhD, ATC, FACSM, and Paul E. Plummer, MA, ATC, contributed to acquisition of the data and drafting, critical revision, and final approval of the article.*

Address correspondence to National Athletic Trainers' Association, Communications Department, 2952 Stemmons Freeway, Dallas, TX 75247.

Objective: To present recommendations for the prevention, recognition, and treatment of exertional heat illnesses and to describe the relevant physiology of thermoregulation.

Background: Certified athletic trainers evaluate and treat heat-related injuries during athletic activity in "safe" and high-risk environments. While the recognition of heat illness has improved, the subtle signs and symptoms associated with heat illness are often overlooked, resulting in more serious problems for affected athletes. The recommendations presented here provide athletic trainers and allied health providers with an integrated scientific and practical approach to the prevention, recognition, and treatment of heat illnesses. These recommendations can be modified based on the environmental conditions of the site, the specific sport, and individual considerations to maximize safety and performance.

Recommendations: Certified athletic trainers and other allied health providers should use these recommendations to establish on-site emergency plans for their venues and athletes. The primary goal of athlete safety is addressed through the prevention and recognition of heat-related illnesses and a well-developed plan to evaluate and treat affected athletes. Even with a heat-illness prevention plan that includes medical screening, acclimatization, conditioning, environmental monitoring, and suitable practice adjustments, heat illness can and does occur. Athletic trainers and other allied health providers must be prepared to respond in an expedient manner to alleviate symptoms and minimize morbidity and mortality.

Key Words: heat cramps, heat syncope, heat exhaustion, heat stroke, hyponatremia, dehydration, exercise, heat tolerance

Heat illness is inherent to physical activity and its incidence increases with rising ambient temperature and relative humidity. Athletes who begin training in the late summer (eg, football, soccer, and cross-country athletes) experience exertional heat-related illness more often than athletes who begin training during the winter and spring.[1-5] Although the hot conditions associated with late summer provide a simple explanation for this difference, we need to understand what makes certain athletes more susceptible and how these illnesses can be prevented.

PURPOSE

This position statement provides recommendations that will enable certified athletic trainers (ATCs) and other allied health providers to (1) identify and implement preventive strategies that can reduce heat-related illnesses in sports, (2) characterize factors associated with the early detection of heat illness, (3) provide on-site first aid and emergency management of athletes with heat illnesses, (4) determine appropriate return-to-play procedures, (5) understand thermoregulation and physiologic responses to heat, and (6) recognize groups with special concerns related to heat exposure.

ORGANIZATION

This position statement is organized as follows:

1. Definitions of exertional heat illnesses, including exercise-associated muscle (heat) cramps, heat syncope, exercise (heat) exhaustion, exertional heat stroke, and exertional hyponatremia;
2. Recommendations for the prevention, recognition, and treatment of exertional heat illnesses;
3. Background and literature review of the diagnosis of exertional heat illnesses; risk factors; predisposing medical conditions; environmental risk factors; thermoregulation, heat acclimatization, cumulative dehydration, and cooling therapies;

Table 1. Signs and Symptoms of Exertional Heat Illnesses

Condition
Sign or Symptom*

Exercise-associated muscle (heat) cramps[6,9–11]
  Dehydration
  Thirst
  Sweating
  Transient muscle cramps
  Fatigue
Heat syncope[10,12]
  Dehydration
  Fatigue
  Tunnel vision
  Pale or sweaty skin
  Decreased pulse rate
  Dizziness
  Lightheadedness
  Fainting
Exercise (heat) exhaustion[6,9,10,13]
  Normal or elevated body-core temperature
  Dehydration
  Dizziness
  Lightheadedness
  Syncope
  Headache
  Nausea
  Anorexia
  Diarrhea
  Decreased urine output
  Persistent muscle cramps
  Pallor
  Profuse sweating
  Chills
  Cool, clammy skin
  Intestinal cramps
  Urge to defecate
  Weakness
  Hyperventilation
Exertional heat stroke[6,9,10,14]
  High body-core temperature ($>40°C$ [$104°F$])
  Central nervous system changes
    Dizziness
    Drowsiness
    Irrational behavior
    Confusion
    Irritability
    Emotional instability
    Hysteria
    Apathy
    Aggressiveness
    Delirium
    Disorientation
    Staggering
    Seizures
    Loss of consciousness
    Coma
  Dehydration
  Weakness
  Hot and wet or dry skin
  Tachycardia (100 to 120 beats per minute)
  Hypotension
  Hyperventilation
  Vomiting
  Diarrhea
Exertional hyponatremia[15–18]
  Body-core temperature $<40°C$ ($104°F$)
  Nausea
  Vomiting

Table 1. Continued

Condition
Sign or Symptom*

  Extremity (hands and feet) swelling
  Low blood-sodium level
  Progressive headache
  Confusion
  Significant mental compromise
  Lethargy
  Altered consciousness
  Apathy
  Pulmonary edema
  Cerebral edema
  Seizures
  Coma

*Not every patient will present with all the signs and symptoms for the suspected condition.

4. Special concerns regarding exertional heat illnesses in pre-pubescent athletes, older athletes, and athletes with spinal-cord injuries;
5. Hospitalization and recovery from exertional heat stroke and resumption of activity after heat-related collapse; and
6. Conclusions.

DEFINITIONS OF EXERTIONAL HEAT ILLNESSES

The traditional classification of heat illness defines 3 categories: heat cramps, heat exhaustion, and heat stroke.[6–8] However, this classification scheme omits several other heat- and activity-related illnesses, including heat syncope and exertional hyponatremia. The signs and symptoms of the exertional heat illnesses are listed in Table 1.

Heat illness is more likely in hot, humid weather but can occur in the absence of hot and humid conditions.

Exercise-Associated Muscle (Heat) Cramps

Exercise-associated muscle (heat) cramps represent a condition that presents during or after intense exercise sessions as an acute, painful, involuntary muscle contraction. Proposed causes include fluid deficiencies (dehydration), electrolyte imbalances, neuromuscular fatigue, or any combination of these factors.[6,9–11,19]

Heat Syncope

Heat syncope, or orthostatic dizziness, can occur when a person is exposed to high environmental temperatures.[19] This condition is attributed to peripheral vasodilation, postural pooling of blood, diminished venous return, dehydration, reduction in cardiac output, and cerebral ischemia.[10,19] Heat syncope usually occurs during the first 5 days of acclimatization, before the blood volume expands,[12] or in persons with heart disease or those taking diuretics.[10] It often occurs after standing for long periods of time, immediately after cessation of activity, or after rapid assumption of upright posture after resting or being seated.

Exercise (Heat) Exhaustion

Exercise (heat) exhaustion is the inability to continue exercise associated with any combination of heavy sweating, dehydration, sodium loss, and energy depletion. It occurs most frequently in hot, humid conditions. At its worst, it is difficult to distinguish from exertional heat stroke without measuring rectal temperature. Other signs and symptoms include pallor, persistent muscular cramps, urge to defecate, weakness, fainting, dizziness, headache, hyperventilation, nausea, anorexia, diarrhea, decreased urine output, and a body-core temperature that generally ranges between 36°C (97°F) and 40°C (104°F).[6,9,10,13,19]

Exertional Heat Stroke

Exertional heat stroke is an elevated core temperature (usually >40°C [104°F]) associated with signs of organ system failure due to hyperthermia. The central nervous system neurologic changes are often the first marker of exertional heat stroke. Exertional heat stroke occurs when the temperature regulation system is overwhelmed due to excessive endogenous heat production or inhibited heat loss in challenging environmental conditions[20] and can progress to complete thermoregulatory system failure.[19,21] This condition is life threatening and can be fatal unless promptly recognized and treated. Signs and symptoms include tachycardia, hypotension, sweating (although skin may be wet or dry at the time of collapse), hyperventilation, altered mental status, vomiting, diarrhea, seizures, and coma.[6,10,14] The risk of morbidity and mortality is greater the longer an athlete's body temperature remains above 41°C (106°F) and is significantly reduced if body temperature is lowered rapidly.[22–24]

Unlike classic heat stroke, which typically involves prolonged heat exposure in infants, elderly persons, or unhealthy, sedentary adults in whom body heat-regulation mechanisms are inefficient,[25–27] exertional heat stroke occurs during physical activity.[28] The pathophysiology of exertional heat stroke is due to the overheating of organ tissues that may induce malfunction of the temperature-control center in the brain, circulatory failure, or endotoxemia (or a combination of these).[29,30] Severe lactic acidosis (accumulation of lactic acid in the blood), hyperkalemia (excessive potassium in the blood), acute renal failure, rhabdomyolysis (destruction of skeletal muscle that may be associated with strenuous exercise), and disseminated intravascular coagulation (a bleeding disorder characterized by diffuse blood coagulation), among other medical conditions, may result from exertional heat stroke and often cause death.[25]

Exertional Hyponatremia

Exertional hyponatremia is a relatively rare condition defined as a serum-sodium level less than 130 mmol/L. Low serum-sodium levels usually occur when activity exceeds 4 hours.[19] Two, often-additive mechanisms are proposed: an athlete ingests water or low-solute beverages well beyond sweat losses (also known as water intoxication), or an athlete's sweat sodium losses are not adequately replaced.[15–18] The low blood-sodium levels are the result of a combination of excessive fluid intake and inappropriate body water retention in the water-intoxication model and insufficient fluid intake and inadequate sodium replacement in the latter. Ultimately, the intravascular and extracellular fluid has a lower solute load than the intracellular fluids, and water flows into the cells, producing intracellular swelling that causes potentially fatal neurologic and physiologic dysfunction. Affected athletes present with a combination of disorientation, altered mental status,

headache, vomiting, lethargy, and swelling of the extremities (hands and feet), pulmonary edema, cerebral edema, and seizures. Exertional hyponatremia can result in death if not treated properly. This condition can be prevented by matching fluid intake with sweat and urine losses and by rehydrating with fluids that contain sufficient sodium.[31,32]

RECOMMENDATIONS

The National Athletic Trainers' Association (NATA) advocates the following prevention, recognition, and treatment strategies for exertional heat illnesses. These recommendations are presented to help ATCs and other allied health providers maximize health, safety, and sport performance as they relate to these illnesses. Athletes' individual responses to physiologic stimuli and environmental conditions vary widely. These recommendations do not guarantee full protection from heat-related illness but should decrease the risk during athletic participation. These recommendations should be considered by ATCs and allied health providers who work with athletes at risk for exertional heat illnesses to improve prevention strategies and ensure proper treatment.

Prevention

1. Ensure that appropriate medical care is available and that rescue personnel are familiar with exertional heat illness prevention, recognition, and treatment. Table 2 provides general guidelines that should be considered.[7] Ensure that ATCs and other health care providers attending practices or events are allowed to evaluate and examine any athlete who displays signs or symptoms of heat illness[33,34] and have the authority to restrict the athlete from participating if heat illness is present.

2. Conduct a thorough, physician-supervised, preparticipation medical screening before the season starts to identify athletes predisposed to heat illness on the basis of risk factors[34–36] and those who have a history of exertional heat illness.

3. Adapt athletes to exercise in the heat (acclimatization) gradually over 10 to 14 days. Progressively increase the intensity and duration of work in the heat with a combination of strenuous interval training and continuous exercise.[6,9,14,33,37–44] Well-acclimatized athletes should train for 1 to 2 hours under the same heat conditions that will be present for their event.[6,45,46] In a cooler environment, an athlete can wear additional clothing during training to induce or maintain heat acclimatization. Athletes should maintain proper hydration during the heat-acclimatization process.[47]

4. Educate athletes and coaches regarding the prevention, recognition, and treatment of heat illnesses[9,33,38,39,42,48–51] and the risks associated with exercising in hot, humid environmental conditions.

5. Educate athletes to match fluid intake with sweat and urine losses to maintain adequate hydration.* (See the "National Athletic Trainers' Association Position Statement: Fluid Replacement in Athletes."[52]) Instruct athletes to drink sodium-containing fluids to keep their urine clear to light yellow to improve hydration[33,34,52–55] and to replace fluids between practices on the same day and on successive days to maintain less than 2% body-weight change. These strategies will lessen the risk of acute and chronic dehydration and decrease the risk of heat-related events.

References 9, 29, 37, 38, 40, 41, 43, 52–66.

Table 2. Prevention Checklist for the Certified Athletic Trainer*

1. Pre-event preparation
 _____Am I challenging unsafe rules (eg, ability to receive fluids, modify game and practice times)?
 _____Am I encouraging athletes to drink before the onset of thirst and to be well hydrated at the start of activity?
 _____Am I familiar with which athletes have a history of a heat illness?
 _____Am I discouraging alcohol, caffeine, and drug use?
 _____Am I encouraging proper conditioning and acclimatization procedures?
2. Checking hydration status
 _____Do I know the preexercise weight of the athletes (especially those at high risk) with whom I work, particularly during hot and humid conditions?
 _____Are the athletes familiar with how to assess urine color? Is a urine color chart accessible?
 _____Do the athletes know their sweat rates and, therefore, know how much to drink during exercise?
 _____Is a refractometer or urine color chart present to provide additional information regarding hydration status in high-risk athletes when baseline body weights are checked?
3. Environmental assessment
 _____Am I regularly checking the wet-bulb globe temperature or temperature and humidity during the day?
 _____Am I knowledgeable about the risk categories of a heat illness based on the environmental conditions?
 _____Are alternate plans made in case risky conditions force rescheduling of events or practices?
4. Coaches' and athletes' responsibilities
 _____Are coaches and athletes educated about the signs and symptoms of heat illnesses?
 _____Am I double checking to make sure coaches are allowing ample rest and rehydration breaks?
 _____Are modifications being made to reduce risk in the heat (eg, decrease intensity, change practice times, allow more frequent breaks, eliminate double sessions, reduce or change equipment or clothing requirements, etc)?
 _____Are rapid weight-loss practices in weight-class sports adamantly disallowed?
5. Event management
 _____Have I checked to make sure proper amounts of fluids will be available and accessible?
 _____Are carbohydrate-electrolyte drinks available at events and practices (especially during twice-a-day practices and those that last longer than 50 to 60 minutes or are extremely intense in nature)?
 _____Am I aware of the factors that may increase the likelihood of a heat illness?
 _____Am I promptly rehydrating athletes to preexercise weight after an exercise session?
 _____Are shaded or indoor areas used for practices or breaks when possible to minimize thermal strain?
6. Treatment considerations
 _____Am I familiar with the most common early signs and symptoms of heat illnesses?
 _____Do I have the proper field equipment and skills to assess a heat illness?
 _____Is an emergency plan in place in case an immediate evacuation is needed?
 _____Is a kiddy pool available in situations of high risk to initiate immediate cold-water immersion of heat-stroke patients?
 _____Are ice bags available for immediate cooling when cold-water immersion is not possible?
 _____Have shaded, air-conditioned, and cool areas been identified to use when athletes need to cool down, recover, or receive treatment?
 _____Are fans available to assist evaporation when cooling?
 _____Am I properly equipped to assess high core temperature (ie, rectal thermometer)?
7. Other situation-specific considerations

*Adapted with permission from Casa.[7]

Table 3. Wet-Bulb Globe Temperature Risk Chart[62–67]*

WBGT	Flag Color	Level of Risk	Comments
<18°C (<65°F)	Green	Low	Risk low but still exists on the basis of risk factors
18–23°C (65–73°F)	Yellow	Moderate	Risk level increases as event progresses through the day
23–28°C (73–82°F)	Red	High	Everyone should be aware of injury potential; individuals at risk should not compete
>28°C (82°F)	Black	Extreme or hazardous	Consider rescheduling or delaying the event until safer conditions prevail; if the event must take place, be on high alert

*Adapted with permission from Roberts.[67]

6. Encourage athletes to sleep at least 6 to 8 hours at night in a cool environment,[41,35,50] eat a well-balanced diet that follows the Food Guide Pyramid and United States Dietary Guidelines,[56–58] and maintain proper hydration status. Athletes exercising in hot conditions (especially during twice-a-day practices) require extra sodium from the diet or rehydration beverages or both.

7. Develop event and practice guidelines for hot, humid weather that anticipate potential problems encountered based on the wet-bulb globe temperature (WBGT) (Table 3) or heat and humidity as measured by a sling psychrometer (Figure 1), the number of participants, the nature of the activity, and other predisposing risk factors.[14,51] If the WBGT is greater than 28°C (82°F, or "very high" as indicated in Table 3, Figure 1), an athletic event should be delayed, rescheduled, or moved into an air-conditioned space, if possible.[69–74] It is important to note that these measures are based on the risk of environmental stress for athletes wearing shorts and a T-shirt; if an

15

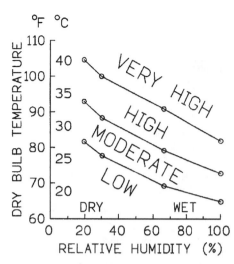

Figure 1. Risk of heat exhaustion or heat stroke while racing in hot environments. However, Figure 2 may be better suited for estimating heat-stroke risk when equipment is worn. Reprinted with permission from Convertino VA, Armstrong LE, Coyle EF, et al. American College of Sports Medicine position stand: exercise and fluid replacement. *Med Sci Sports Exerc.* 1996;28:i–vii.[31]

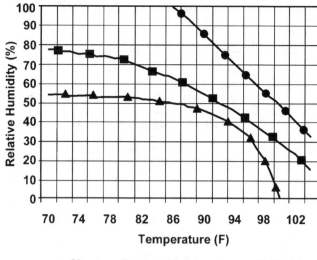

—●—Shorts only   —■—Light pads   —▲—Full pads

Figure 2. Heat stress risk temperature and humidity graph. Heat-stroke risk rises with increasing heat and relative humidity. Fluid breaks should be scheduled for all practices and scheduled more frequently as the heat stress rises. Add 5° to temperature between 10 AM and 4 PM from mid May to mid September on bright, sunny days. Practices should be modified for the safety of the athletes to reflect the heat-stress conditions. Regular practices with full practice gear can be conducted for conditions that plot to the left of the triangles. Cancel all practices when the temperature and relative humidity plot is to the right of the circles; practices may be moved into air-conditioned spaces or held as walk-through sessions with no conditioning activities.

Conditions that plot between squares and circles: increase rest-to-work ratio with 5- to 10-minute rest and fluid breaks every 15 to 20 minutes; practice should be in shorts only with all protective equipment removed.

Conditions that plot between triangles and squares: increase rest-to-work ratio with 5- to 10-minute rest and fluid breaks every 20 to 30 minutes; practice should be in shorts with helmets and shoulder pads (not full equipment).

Adapted with permission from Kulka J, Kenney WL. Heat balance limits in football uniforms: how different uniform ensembles alter the equation. *Physician Sportsmed.* 2002;30(7):29–39.[68]

athlete is wearing additional clothing (ie, football uniform, wetsuit, helmet), a lower WBGT value could result in comparable risk of environmental heat stress (Figure 2).[75,76] If the event or practice is conducted in hot, humid conditions, then use extreme caution in monitoring the athletes and be proactive in taking preventive steps. In addition, be sure that emergency supplies and equipment are easily accessible and in good working order. The most important factors are to limit intensity and duration of activity, limit the amount of clothing and equipment worn, increase the number and length of rest breaks, and encourage proper hydration.

Modify activity under high-risk conditions to prevent exertional heat illnesses.[19,21] Identify individuals who are susceptible to heat illnesses. In some athletes, the prodromal signs and symptoms of heat illnesses are not evident before collapse, but in many cases, adept medical supervision will allow early intervention.

8. Check the environmental conditions before and during the activity, and adjust the practice schedule accordingly.[29,38,41,42,60] Schedule training sessions to avoid the hottest part of the day (10 AM to 5 PM) and to avoid radiant heating from direct sunlight, especially in the acclimatization during the first few days of practice sessions.[9,29,33,34,38,40,50,60]

9. Plan rest breaks to match the environmental conditions and the intensity of the activity.[33,34] Exercise intensity and environmental conditions should be the major determinants in deciding the length and frequency of rest breaks. If possible, cancel or postpone the activity or move it indoors (if air conditioned) if the conditions are "extreme or hazardous" (see Table 3) or "very high" (see Figure 1) or to the right of the circled line (see Figure 2). General guidelines during intense exercise would include a work:rest ratio of 1:1, 2:1, 3:1, and 4:1 for "extreme or hazardous" (see Table 3) or "very high" (see Figure 1), "high," "moderate," or "low" environmental risk, respectively.[41,77] For activities such as football in which equipment must be considered, please refer to Figure 2 for equipment modifications and appropriate work:rest ratios for various environmental conditions. Rest breaks should occur in the shade if possible, and hydration during rest breaks should be encouraged.

10. Implement rest periods at mealtime by allowing 2 to 3 hours for food, fluids, nutrients, and electrolytes (sodium and potassium) to move into the small intestine and bloodstream before the next practice.[34,50,77]

11. Provide an adequate supply of proper fluids (water or sports drinks) to maintain hydration[9,34,38,40,50,60] and institute a hydration protocol that allows the maintenance of hydration status.[34,49] Fluids should be readily available and served in containers that allow adequate volumes to be ingested with ease and with minimal interruption of exercise.[49,52] The goal should be to lose no more than 2% to 3% of body weight during the practice session (due to sweat and urine losses).[78–82] (See the "National Athletic Trainers' Association Position Statement: Fluid Replacement in Athletes."[52])

12. Weigh high-risk athletes (in high-risk conditions, weigh all athletes) before and after practice to estimate the amount of body water lost during practice and to ensure a return to prepractice weight before the next practice. Following exercise athletes should consume approximately 1–1.25 L (16 oz) of fluid for each kilogram of body water lost during exercise.†

---

†*References 6, 9, 29, 33, 38, 40, 49, 60, 77, 83.*

13. Minimize the amount of equipment and clothing worn by the athlete in hot or humid (or both) conditions. For example, a full football uniform prevents sweat evaporation from more than 60% of the body.[29,33,40,51,77] Consult Figure 2 for possible equipment and clothing recommendations. When athletes exercise in the heat, they should wear loose-fitting, absorbent, and light-colored clothing; mesh clothing and new-generation cloth blends have been specially designed to allow more effective cooling.‡

14. Minimize warm-up time when feasible, and conduct warm-up sessions in the shade when possible to minimize the radiant heat load in "high" or "very high" or "extreme or hazardous" (see Table 3, Figure 1) conditions.[77]

15. Allow athletes to practice in shaded areas and use electric or cooling fans to circulate air whenever feasible.[66]

16. Include the following supplies on the field, in the locker room, and at various other stations:

- A supply of cool water or sports drinks or both to meet the participants' needs (see the "National Athletic Trainers' Association Position Statement: Fluid Replacement in Athletes"[52] for recommendations regarding the appropriate composition of rehydration beverages based on the length and intensity of the activity)[29,34,38]
- Ice for active cooling (ice bags, tub cooling) and to keep beverages cool during exercise[29,38]
- Rectal thermometer to assess body-core temperature[39,74,75,87,88]
- Telephone or 2-way radio to communicate with medical personnel and to summon emergency medical transportation[38,39,48]
- Tub, wading pool, kiddy pool, or whirlpool to cool the trunk and extremities for immersion cooling therapy[35,65]

17. Notify local hospital and emergency personnel before mass participation events to inform them of the event and the increased possibility of heat-related illnesses.[41,89]

18. Mandate a check of hydration status at weigh-in to ensure athletes in sports requiring weight classes (eg, wrestling, judo, rowing) are not dehydrated. Any procedures used to induce dramatic dehydration (eg, diuretics, rubber suits, exercising in a sauna) are strictly prohibited.[52] Dehydrated athletes exercising at the same intensity as euhydrated athletes are at increased risk for thermoregulatory strain (see the "National Athletic Trainers' Association Position Statement: Fluid Replacement in Athletes"[52]).

Recognition and Treatment

19. Exercise-associated muscle (heat) cramps:

- An athlete showing signs or symptoms including dehydration, thirst, sweating, transient muscle cramps, and fatigue is likely experiencing exercise-associated muscle (heat) cramps.
- To relieve muscle spasms, the athlete should stop activity, replace lost fluids with sodium-containing fluids, and begin mild stretching with massage of the muscle spasm.
- Fluid absorption is enhanced with sports drinks that contain sodium.[52,60,87] A high-sodium sports product may be added to the rehydration beverage to prevent or relieve cramping in athletes who lose large amounts of sodium in their sweat.[19] A simple salted fluid consists of two 10-grain salt

‡References 8, 9, 29, 33, 38, 40, 53, 59, 84–86.

tablets dissolved in 1 L (34 oz) of water. Intravenous fluids may be required if nausea or vomiting limits oral fluid intake; these must be ordered by a physician.[6,7,52,90,91]
- A recumbent position may allow more rapid redistribution of blood flow to cramping leg muscles.

20. Heat syncope:

- If an athlete experiences a brief episode of fainting associated with dizziness, tunnel vision, pale or sweaty skin, and a decreased pulse rate but has a normal rectal temperature (for exercise, 36°C to 40°C [97°F to 104°F]), then heat syncope is most likely the cause.[19]
- Move the athlete to a shaded area, monitor vital signs, elevate the legs above the level of the head, and rehydrate.

21. Exercise (heat) exhaustion:

- Cognitive changes are usually minimal, but assess central nervous system function for bizarre behavior, hallucinations, altered mental status, confusion, disorientation, or coma (see Table 1) to rule out more serious conditions.
- If feasible, measure body-core temperature (rectal temperature) and assess cognitive function (see Table 1) and vital signs.[19] Rectal temperature is the most accurate method possible in the field to monitor body-core temperature.[34,74,75,87,88] The ATC should not rely on the oral, tympanic, or axillary temperature for athletes because these are inaccurate and ineffective measures of body-core temperature during and after exercise.[75,89,92]
- If the athlete's temperature is elevated, remove his or her excess clothing to increase the evaporative surface and to facilitate cooling.[6,93]
- Cool the athlete with fans,[94] ice towels,[29,38] or ice bags because these may help the athlete with a temperature of more than 38.8°C (102°F) to feel better faster.
- Remove the athlete to a cool or shaded environment if possible.
- Start fluid replacement.[6,52,93,95]
- Transfer care to a physician if intravenous fluids are needed[6,52,90,91,96] or if recovery is not rapid and uneventful.

22. Exertional heat stroke:

- Measure the rectal temperature if feasible to differentiate between heat exhaustion and heat stroke. With heat stroke, rectal temperature is elevated (generally higher than 40°C [104°F]).[19]
- Assess cognitive function, which is markedly altered in exertional heat stroke (see Table 1).
- Lower the body-core temperature as quickly as possible.[34,70,77] The fastest way to decrease body temperature is to remove clothes and equipment and immerse the body (trunk and extremities) into a pool or tub of cold water (approximately 1°C to 15°C [35°F to 59°F]).[32,91,92,97–99] Aggressive cooling is the most critical factor in the treatment of exertional heat stroke. Circulation of the tub water may enhance cooling.
- Monitor the temperature during the cooling therapy and recovery (every 5 to 10 minutes).[39,87] Once the athlete's rectal temperature reaches approximately 38.3°C to 38.9°C (101°F to 102°F), he or she should be removed from the pool or tub to avoid overcooling.[40,100]
- If a physician is present to manage the athlete's medical care on site, then initial transportation to a medical facility may not be necessary so immersion can continue uninterrupted.

If a physician is not present, aggressive first-aid cooling should be initiated on site and continued during emergency medical system transport and at the hospital until the athlete is normothermic.

- Activate the emergency medical system.
- Monitor the athlete's vital signs and other signs and symptoms of heat stroke (see Table 1).[34,95]
- During transport and when immersion is not feasible, other methods can be used to reduce body temperature: removing the clothing; sponging down the athlete with cool water and applying cold towels; applying ice bags to as much of the body as possible, especially the major vessels in the armpit, groin, and neck; providing shade; and fanning the body with air.[39,95]
- In addition to cooling therapies, first-aid emergency procedures for heat stroke may include airway management. Also a physician may decide to begin intravenous fluid replacement.[87]
- Monitor for organ-system complications for at least 24 hours.

23. Exertional hyponatremia:

- Attempt to differentiate between hyponatremia and heat exhaustion. Hyponatremia is characterized by increasing headache, significant mental compromise, altered consciousness, seizures, lethargy, and swelling in the extremities. The athlete may be dehydrated, normally hydrated, or overhydrated.[19]
- Attempt to differentiate between hyponatremia and heat stroke. In hyponatremia, hyperthermia is likely to be less (rectal temperature less than 40°C [104°F]).[19] The plasma-sodium level is less than 130 mEq/L and can be measured with a sodium analyzer on site if the device is available.
- If hyponatremia is suspected, immediate transfer to an emergency medical center via the emergency medical system is indicated. An intravenous line should be placed to administer medication as needed to increase sodium levels, induce diuresis, and control seizures.
- An athlete with suspected hyponatremia should not be administered fluids until a physician is consulted.

24. Return to activity

In cases of exercise-associated muscle (heat) cramps or heat syncope, the ATC should discuss the athlete's case with the supervising physician. The cases of athletes with heat exhaustion who were not transferred to the physician's care should also be discussed with the physician. After exertional heat stroke or exertional hyponatremia, the athlete must be cleared by a physician before returning to athletic participation.[92] The return to full activity should be gradual and monitored.[8,87]

BACKGROUND AND LITERATURE REVIEW

Diagnosis

To differentiate heat illnesses in athletes, ATCs and other on-site health care providers must be familiar with the signs and symptoms of each condition (see Table 1). Other medical conditions (eg, asthma, status epilepticus, drug toxicities) may also present with similar signs and symptoms. It is important to realize, however, that an athlete with a heat illness will not exhibit all the signs and symptoms of a specific condition, increasing the need for diligent observation during athletic activity.

Nonenvironmental Risk Factors

Athletic trainers and other health care providers should be sensitive to the following nonenvironmental risk factors, which could place athletes at risk for heat illness.

Dehydration. Sweating, inadequate fluid intake, vomiting, diarrhea, certain medications,[89,101–103] and alcohol[104,105] or caffeine[106] use can lead to fluid deficit. Body-weight change is the preferred method to monitor for dehydration in the field, but a clinical refractometer is another accurate method (specific gravity should be no more than 1.020).[34,49,107–110] Dehydration can also be identified by monitoring urine color or body-weight changes before, during, and after a practice or an event and across successive days.[53,54]

The signs and symptoms of dehydration are thirst, general discomfort, flushed skin, weariness, cramps, apathy, dizziness, headache, vomiting, nausea, heat sensations on the head or neck, chills, decreased performance, and dyspnea.[52] Water loss that is not regained by the next practice increases the risk for heat illness.[110]

Barriers to Evaporation. Athletic equipment and rubber or plastic suits used for "weight loss" do not allow water vapor to pass through and inhibit evaporative, convective, and radiant heat loss.[111,112] Participants who wear equipment that does not allow for heat dissipation are at an increased risk for heat illness.[113] Helmets are also limiting because a significant amount of heat is dissipated through the head.

Illness. Athletes who are currently or were recently ill may be at an increased risk for heat illness because of fever or dehydration.[114–116]

History of Heat Illness. Some individuals with a history of heat illness are at greater risk for recurrent heat illness.[8,117]

Increased Body Mass Index (Thick Fat Layer or Small Surface Area). Obese individuals are at an increased risk for heat illness because the fat layer decreases heat loss.[118] Obese persons are less efficient and have a greater metabolic heat production during exercise. Conversely, muscle-bound individuals have increased metabolic heat production and a lower ratio of surface area to mass, contributing to a decreased ability to dissipate heat.[119–121]

Wet-Bulb Globe Temperature on Previous Day and Night. When the WBGT is high to extreme (see Table 3), the risk of heat-related problems is greater the next day; this appears to be one of the best predictors of heat illness.[121] Athletes who sleep in cool or air-conditioned quarters are at less risk.

Poor Physical Condition. Individuals who are untrained are more susceptible to heat illness than are trained athletes. As the $\dot{V}O_2max$ of an individual improves, the ability to withstand heat stress improves independent of acclimatization and heat adaptation.[122] High-intensity work can easily produce 1000 kcal/h and elevate the core temperature of at-risk individuals (those who are unfit, overweight, or unacclimatized) to dangerous levels within 20 to 30 minutes.[123]

Excessive or Dark-Colored Clothing or Equipment. Excessive clothing or equipment decreases the ability to thermoregulate, and dark-colored clothing or equipment may cause a greater absorption of heat from the environment. Both should be avoided.[113]

Overzealousness. Overzealous athletes are at a higher risk for heat illness because they override the normal behavioral adaptations to heat and decrease the likelihood of subtle cues being recognized.

Lack of Acclimatization to Heat. An athlete with no or minimal physiologic acclimatization to hot conditions is at an increased risk of heat-related illness.[8,37,83,124]

Medications and Drugs. Athletes who take certain medications or drugs, particularly medications with a dehydrating effect, are at an increased risk for a heat illness.[101-106,125-136] Alcohol, caffeine, and theophylline at certain doses are mild diuretics.[106,137,138] Caffeine is found in coffee, tea, soft drinks, chocolate, and several over-the-counter and prescription medications.[139] Theophylline is found mostly in tea and anti-asthma medications.[140]

Electrolyte Imbalance. Electrolyte imbalances do not usually occur in trained, acclimatized individuals who engage in physical activity and eat a normal diet.[141] Most sodium and chloride losses in athletes occur through the urine, but athletes who sweat heavily, are salty sweaters, or are not heat acclimatized can lose significant amounts of sodium during activity.[142] Electrolyte imbalances often contribute to heat illness in older athletes who use diuretics.[143,144]

Predisposing Medical Conditions

The following predisposing medical conditions add to the risk of heat illness.

Malignant Hyperthermia. Malignant hyperthermia is caused by an autosomal dominant trait that causes muscle rigidity, resulting in elevation of body temperature due to the accelerated metabolic rate in the skeletal muscle.[145-147]

Neuroleptic Malignant Syndrome. Neuroleptic malignant syndrome is associated with the use of neuroleptic agents and antipsychotic drugs and an unexpected idiopathic increase in core temperature during exercise.[148-151]

Arteriosclerotic Vascular Disease. Arteriosclerotic vascular disease compromises cardiac output and blood flow through the vascular system by thickening the arterial walls.[115,152]

Scleroderma. Scleroderma is a skin disorder that decreases sweat production, thereby decreasing heat transfer.[149,153]

Cystic Fibrosis. Cystic fibrosis causes increased salt loss in sweat and can increase the risk for hyponatremia.[154,155]

Sickle Cell Trait. Sickle cell trait limits blood-flow distribution and decreases oxygen-carrying capacity. The condition is exacerbated by exercise at higher altitudes.[156,157]

Environmental Risk Factors

When the environmental temperature is above skin temperature, athletes begin to absorb heat from the environment and depend entirely on evaporation for heat loss.[113,158,159] High relative humidity inhibits heat loss from the body through evaporation.[61]

The environmental factors that influence the risk of heat illness include the ambient air temperature, relative humidity (amount of water vapor in the air), air motion, and the amount of radiant heat from the sun or other sources.[2,9,41] The relative risk of heat illness can be calculated using the WBGT equation.[2,43,50,69,77,160,161] Using the WBGT index to modify activity in high-risk settings has virtually eliminated heat-stroke deaths in United States Marine Corps recruits.[159] Wet-bulb globe temperature is calculated using the wet-bulb (wb), dry-bulb (db), and black-globe (bg) temperature with the following equation[49,62,85,162,163]:

$$\text{WBGT} = 0.7T_{wb} + 0.2T_{bg} + 0.1T_{db}$$

When there is no radiant heat load, $T_{db} = T_{bg}$, and the equation is reduced[62] to

$$\text{WBGT} = 0.7T_{wb} + 0.3T_{db}$$

This equation is used to estimate risk as outlined in Table 3.[13,40,50,61,85] This index was determined for athletes wearing a T-shirt and light pants.[158] The WBGT calculation can be performed using information obtained from electronic devices[42] or the local meteorologic service, but conversion tables for relative humidity and T_{db} are needed to calculate the wet-bulb temperature.[50,162] The predictive value from the meteorologic service is not as accurate as site-specific data for representing local heat load but will suffice in most situations. When WBGT measures are not possible, environmental heat stress can be estimated using a sling psychrometer (see Figures 1, 2).

Several recommendations have been published for distance running, but these can also be applied to other continuous activity sports. The Canadian Track and Field Association recommended that a distance race should be cancelled if the WBGT is greater than 26.7°C (80°F).[39] The American College of Sports Medicine guidelines from 1996 recommended that a race should be delayed or rescheduled when the WBGT is greater than 27.8°C (82°F).[31,72,73] In some instances, the event will go on regardless of the WBGT; ATCs should then have an increased level of suspicion for heat stroke and focus on hydration, emergency supplies, and detection of exertional heat illnesses.

Thermoregulation

Thermoregulation is a complex interaction among the central nervous system (CNS), the cardiovascular system, and the skin to maintain a body-core temperature of 37°C.[9,43,51,164] The CNS temperature-regulation center is located in the hypothalamus and is the site where the core temperature setpoint is determined.[9,43,82,158,164-166] The hypothalamus receives information regarding body-core and shell temperatures from peripheral skin receptors and the circulating blood; body-core temperature is regulated through an open-ended feedback loop similar to that in a home thermostat system.[158,165,167,168] Body responses for heat regulation include cutaneous vasodilation, increased sweating, increased heart rate, and increased respiratory rate.[38,43,51,164,165]

Body-core temperature is determined by metabolic heat production and the transfer of body heat to and from the surrounding environment using the following heat-production and heat-storage equation[166,167]:

$$S = M \pm R \pm K \pm Cv - E$$

where S is the amount of stored heat, M is the metabolic heat production, R is the heat gained or lost by radiation, K is the conductive heat lost or gained, Cv is the convective heat lost or gained, and E is the evaporative heat lost.

Basal metabolic heat production fasting and at absolute rest is approximately 60 to 70 kcal/h for an average adult, with 50% of the heat produced by the internal organs. Metabolic heat produced by intense exercise may approach 1000 kcal/h,[51,164] with greater than 90% of the heat resulting from muscle metabolism.[9,40,42,166]

Heat is gained or lost from the body by one or more of the following mechanisms[9,85]:

Table 4. Physiologic Responses After Heat Acclimatization Relative to Nonacclimatized State

Physiologic Variable	After Acclimatization (10–14 Days' Exposure)
Heart rate	Decreases[46,145]
Stroke volume	Increases[145,147]
Body-core temperature	Decreases[145]
Skin temperature	Decreases[152]
Sweat output/rate	Increases[46,47,149]
Onset of sweat	Earlier in training[46,145]
Evaporation of sweat	Increases[47,152]
Salt in sweat	Decreases[9,50]
Work output	Increases[46,50]
Subjective discomfort (rating of perceived exertion [RPE])	Decreases[50,145]
Fatigue	Decreases[50]
Capacity for work	Increases[46,50]
Mental disturbance	Decreases[50]
Syncopal response	Decreases[9,50]
Extracellular fluid volume	Increases[50]
Plasma volume	Increases[50,150]

Radiation. The energy is transferred to or from an object or body via electromagnetic radiation from higher to lower energy surfaces.[9,43,51,85,166]

Conduction. Heat transfers from warmer to cooler objects through direct physical contact.[9,43,51,85,166] Ice packs and cold-water baths are examples of conductive heat exchange.

Convection. Heat transfers to or from the body to surrounding moving fluid (including air).[9,43,51,85,166] Moving air from a fan, cycling, or windy day produces convective heat exchange.

Evaporation. Heat transfers via the vaporization of sweat§ and is the most efficient means of heat loss.[51,158,169] The evaporation of sweat from the skin depends on the water saturation of the air and the velocity of the moving air.[170–172] The effectiveness of this evaporation for heat loss from the body diminishes rapidly when the relative humidity is greater than 60%.[9,20,164]

Cognitive performance and associated CNS functions deteriorate when brain temperature rises. Signs and symptoms include dizziness, confusion, behavior changes, coordination difficulties, decreased physical performance, and collapse due to hyperthermia.[168,173] The residual effects of elevated brain temperature depend on the duration of the hyperthermia. Heat stroke rarely leads to permanent neurologic deficits[51]; however, some sporadic symptoms of frontal headache and sleep disturbances have been noted for up to 4 months.[168,174,175] When permanent CNS damage occurs, it is associated with cerebellar changes, including ataxia, marked dysarthria, and dysmetria.[174]

Heat Acclimatization

Heat acclimatization is the physiologic response produced by repeated exposures to hot environments in which the capacity to withstand heat stress is improved.[14,43,75,176,177] Physiologic responses to heat stress are summarized in Table 4. Exercise heat exposure produces progressive changes in thermoregulation that involve sweating, skin circulation, thermoregulatory setpoint, cardiovascular alterations, and endocrine

§References 9, 40, 43, 50, 51, 85, 159, 165, 166.

adjustments.[29,43,178] Individual differences affect the onset and decay of acclimatization.[29,45,179] The rate of acclimatization is related to aerobic conditioning and fitness; more conditioned athletes acclimatize more quickly.[43,45,180] The acclimatization process begins with heat exposure and is reasonably protective after 7 to 14 days, but maximum acclimatization may take 2 to 3 months.[45,181,182] Heat acclimatization diminishes by day 6 when heat stress is no longer present.[180,183] Fluid replacement improves the induction and effect of heat acclimatization.[184–187] Extra salt in the diet during the first few days of heat exposure also improves acclimatization; this can be accomplished by encouraging the athlete to eat salty foods and to use the salt shaker liberally during meals.

Cumulative Dehydration

Cumulative dehydration develops insidiously over several days and is typically observed during the first few days of a season during practice sessions or in tournament competition. Cumulative dehydration can be detected by monitoring daily prepractice and postpractice weights. Even though a small decrease in body weight (less than 1%) may not have a detrimental effect on the individual, the cumulative effect of a 1% fluid loss per day occurring over several days will create an increased risk for heat illness and a decrease in performance.[110]

During intense exercise in the heat, sweat rates can be 1 to 2.5 L/h (about 1 to 2.25 kilograms [2 to 5 pounds] of body weight per hour) or more, resulting in dehydration. Unfortunately, the volume of fluid that most athletes drink voluntarily during exercise replaces only about 50% of body-fluid losses.[188] Ideally, rehydration involves drinking at a rate sufficient to replace all of the water lost through sweating and urination.[60,77] If the athlete is not able to drink at this rate, he or she should drink the maximum tolerated. Use caution to ensure that athletes do not overhydrate and put themselves at risk for the development of hyponatremia. However, hydration before an event is essential to help decrease the incidence of heat illnesses. For more information on this topic, see the "National Athletic Trainers' Association Position Statement: Fluid Replacement in Athletes."[52]

Cooling Therapies

The fastest way to decrease body-core temperature is immersion of the trunk and extremities into a pool or tub filled with cold water (between 1°C [35°F] and 15°C [59°F]).[39,88,91,97] Conditions that have been associated with immersion therapy include shivering and peripheral vasoconstriction; however, the potential for these should not deter the medical staff from using immersion therapy for rapid cooling. Shivering can be prevented if the athlete is removed from the water once rectal temperature reaches 38.3°C to 38.9°C (101°F to 102°F). Peripheral vasoconstriction may occur, but the powerful cooling potential of immersion outweighs any potential concerns. Cardiogenic shock has also been a proposed consequence of immersion therapy, but this connection has not been proven in cooling heat-stroke patients.[39] Cold-water immersion therapy was associated with a zero percent fatality rate in 252 cases of exertional heat stroke in the military.[89] Other forms of cooling (water spray; ice packs covering the body; ice packs on axillae, groin, and neck; or blowing air) decrease body-core temperature at a slower rate compared with cold-water immersion.[97] If immersion cooling is not being used, cooling with ice bags should be directed to as much of the body as possible, especially the major vessels in the armpit, groin, and neck regions (and likely the hands and feet), and cold towels may be applied to the head and trunk because these areas have been demonstrated on thermography[173,189] to have the most rapid heat loss.

SPECIAL CONCERNS

Most research related to heat illness has been performed on normal, healthy adults. Child athletes, older athletes, and athletes with spinal-cord injuries have been studied less frequently. The following are suggestions for special populations or those with special conditions.

Children (Prepubescents)

Exercise in hot environments and heat tolerance are affected by many physiologic factors in children. These include decreased sweat gland activity,[190] higher skin temperatures,[191–193] decreased cardiac output (increased heart rate and lower stroke volume) due to increased peripheral circulation,[194] decreased exercise economy,[195] decreased ability to acclimatize to heat (slower and takes longer),[192] smaller body size (issues related to body surface-to-mass ratio), maturational differences,[190] and predisposing conditions (obesity, hypohydration, childhood illnesses, and other disease states).[190,192,196]

- Decrease the intensity of activities that last longer than 30 minutes,[197] and have the athlete take brief rests[50] if the WBGT is between 22.8°C and 27.8°C (73°F and 82°F); cancel or modify the activity if the WBGT is greater than 27.8°C (82°F).[31,69–73] Modification could involve longer and more frequent rest breaks than are usually permitted within the rules of the sport (eg, insert a rest break before halftime).
- Encourage children to ingest some fluids at least every 15 to 30 minutes during activity to maintain hydration, even if they are not thirsty.[197]
- Use similar precautions as listed earlier for adults.

Older Athletes (>50 Years Old)

The ability of the older athlete to adapt is partly a function of age and also depends on functional capacity and physiologic health status.[198–206]

- The athlete should be evaluated by a physician before exercise, with the potential consequences of predisposing medical conditions and illnesses addressed.[9,34–36] An increase has been shown in the exercise heart rate of 1 beat per minute for each 1°C (1.8°F) increase in ambient temperature above neutral (23.9°C [75°F]).[207] Athletes with known or suspected heart disease should curtail activities at lower temperatures than healthy athletes and should have cardiovascular stress testing before participating in hot environments.
- Older athletes have a decreased ability to maintain an adequate plasma volume and osmolality during exercise,[198,208] which may predispose them to dehydration. Regular fluid intake is critical to avoid hyperthermia.

Athletes with Spinal-Cord Injuries

As sport participation for athletes with spinal-cord injuries increases from beginner to elite levels, understanding the dis-

ability,[209,210] training methods, and causes of heat injury will help make competition safer.[211] For example, the abilities to regulate heart rate, circulate the blood volume, produce sweat, and transfer heat to the surface vary with the level and severity of the spinal-cord lesion.[208,212–218]

- Monitor these athletes closely for heat-related problems. One technique for determining hyperthermia is to feel the skin under the arms of the distressed athlete.[211] Rectal temperature may not be as accurate for measuring core temperature as in other athletes due to decreased ability to regulate blood flow beneath the spinal-cord lesion.[218–220]
- If the athlete is hyperthermic, provide more water, lighter clothing, or cooling of the trunk,[211,213] legs,[211] and head.[213]

HOSPITALIZATION AND RECOVERY

After an episode of heat stroke, the athlete may experience impaired thermoregulation, persistent CNS dysfunction,[221,222] hepatic insufficiency, and renal insufficiency.[39,223] For persons with exertional heat stroke and associated multisystem tissue damage, the rate of recovery is highly individualized, ranging up to more than 1 year.[8,86,221] In one study, 9 of 10 patients exhibited normal heat-acclimatization responses, thermoregulation, whole-body sodium and potassium balance, sweat-gland function, and blood values about 2 months after the heat stroke.[8] Transient or persistent heat intolerance was found in a small percentage of patients.[83] For some athletes, a history of exertional heat stroke increases the chance of experiencing subsequent episodes.[39]

An athlete who experiences heat stroke may have compromised heat tolerance and heat acclimatization after physician clearance.[35,224,225] Decreased heat tolerance may affect 15% to 20% of persons after a heat stroke-related collapse,[226,227] and in a few individuals, decreased heat tolerance has persisted up to 5 years.[35,224,228] Additional heat stress may reduce the athlete's ability to train and compete due to impaired cardiovascular and thermoregulatory responses.[115,228–230]

After recovery from an episode of heat stroke or hyponatremia, an athlete's physical activity should be restricted[8,86] and the gradual return to sport individualized by his or her physician. The athlete should be monitored on a daily basis by the ATC during exercise.[86] During the return-to-exercise phase, an athlete may experience some detraining and deconditioning not directly related to the heat exposure.[8,86] Evaluate the athlete over time to determine whether there has been a complete recovery of exercise and heat tolerance.[8,86]

CONCLUSIONS

Athletic trainers and other allied health providers must be able to differentiate exercise-associated muscle (heat) cramps, heat syncope, exercise (heat) exhaustion, exertional heat stroke, and exertional hyponatremia in athletes.

This position statement outlines the NATA's current recommendations to reduce the incidence, improve the recognition, and optimize treatment of heat illness in athletes. Education and increased awareness will help to reduce both the frequency and the severity of heat illness in athletes.

ACKNOWLEDGMENTS

This pronouncement was reviewed for the NATA by the Pronouncements Committee, Edward R. Eichner, MD, FACSM, and William O. Roberts, MD, MS, FACSM. T. Kyle Eubanks, MA, ATC, and Paul C. Miller, PhD, provided assistance in the preparation of the manuscript.

REFERENCES

1. Hawley DA, Slentz K, Clark MA, Pless JE, Waller BF. Athletic fatalities. *Am J Forensic Med Pathol*. 1990;11:124–129.
2. Mueller FO, Schindler RD. Annual survey of football injury research 1931–1984. *Athl Train J Natl Athl Train Assoc*. 1985;20:213–218.
3. Bijur PE, Trumble A, Harel Y, Overpeck MD, Jones D, Scheidt PC. Sports and recreation injuries in US children and adolescents. *Arch Pediatr Adolesc Med*. 1995;149:1009–1016.
4. Tucker AM. Common soccer injuries: diagnosis, treatment and rehabilitation. *Sports Med*. 1997;23:21–32.
5. Martin DE. Influence of elevated climatic heat stress on athletic competition in Atlanta, 1996. *New Stud Athl*. 1997;12:65–78.
6. Rich B. Environmental concerns: heat. In: Sallis RE, Massimino F, eds. *Essentials of Sports Medicine*. St Louis, MO: Mosby Year Book; 1997: 129–133.
7. Casa DJ. Exercise in the heat, II: critical concepts in rehydration, exertional heat illnesses, and maximizing athletic performance. *J Athl Train*. 1999;34:253–262.
8. Armstrong LE, De Luca JP, Hubbard RW. Time course of recovery and heat acclimation ability of prior exertional heatstroke patients. *Med Sci Sports Exerc*. 1990;22:36–48.
9. Brewster SJ, O'Connor FG, Lillegard WA. Exercise-induced heat injury: diagnosis and management. *Sports Med Arthrosc Rev*. 1995;3:206–266.
10. Knochel JP. Environmental heat illness: an eclectic review. *Arch Intern Med*. 1974;133:841–864.
11. Bergeron MF. Heat cramps during tennis: a case report. *Int J Sport Nutr*. 1996;6:62–68.
12. Hubbard R, Gaffin S, Squire D. Heat-related illness. In: Auerbach PS, ed. *Wilderness Medicine*. 3rd ed. St Louis, MO: Mosby Year Book; 1995:167–212.
13. Armstrong LE, Hubbard RW, Kraemer WJ, DeLuca JP, Christensen EL. Signs and symptoms of heat exhaustion during strenuous exercise. *Ann Sports Med*. 1987;3:182–189.
14. Epstein Y. Exertional heatstroke: lessons we tend to forget. *Am J Med Sports*. 2000;2:143–152.
15. Epstein Y, Armstrong LE. Fluid-electrolyte balance during labor and exercise: concepts and misconceptions. *Int J Sport Nutr*. 1999;9:1–12.
16. Maughan RJ. Optimizing hydration for competitive sport. In: Lamb DR, Murray R, eds. *Optimizing Sport Performance*. Carmel, IN: Cooper Publishing; 1997:139–183.
17. Armstrong LE, Curtis WC, Hubbard RW, Francesconi RP, Moore R, Askew W. Symptomatic hyponatremia during prolonged exercise in the heat. *Med Sci Sports Exerc*. 1993;25:543–549.
18. Garigan T, Ristedt DE. Death from hyponatremia as a result of acute water intoxication in an Army basic trainee. *Mil Med*. 1999;164:234–238.
19. Casa DJ, Roberts WO. Considerations for the medical staff in preventing, identifying and treating exertional heat illnesses. In: Armstrong LE, ed. *Exertional Heat Illnesses*. Champaign, IL: Human Kinetics; 2003. In press.
20. Cabanac M, White MD. Core temperature thresholds of hyperpnea during passive hyperthermia in humans. *Eur J Appl Physiol Occup Physiol*. 1995;71:71–76.
21. Casa DJ, Armstrong LE. Heatstroke: a medical emergency. In: Armstrong LE, ed. *Exertional Heat Illnesses*. Champaign, IL: Human Kinetics: 2003. In press.
22. Vicario SJ, Okabajue R, Haltom T. Rapid cooling in classic heatstroke: effect on mortality rates. *Am J Emerg Med*. 1986;4:394–398.
23. Assia E, Epstein Y, Shapiro Y. Fatal heatstroke after a short march at night: a case report. *Aviat Space Environ Med*. 1985;56:441–442.
24. Graham BS, Lichtenstein MJ, Hinson JM, Theil GB. Nonexertional heatstroke: physiologic management and cooling in 14 patients. *Arch Intern Med*. 1986;146:87–90.
25. Hart GR, Anderson RJ, Crumpler CP, Shulkin A, Reed G, Knochel JP. Epidemic classical heat stroke: clinical characteristics and course of 28 patients. *Medicine (Baltimore)*. 1982;61:189–197.
26. Thomas C, ed. *Taber's Cyclopedic Medical Dictionary*. Philadelphia, PA: FA Davis; 1993.
27. Akhtar MJ, Al-Nozha M, al-Harthi S, Nouh MS. Electrocardiographic abnormalities in patients with heat stroke. *Chest*. 1993;104:411–414.
28. Partin N. Internal medicine: exertional heatstroke. *Athl Train J Natl Athl Train Assoc*. 1990;25:192–194.
29. Knochel J. Management of heat conditions. *Athl Ther Today*. 1996;1: 30–34.
30. Hubbard RW, Armstrong LE. Hyperthermia: new thoughts on an old problem. *Physician Sportsmed*. 1989;17(6):97–98,101,104,107–108,111–113.
31. Convertino VA, Armstrong LE, Coyle EF, et al. American College of Sports Medicine position stand: exercise and fluid replacement. *Med Sci Sports Exerc*. 1996;28:i–vii.
32. Armstrong LE, Casa DJ, Watson G. Exertional hyponatremia: unanswered questions and etiological perspectives. *Int J Sport Nutr Exerc Metab*. In press.
33. Francis K, Feinstein R, Brasher J. Optimal practice times for the reduction of the risk of heat illness during fall football practice in the Southeastern United States. *Athl Train J Natl Athl Train Assoc*. 1991;26:76–78,80.
34. Shapiro Y, Seidman DS. Field and clinical observations of exertional heat stroke patients. *Med Sci Sports Exerc*. 1990;22:6–14.
35. Epstein Y, Shapiro Y, Brill S. Role of surface area-to-mass ratio and work efficiency in heat intolerance. *J Appl Physiol*. 1983;54:831–836.
36. Kenney WL. Physiological correlates of heat intolerance. *Sports Med*. 1985;2:279–286.
37. Mitchell D, Senay LC, Wyndham CH, van Rensburg AJ, Rogers GG, Strydom NB. Acclimatization in a hot, humid environment: energy exchange, body temperature, and sweating. *J Appl Physiol*. 1976;40:768–778.
38. Davidson M. Heat illness in athletics. *Athl Train J Natl Athl Train Assoc*. 1985;20:96–101.
39. Brodeur VB, Dennett SR, Griffin LS. Exertional hyperthermia, ice baths, and emergency care at the Falmouth Road Race. *J Emerg Nurs*. 1989; 15:304–312.
40. Allman FL Jr. The effects of heat on the athlete. *J Med Assoc Ga*. 1992; 81:307–310.
41. Bernard TE. Risk management for preventing heat illness in athletes. *Athl Ther Today*. 1996;1:19–21.
42. Delaney KA. Heatstroke: underlying processes and lifesaving management. *Postgrad Med*. 1992;91:379–388.
43. Haymes EM, Wells CL. *Environment and Human Performance*. Champaign, IL: Human Kinetics; 1986:1–41.
44. Gisolfi C, Robinson S. Relations between physical training, acclimatization, and heat tolerance. *J Appl Physiol*. 1969;26:530–534.
45. Armstrong LE, Maresh CM. The induction and decay of heat acclimatisation in trained athletes. *Sports Med*. 1991;12:302–312.
46. Fortney SM, Vroman NB. Exercise, performance and temperature control: temperature regulation during exercise and implications for sports performance and training. *Sports Med*. 1985;2:8–20.
47. Dawson B. Exercise training in sweat clothing in cool conditions to improve heat tolerance. *Sports Med*. 1994;17:233–244.
48. Kleiner DM, Glickman SE. Medical considerations and planning for short distance road races. *J Athl Train*. 1994;29:145–146,149–151.
49. Murray B. Fluid replacement: the American College of Sports Medicine position stand. *Sport Sci Exch*. 1996;9(4S):63.
50. Elias SR, Roberts WO, Thorson DC. Team sports in hot weather: guidelines for modifying youth soccer. *Physician Sportsmed*. 1991;19(5):67–68,72–74,77,80.
51. Knochel JP. Heat stroke and related heat stress disorders. *Dis Month*. 1989;35:301–377.
52. Casa DJ, Armstrong LE, Hillman SK, et al. National Athletic Trainers' Association position statement: fluid replacement for athletes. *J Athl Train*. 2000;35:212–224.
53. Armstrong LE, Maresh CM, Castellani JW, et al. Urinary indices of hydration status. *Int J Sport Nutr*. 1994;4:265–279.
54. Armstrong LE, Soto JA, Hacker FT Jr, Casa DJ, Kavouras SA, Maresh

CM. Urinary indices during dehydration exercise and rehydration. *Int J Sport Nutr*. 1997;8:345–355.

55. Heat and humidity. In: Armstrong LE. *Performing in Extreme Environments*. Champaign, IL: Human Kinetics; 2000:15–70.

56. Nadel ER, Fortney SM, Wenger CB. Effect of hydration state on circulatory and thermal regulations. *J Appl Physiol*. 1980;49:715–721.

57. Keithley JK, Keller A, Vazquez MG. Promoting good nutrition: using the food guide pyramid in clinical practice. *Medsurg Nurs*. 1996;5:397–403.

58. Achterberg C, McDonnell E, Bagby R. How to put the Food Guide Pyramid into practice. *J Am Diet Assoc*. 1994;94:1030–1035.

59. Laywell P. Guidelines for pre-event eating. *Texas Coach*. 1981;25:40–41,59.

60. Terrados N, Maughan RJ. Exercise in the heat: strategies to minimize the adverse effects on performance. *J Sports Sci*. 1995;13(suppl):55–62.

61. Armstrong LE, Hubbard RW, Szlyk PC, Matthew WT, Sils IV. Voluntary dehydration and electrolyte losses during prolonged exercise in the heat. *Aviat Space Environ Med*. 1985;56:765–770.

62. Sandor RP. Heat illness: on-site diagnosis and cooling. *Physician Sportsmed*. 1997;25(6):35–40.

63. Squire DL. Heat illness: fluid and electrolyte issues for pediatric and adolescent athletes. *Pediatr Clin North Am*. 1990;37:1085–1109.

64. Murray R. Fluid needs in hot and cold environments. *Int J Sports Nutr*. 1995;5(suppl):62–73.

65. Gisolfi CV. Fluid balance for optimal performance. *Nutr Rev*. 1996;54(4 Pt 2, suppl):159–168.

66. Sawka MN, Coyle EF. Influence of body water and blood volume on thermoregulation and exercise performance in the heat. *Exerc Sport Sci Rev*. 1999;27:167–218.

67. Roberts WO. Medical management and administration manual for long distance road racing. In: Brown CH, Gudjonsson B, eds. *IAAF Medical Manual for Athletics and Road Racing Competitions: A Practical Guide*. Monaco: International Amateur Athletic Federation Publications; 1998: 39–75.

68. Kulka TJ, Kenney WL. Heat balance limits in football uniforms: how different uniform ensembles alter the equation. *Physician Sportsmed*. 2002;30(7):29–39.

69. Department of the Army. *Prevention Treatment and Control of Heat Injury*. Washington, DC: Department of the Army; 1980. Technical bulletin TBMED 507:1–21.

70. Hughson RL, Staudt LA, Mackie JM. Monitoring road racing in the heat. *Physician Sportsmed*. 1983;11(5):94–102.

71. American College of Sports Medicine. ACSM position statement: prevention of thermal injuries during distance running. *Med Sci Sports Exerc*. 1987;19:529–533.

72. Armstrong LE, Epstein Y, Greenleaf JE, et al. American College of Sports Medicine position stand: heat and cold illnesses during distance running. *Med Sci Sports Exerc*. 1996;28:i–x.

73. Rozycki TJ. Oral and rectal temperatures in runners. *Physician Sportsmed*. 1984;12(6):105–110.

74. Knight JC, Casa DJ, McClung JM, Caldwell KA, Gilmer AM, Meenan PM, Goss PJ. Assessing if two tympanic temperature instruments are valid predictors of core temperature in hyperthermic runners and does drying the ear canal help [abstract]. *J Athl Train*. 2000;35(suppl):S21.

75. Shapiro Y, Pandolf KB, Goldman RF. Predicting sweat loss response to exercise, environment and clothing. *Eur J Appl Physiol Occup Physiol*. 1982;48:83–96.

76. Shvartz E, Saar E, Benor D. Physique and heat tolerance in hot dry and hot humid environments. *J Appl Physiol*. 1973;34:799–803.

77. Murray R. Dehydration, hyperthermia, and athletes: science and practice. *J Athl Train*. 1996;31:248–252.

78. Pichan G, Gauttam RK, Tomar OS, Bajaj AC. Effects of primary hypohydration on physical work capacity. *Int J Biometerorol*. 1988;32:176–180.

79. Walsh RM, Noakes TD, Hawley JA, Dennis SC. Impaired high-intensity cycling performance time at low levels of dehydration. *Int J Sports Med*. 1994;15:392–398.

80. Cheung SS, McLellan TM. Heat acclimation, aerobic fitness, and hy-

dration effects on tolerance during uncompensable heat stress. *J Appl Physiol*. 1998;84:1731–1739.

81. Bijlani R, Sharma KN. Effect of dehydration and a few regimes of rehydration on human performance. *Indian J Physiol Pharmacol*. 1980; 24:255–266.

82. Nielsen B. Solar heat load: heat balance during exercise in clothed subjects. *Eur J Appl Physiol Occup Physiol*. 1990;60:452–456.

83. Maughan RJ, Shirreffs SM. Preparing athletes for competition in the heat: developing an effective acclimatization strategy. *Sports Sci Exchange*. 1997;10:1–4.

84. Lloyd EL. ABC of sports medicine: temperature and performance—II: heat. *BMJ*. 1994;309:587–589.

85. Pascoe DD, Shanley LA, Smith EW. Clothing and exercise, I: biophysics of heat transfer between the individual clothing and environment. *Sports Med*. 1994;18:38–54.

86. Anderson MK, Hall SJ. *Sports Injury Management*. Philadelphia, PA: Williams & Wilkins; 1995:66–75.

87. Roberts WO. Assessing core temperature in collapsed athletes: what's the best method? *Physician Sportsmed*. 1994;22(8):49–55.

88. Armstrong LE, Maresh CM, Crago AE, Adams R, Roberts RO. Interpretation of aural temperatures during exercise, hyperthermia, and cooling therapy. *Med Exerc Nutr Health*. 1994;3:9–16.

89. Adner MM, Scarlet JJ, Casey J, Robinson W, Jones BH. The Boston Marathon medical care team: ten years of experience. *Physician Sportsmed*. 1988;16(7):99–108.

90. Casa DJ, Maresh CM, Armstrong LE, et al. Intravenous versus oral rehydration during a brief period: responses to subsequent exercise in the heat. *Med Sci Sports Exerc*. 2000;32:124–133.

91. Noakes T. Failure to thermoregulate. In: Sutton J, Thompson M, Torode M, eds. *Exercise and Thermoregulation*. Sydney, Australia: The University of Sydney; 1995:37.

92. Deschamps A, Levy RD, Coslo MG, Marliss EB, Magder S. Tympanic temperature should not be used to assess exercise-induced hyperthermia. *Clin J Sport Med*. 1992;2:27–32.

93. Gonzalez-Alonso J, Mora-Rodriguez R, Coyle EF. Supine exercise restores arterial blood pressure and skin blood flow despite dehydration and hyperthermia. *Am J Physiol*. 1999;277(2 Pt 2):H576–H583.

94. Germain M, Jobin M, Cabanac M. The effect of face fanning during the recovery from exercise hyperthermia. *Can J Physiol Pharmacol*. 1987; 65:87–91.

95. Roberts WO. Exercise-associated collapse in endurance events: a classification system. *Physician Sportsmed*. 1989;17(5):49–55.

96. Matthew CB. Treatment of hyperthermia and dehydration with hypertonic saline in dextran. *Shock*. 1994;2:216–221.

97. Armstrong LE, Crago AE, Adams R, Roberts WO, Maresh CM. Whole-body cooling of hyperthermic runners: comparison to two field therapies. *Am J Emerg Med*. 1996;14:355–358.

98. Marino F, Booth J. Whole body cooling by immersion in water at moderate temperature. *J Sci Med Sport*. 1998;1:73–82.

99. Clements JM, Casa DJ, Knight JC, et al. Ice-water immersion and cold-water immersion provide similar cooling rates in runners with exercise-induced hyperthermia. *J Athl Train*. 2002;37:146–150.

100. Ash CJ, Cook JR, McMurry TA, Auner CR. The use of rectal temperature to monitor heat stroke. *Mo Med*. 1992;89:283–288.

101. Brechue WF, Stager JM. Acetazolamide alters temperature regulation during submaximal exercise. *J Appl Physiol*. 1990;69:1402–1407.

102. Kubica R, Nielsen B, Bonnesen A, Rasmussen IB, Stoklosa J, Wilk B. Relationship between plasma volume reduction and plasma electrolyte changes after prolonged bicycle exercise, passive heating and diuretic dehydration. *Acta Physiol Pol*. 1983;34:569–579.

103. Claremont AD, Costill DL, Fink W, Van Handel P. Heat tolerance following diuretic induced dehydration. *Med Sci Sports*. 1976;8:239–243.

104. Desruelle AV, Boisvert P, Candas V. Alcohol and its variable effect on human thermoregulatory response to exercise in a warm environment. *Eur J Appl Physiol Occup Physiol*. 1996;74:572–574.

105. Kalant H, Le AD. Effect of ethanol on thermoregulation. *Pharmacol Ther*. 1983;23:313–364.

106. Vanakoski J, Seppala T. Heat exposure and drugs: a review of the effects

of hyperthermia on pharmacokinetics. *Clin Pharmacokinet*. 1998;34:311–322.

107. Shirreffs SM, Maughan RJ. Urine osmolality and conductivity as indices of hydration status in athletes in the heat. *Med Sci Sports Exerc*. 1998;30:1598–1602.

108. Kaplan A, Szabo LL, Opheim KE. *Clinical Chemistry: Interpretations and Techniques*. 2nd ed. Philadelphia, PA: Lea & Febiger; 1983.

109. Ross D, Neely AE. *Textbook of Urinalysis and Body Fluids*. Norwalk, CT: Appleton-Century-Crofts; 1983.

110. Armstrong L. The impact of hyperthermia and hypohydration on circulation strength endurance and health. *J Appl Sport Sci Res*. 1998;2:60–65.

111. Montain SJ, Sawka MN, Cadarette BS, Quigley MD, McKay JM. Physiological tolerance to uncompensable heat stress: effects of exercise intensity, protective clothing, and climate. *J Appl Physiol*. 1994;77:216–222.

112. Kenney WL, Hyde DE, Bernard TE. Physiological evaluation of liquid-barrier, vapor-permeable protective clothing ensembles for work in hot environments. *Am Ind Hyg Assoc J*. 1993;54:397–402.

113. Mathews DK, Fox EL, Tanzi D. Physiological responses during exercise and recovery in a football uniform. *J Appl Physiol*. 1969;26:611–615.

114. Armstrong LE. The nature of heatstroke during exercise. *Natl Strength Condition J*. 1992;14:80.

115. Wetterhall SF, Coulombier DM, Herndon JM, Zaza S, Cantwell JD. Medical care delivery at the 1996 Olympic Games: Centers for Disease Control and Prevention Olympics Surveillance Unit. *JAMA*. 1998;279:1463–1468.

116. Cooper KE. Some responses of the cardiovascular system to heat and fever. *Can J Cardiol*. 1994;10:444–448.

117. Epstein Y. Heat intolerance: predisposing factor or residual injury? *Med Sci Sports Exerc*. 1990;22:29–35.

118. Chung NK, Pin CH. Obesity and the occurrence of heat disorders. *Mil Med*. 1996;161:739–742.

119. Gardner JW, Kark JA, Karnei K, et al. Risk factors predicting exertional heat illness in male Marine Corps recruits. *Med Sci Sports Exerc*. 1996;28:939–944.

120. Hayward JS, Eckerson JD, Dawson BT. Effect of mesomorphy on hyperthermia during exercise in a warm, humid environment. *Am J Phys Anthropol*. 1986;70:11–17.

121. Kark JA, Burr PQ, Wenger CB, Gastaldo E, Gardner JW. Exertional heat illness in Marine Corps recruit training. *Aviat Space Environ Med*. 1996;67:354–360.

122. Piwonka RW, Robinson S, Gay VL, Manalis RS. Preacclimatization of men to heat by training. *J Appl Physiol*. 1965;20:379–384.

123. Noakes TD, Myburgh KH, du Plessis J, et al. Metabolic rate, not percent dehydration, predicts rectal temperature in marathon runners. *Med Sci Sports Exerc*. 1991;23:443–449.

124. Nadel ER, Pandolf KB, Roberts MF, Stolwijk JA. Mechanisms of thermal acclimation to exercise and heat. *J Appl Physiol*. 1974;37:515–520.

125. Walter FF, Bey TA, Ruschke DS, Benowitz NL. Marijuana and hyperthermia. *J Toxicol Clin Toxicol*. 1996;34:217–221.

126. Watson JD, Ferguson C, Hinds CJ, Skinner R, Coakley JH. Exertional heat stroke induced by amphetamine analogues: does dantrolene have a place? *Anaesthesia*. 1993;48:1057–1060.

127. Epstein Y, Albukrek D, Kalmovitc B, Moran DS, Shapiro Y. Heat intolerance induced by antidepressants. *Ann N Y Acad Sci*. 1997;813:553–558.

128. Stadnyk AN, Glezos JD. Drug-induced heat stroke. *Can Med Assoc J*. 1983;128:957–959.

129. Forester D. Fatal drug-induced heat stroke. *JACEP*. 1978;7:243–244.

130. Sarnquist F, Larson CP Jr. Drug-induced heat stroke. *Anesthesiology*. 1973;39:348–350.

131. Zelman S, Guillan R. Heat stroke in phenothiazine-treated patients: a report of three fatalities. *Am J Psychiatry*. 1970;126:1787–1790.

132. Gordon NF, Duncan JJ. Effect of beta-blockers on exercise physiology: implications for exercise training. *Med Sci Sports Exerc*. 1991;23:668–676.

133. Freund BJ, Joyner MJ, Jilka SM, et al. Thermoregulation during prolonged exercise in heat: alterations with beta-adrenergic blockade. *J Appl Physiol*. 1987;63:930–936.

134. Kew MC, Hopp M, Rothberg A. Fatal heat-stroke in a child taking appetite-suppressant drugs. *S Afr Med J*. 1982;62:905–906.

135. Lomax P, Daniel KA. Cocaine and body temperature: effect of exercise at high ambient temperature. *Pharmacology*. 1993;46:164–172.

136. Chen WL, Huang WS, Lin YF, Shieh SD. Changes in thyroid hormone metabolism in exertional heat stroke with or without acute renal failure. *J Clin Endocrinol Metab*. 1996;81:625–629.

137. Wemple RD, Lamb DR, McKeever KH. Caffeine vs caffeine-free sports drinks: effect on urine production at rest and during prolonged exercise. *Int J Sports Med*. 1997;18:40–46.

138. Odlind B. Site and mechanism of the action of diuretics. *Acta Pharmacol Toxicol (Copenh)*. 1984;54(suppl 1):5–15.

139. Stookey JD. The diuretic effects of alcohol and caffeine and total water intake misclassification. *Eur J Epidemiol*. 1999;15:181–188.

140. Schlaeffer F, Engelberg I, Kaplanski J, Danon A. Effect of exercise and environmental heat on theophylline kinetics. *Respiration*. 1984;45:438–442.

141. Armstrong LE, Hubbard RW, Askew EW, et al. Responses to moderate and low sodium diets during exercise-heat acclimation. *Int J Sport Nutr*. 1993;3:207–221.

142. Armstrong LE, Szlyk PC, DeLuca JP, Sils IV, Hubbard RW. Fluid-electrolyte losses in uniforms during prolonged exercise at 30 degrees C. *Aviat Space Environ Med*. 1992;63:351–355.

143. Mendyka BE. Fluid and electrolyte disorders caused by diuretic therapy. *AACN Clin Issues Crit Care Nurs*. 1992;3:672–680.

144. Melby JC. Selected mechanisms of diuretic-induced electrolyte changes. *Am J Cardiol*. 1986;58:1A–4A.

145. Bourdon L, Canini F. On the nature of the link between malignant hyperthermia and exertional heatstroke. *Med Hypotheses*. 1995;45:268–270.

146. Dixit SN, Bushara KO, Brooks BR. Epidemic heat stroke in midwest community: risk factors, neurological complications, and sequelae. *Wis Med J*. 1997;96:39–41.

147. Hunter SL, Rosenberg H, Tuttle GH, DeWalt JL, Smodie R, Martin J. Malignant hyperthermia in a college football player. *Physician Sportsmed*. 1987;15(12):77–81.

148. Lazarus A. Differentiating neuroleptic-related heatstroke from neuroleptic malignant syndrome. *Psychosomatics*. 1989;30:454–456.

149. Rampertaap MP. Neuroleptic malignant syndrome. *South Med J*. 1986;79:331–336.

150. Addonizio G, Susman V. Neuroleptic malignant syndrome and heat stroke. *Br J Psychiatry*. 1984;145:556–557.

151. Martin ML, Lucid EJ, Walker RW. Neuroleptic malignant syndrome. *Ann Emerg Med*. 1985;14:354–358.

152. Virmani R, Robinowitz M. Cardiac pathology and sports medicine. *Hum Pathol*. 1987;18:493–501.

153. Buchwald I, Davis PJ. Scleroderma with fatal heat stroke. *JAMA*. 1967;201:270–271.

154. Smith HR, Dhatt GS, Melia WM, Dickinson JG. Cystic fibrosis presenting as hyponatraemic heat exhaustion. *BMJ*. 1995;310:579–580.

155. Andrews C, Mango M, Venuto RC. Cystic fibrosis in adults. *Ann Intern Med*. 1978;88:128–129.

156. Kerle KK, Nishimura KD. Exertional collapse and sudden death associated with sickle cell trait. *Am Fam Physician*. 1996;54:237–240.

157. Gardner JW, Kark JA. Fatal rhabdomyolysis presenting as mild heat illness in military training. *Mil Med*. 1994;159:160–163.

158. Kenney WL. Thermoregulation during exercise in the heat. *Athl Ther Today*. 1996;1:13–16.

159. Tilley RI, Standerwick JM, Long GJ. Ability of the Wet Bulb Globe Temperature Index to predict heat stress in men wearing NBC protective clothing. *Mil Med*. 1987;152:554–556.

160. Rasch W, Cabanac M. Selective brain cooling is affected by wearing headgear during exercise. *J Appl Physiol*. 1993;74:1229–1233.

161. Sheffield-Moore M, Short KR, Kerr CG, Parcell AC, Bolster DR, Costill DL. Thermoregulatory responses to cycling with and without a helmet. *Med Sci Sports Exerc*. 1997;29:755–761.

162. Shapiro Y, Pandolf KB, Avellini BA, Pimental NA, Goldman RF. Phys-

iological responses of men and women to humid and dry heat. *J Appl Physiol*. 1980;49:1–8.

163. Yaglou CP, Minard D. Control of heat casualties at military training centers. *Arch Ind Health*. 1957;16:302–305.

164. Bracker MO. Hyperthermia: man's adaptation to a warm climate. *Sports Med Dig*. 1991;13:1–2.

165. Johnson SC, Ruhling RO. Aspirin in exercise-induced hyperthermia: evidence for and against its role. *Sports Med*. 1985;2:1–7.

166. Werner J. Central regulation of body temperature. In: Gisolfi C, ed. *Exercise, Heat, and Thermoregulation*. Carmel, IN: Cooper Publishing; 1993:7–35.

167. Galaski MJ. Hyperthermia. *J Can Athl Ther*. 1985;12:23–26.

168. Yaqub BA. Neurologic manifestations of heatstroke at the Mecca pilgrimage. *Neurology*. 1987;37:1004–1006.

169. Armstrong LE. *Keeping Your Cool in Barcelona: The Effects of Heat Humidity and Dehydration on Athletic Performance Strength and Endurance*. Colorado Springs, CO: United States Olympic Committee Sports Sciences Division; 1992:1–29.

170. Anderson GS, Meneilly GS, Mekjavic IB. Passive temperature lability in the elderly. *Eur J Appl Physiol Occup Physiol*. 1996;73:278–286.

171. Candas V, Libert JP, Vogt JJ. Influence of air velocity and heat acclimation on human skin wettedness and sweating efficiency. *J Appl Physiol*. 1979;47:1194–2000.

172. Berglund LG, Gonzalez RR. Evaporation of sweat from sedentary man in humid environments. *J Appl Physiol*. 1977;42:767–772.

173. Gabrys J, Pieniazek W, Olejnik I, Pogorzelska T, Karpe J. Effects of local cooling of neck circulatory responses in men subjected to physical exercise in hyperthermia. *Biol Sport*. 1993;10:167–171.

174. Royburt M, Epstein Y, Solomon Z, Shemer J. Long-term psychological and physiological effects of heat stroke. *Physiol Behav*. 1993;54:265–267.

175. Mehta AC, Baker RN. Persistent neurological deficits in heat stroke. *Neurology*. 1970;20:336–340.

176. McArdle WD, Katch FI, Katch VL. *Exercise Physiology*. 3rd ed. Philadelphia, PA: Lea & Febiger; 1991:556–570.

177. Avellini BA, Kamon E, Krajewski JT. Physiological responses of physically fit men and women to acclimation to humid heat. *J Appl Physiol*. 1980;49:254–261.

178. Geor RJ, McCutcheon LJ. Thermoregulatory adaptations associated with training and heat acclimation. *Vet Clin North Am Equine Pract*. 1988; 14:97–120.

179. Nielsen B. Heat stress and acclimation. *Ergonomics*. 1994;37:49–58.

180. Gisolfi CV, Wenger CB. Temperature regulation during exercise: old concepts, new ideas. *Exerc Sport Sci Rev*. 1984;12:339–372.

181. Morimoto T, Miki K, Nose H, Yamada S, Hirakawa K, Matsubara D. Changes in body fluid and its composition during heavy sweating and effect of fluid and electrolyte replacement. *Jpn J Biometeorol*. 1981;18: 31–39.

182. Pandolf KB, Cadarette BS, Sawka MN, Young AJ, Francesconi RP, Gonzalez RR. Thermoregulatory responses of middle-aged and young men during dry-heat acclimation. *J Appl Physiol*. 1998;65:65–71.

183. Pandolf KB, Burse RL, Goldman RF. Role of physical fitness in heat acclimatisation, decay and reinduction. *Ergonomics*. 1977;20:399–408.

184. Cadarette BS, Sawka MN, Toner MM, Pandolf KB. Aerobic fitness and the hypohydration response to exercise-heat stress. *Aviat Space Environ Med*. 1984;55:507–512.

185. Buskirk ER, Iampietro PF, Bass DE. Work performance after dehydration: effects of physical conditioning and heat acclimatization. *J Appl Physiol*. 1958;12:789–794.

186. Adams J, Fox R, Grimby G, Kidd D, Wolff H. Acclimatization to heat and its rate of decay in man. *J Physiol*. 1960;152:26P–27P.

187. Czerkawski JT, Meintod A, Kleiner DM. Exertional heat illness: teaching patients when to cool it. *Your Patient Fitness*. 1996;10:13–20.

188. Wyndham C, Strydom N, Cooks H, et al. Methods of cooling subjects with hyperpyrexia. *J Appl Physiol*. 1959;14:771–776.

189. Hayward JS, Collis M, Eckerson JD. Thermographic evaluation of relative heat loss areas of man during cold water immersion. *Aerosp Med*. 1973;44:708–711.

190. Tsuzuki-Hayakawa K, Tochihara Y, Ohnaka T. Thermoregulation during

heat exposure of young children compared to their mothers. *Eur J Appl Physiol Occup Physiol*. 1995;72:12–17.

191. Bar-Or O. Children's responses to exercise in hot climates: implications for performance and health. *Sports Sci Exerc*. 1994;7:1–5.

192. Davies CT. Thermal responses to exercise in children. *Ergonomics*. 1981;24:55–61.

193. Docherty D, Eckerson JD, Hayward JS. Physique and thermoregulation in prepubertal males during exercise in a warm, humid environment. *Am J Phys Anthropol*. 1986;70:19–23.

194. Armstrong LE, Maresh CM. Exercise-heat tolerance of children and adolescents. *Pediatr Exerc Sci*. 1995;7:239–252.

195. Gutierrez GG. Solar injury and heat illness: treatment and prevention in children. *Physician Sportsmed*. 1995;23(7):43–48.

196. Nash HL. Hyperthermia: risks greater in children. *Physician Sportsmed*. 1987;15(2):29.

197. American Academy of Pediatrics Committee on Sports Medicine. Climatic heat stress and the exercising child. *Pediatrics*. 1982;69:808–809.

198. Kenney WL, Hodgson JL. Heat tolerance, thermoregulation, and ageing. *Sports Med*. 1987;4:446–456.

199. Wagner JA, Robinson S, Tzankoff SP, Marino RP. Heat tolerance and acclimatization to work in the heat in relation to age. *J Appl Physiol*. 1972;33:616–622.

200. Pandolf KB. Heat tolerance and aging. *Exp Aging Res*. 1994;20:275–284.

201. Pandolf KB. Aging and human heat tolerance. *Exp Aging Res*. 1997;23: 69–105.

202. Kenney W. The older athlete: exercise in hot environments. *Sports Sci Exerc*. 1993;6:1–4.

203. Inoue Y, Shibasaki M, Hirata K, Araki T. Relationship between skin blood flow and sweating rate and age related regional differences. *Eur J Appl Physiol Occup Physiol*. 1998;79:17–23.

204. Sagawa S, Shiraki K, Yousef MK, Miki K. Sweating and cardiovascular responses of aged men to heat exposure. *J Gerontol*. 1988;43:M1–M8.

205. Inoue Y, Shibasaki M. Regional differences in age-related decrements of the cutaneous vascular and sweating responses to passive heating. *Eur J Appl Physiol Occup Physiol*. 1996;74:78–84.

206. Inoue Y, Shibasaki M, Ueda H, Ishizashi H. Mechanisms underlying the age-related decrement in the human sweating response. *Eur J Appl Physiol Occup Physiol*. 1999;79:121–126.

207. Pandolf KB, Cafarelli E, Noble BJ, Metz KF. Hyperthermia: effect on exercise prescription. *Arch Phys Med Rehabil*. 1975;56:524–526.

208. Zappe DH, Bell GW, Swartzentruber H, Wideman RF, Kenney WL. Age and regulation of fluid and electrolyte balance during repeated exercise sessions. *Am J Physiol*. 1996;207(1 Pt 2):R71–R79.

209. Binkhorst RA, Hopman MT. Heat balance in paraplegic individuals during arm exercise at 10 and 35°C. *Med Sci Sports Exerc*. 1995;27(suppl): 83.

210. Clark MW. The physically challenged athlete. *Adolesc Med*. 1998;9: 491–499.

211. Bloomquist LE. Injuries to athletes with physical disabilities: prevention implications. *Physician Sportsmed*. 1986;14(9):96–100,102,105.

212. Hopman MT, Binkhourst RA. Spinal cord injury and exercise in the heat. *Sports Sci Exerc*. 1997;10:1–4.

213. Armstrong LE, Maresh CM, Riebe D, et al. Local cooling in wheelchair athletes during exercise-heat stress. *Med Sci Sports Exerc*. 1995;27:211–216.

214. Sawka MN, Latzka WA, Pandolf KB. Temperature regulation during upper body exercise: able-bodied and spinal cord injured. *Med Sci Sports Exerc*. 1989;21(5 suppl):132–140.

215. Hopman MT, Oeseburg B, Binkhorst RA. Cardiovascular responses in persons with paraplegia to prolonged arm exercise and thermal stress. *Med Sci Sports Exerc*. 1993;25:577–583.

216. Petrofsky JS. Thermoregulatory stress during rest and exercise in heat in patients with a spinal cord injury. *Eur J Appl Physiol Occup Physiol*. 1992;64:503–507.

217. Bracker MD. Environmental and thermal injury. *Clin Sports Med*. 1992; 11:419–436.

218. Hopman MT. Circulatory responses during arm exercise in individuals with paraplegia. *Int J Sports Med*. 1994;15:126–131.

219. Yamaski M, Kim KT, Choi SW, Muraki S, Shiokawa M, Kurokawa T. Characteristics of body heat balance of paraplegics during exercise in a hot environment. *J Physiol Anthropol Appl Human Sci*. 2001;20:227–232.

220. Gass GC, Camp EM, Nadel ER, Gwinn TH, Engel P. Rectal and rectal vs. esophageal temperatures in paraplegic men during prolonged exercise. *J Appl Physiol*. 1998;64:2265–2271.

221. Yaqub BA, Al-Harthi SS, Al-Orainey IO, Laajam MA, Obeid MT. Heat stroke at the Mekkah pilgrimage: clinical characteristics and course of 30 patients. *Q J Med*. 1986;59:523–530.

222. Hubbard RW. The role of exercise in the etiology of exertional heatstroke. *Med Sci Sports Exerc*. 1990;22:2–5.

223. Holman ND, Schneider AJ. Multi-organ damage in exertional heat stroke. *Neth J Med*. 1989;35:38–43.

224. Shibolet S, Coll R, Gilat T, Sohar E. Heatstroke: its clinical picture and mechanism in 36 cases. *Q J Med*. 1965;36:525–548.

225. Gummaa K, El-Mahrouky S, Mahmoud H, Mustafa K, Khogall M. The metabolic status of heat stroke patients: the Makkah experience. In: Khogali M, Hale JR, eds. *Heat Stroke and Temperature Regulation*. New York, NY: Academic Press; 1983:157–169.

226. Garcia-Rubira JC, Aguilar J, Romero D. Acute myocardial infarction in a young man after heat exhaustion. *Int J Cardiol*. 1995;47:297–300.

227. Senay LC, Kok R. Body fluid responses of heat-tolerant and intolerant men to work in a hot wet environment. *J Appl Physiol*. 1976;40:55–59.

228. Shvartz E, Shibolet S, Merez A, Magazanik A, Shapiro Y. Prediction of heat tolerance from heart rate and rectal temperature in a temperate environment. *J Appl Physiol*. 1977;43:684–688.

229. Strydom NB. Heat intolerance: its detection and elimination in the mining industry. *S Afr J Sci*. 1980;76:154–156.

230. Robergs RA, Roberts SO. *Exercise Physiology: Exercise, Performance, and Clinical Applications*. St Louis, MO: Mosby; 1997:653–662.

Exertional Heat Illness Review Questions:

1. What causes an athlete to have exertional heat stroke? Can you do anything to prevent it? Answer for each type of heat illness.

2. How do you recognize/assess an exertional heat stroke? Answer for each type of heat illness.

3. What would you tell a fellow athletic trainer about our current knowledge regarding temperature assessment of a suspected exertional heat stroke victim?

4. Please explain the best way to treat a victim of exertional heat stroke and any helpful hints regarding this process.

5. What factors need to be considered when altering/cancelling practice based on WBGT?

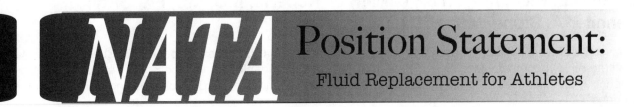

NATA Position Statement:
Fluid Replacement for Athletes

In This Section: Dehydration is a major contributor to heat illness and can greatly affect athletic performance. The following position statement provides guidance for athletic trainers in educating their athletes about the importance of proper hydration and describes how to develop individual fluid replacement practices before, during and after physical activity.

National Athletic Trainers' Association Position Statement: Fluid Replacement for Athletes

Douglas J. Casa, PhD, ATC, CSCS (Chair)*;
Lawrence E. Armstrong, PhD, FACSM*; Susan K. Hillman, MS, MA, ATC, PT†;
Scott J. Montain, PhD, FACSM‡; Ralph V. Reiff, MEd, ATC§;
Brent S.E. Rich, MD, ATC‖; William O. Roberts, MD, MS, FACSM¶;
Jennifer A. Stone, MS, ATC#

*University of Connecticut, Storrs, CT; †Arizona School of Health Sciences, Phoenix, AZ; ‡US Army Research Institute of Environmental Medicine, Natick, MA; §St. Vincent Hospital, Indianapolis, IN; ‖Arizona State University, Phoenix, AZ; ¶MinnHealth Family Physicians, White Bear Lake, MN; #US Olympic Training Center, Colorado Springs, CO

Objective: To present recommendations to optimize the fluid-replacement practices of athletes.

Background: Dehydration can compromise athletic performance and increase the risk of exertional heat injury. Athletes do not voluntarily drink sufficient water to prevent dehydration during physical activity. Drinking behavior can be modified by education, increasing accessibility, and optimizing palatability. However, excessive overdrinking should be avoided because it can also compromise physical performance and health. We provide practical recommendations regarding fluid replacement for athletes.

Recommendations: Educate athletes regarding the risks of dehydration and overhydration on health and physical performance. Work with individual athletes to develop fluid-replacement practices that optimize hydration status before, during, and after competition.

Key Words: athletic performance, dehydration, heat illness, hydration protocol, hydration status, oral rehydration solution, rehydration

During exercise, evaporation is usually the primary mechanism of heat dissipation. The evaporation of sweat from the skin's surface assists the body in regulating core temperature. If the body cannot adequately evaporate sweat from the skin's surface, core temperature rises rapidly. A side effect of sweating is the loss of valuable fluids from the finite reservoir within the body, the rate being related to exercise intensity, individual differences, environmental conditions, acclimatization state, clothing, and baseline hydration status. Athletes whose sweat loss exceeds fluid intake become dehydrated during activity. Therefore, a person with a high sweat rate who undertakes intense exercise in a hot, humid environment can rapidly become dehydrated. Dehydration of 1% to 2% of body weight begins to compromise physiologic function and negatively influence performance. Dehydration of greater than 3% of body weight further disturbs physiologic function and increases an athlete's risk of developing an exertional heat illness (ie, heat cramps, heat exhaustion, or heat stroke). This level of dehydration is common in sports; it can be elicited in just an hour of exercise or even

more rapidly if the athlete enters the exercise session dehydrated. The onset of significant dehydration is preventable, or at least modifiable, when hydration protocols are followed to assure all athletes the most productive and the safest athletic experience.

The purpose of this position stand is to 1) provide useful recommendations to optimize fluid replacement for athletes, 2) emphasize the physiologic, medical, and performance considerations associated with dehydration, and 3) identify factors that influence optimal rehydration during and after athletic participation.

RECOMMENDATIONS

The National Athletic Trainers' Association (NATA) recommends the following practices regarding fluid replacement for athletic participation:

1. Establish a hydration protocol for athletes, including a rehydration strategy that considers the athlete's sweat rate, sport dynamics (eg, rest breaks, fluid access), environmental factors, acclimatization state, exercise duration, exercise intensity, and individual preferences (see Table 1 for examples of potential outcomes).

Address correspondence to National Athletic Trainers' Association, Communications Department, 2952 Stemmons Freeway, Dallas, TX 75247.

2. A proper hydration protocol considers each sport's unique features. If rehydration opportunities are frequent (eg, baseball, football, track and field), the athlete can consume smaller volumes at a convenient pace based on sweat rate and environmental conditions. If rehydration must occur at specific times (eg, soccer, lacrosse, distance running), the athlete must consume fluids to maximize hydration within the sport's confines and rules.

3. Fluid-replacement beverages should be easily accessible in individual fluid containers and flavored to the athlete's preference. Individual containers permit easier monitoring of fluid intake. Clear water bottles marked in 100-mL (3.4-fl oz) increments provide visual reminders to athletes to drink beyond thirst satiation or the typical few gulps. Carrying water bottles or other hydration systems, when practical, during exercise encourages greater fluid volume ingestion.

4. Athletes should begin all exercise sessions well hydrated. Hydration status can be approximated by athletes and athletic trainers in several ways (Table 2). Assuming proper hydration, pre-exercise body weight should be relatively consistent across exercise sessions. Determine the percentage difference between the current body weight and the hydrated baseline body weight. Remember that body weight is dynamic. Frequent exercise sessions can induce nonfluid-related weight loss influenced by timing of meals and defecation, time of day, and calories expended in exercise. The simplest method is comparison of urine color (from a sample in a container) with a urine color chart (Figure). Measuring urine specific gravity (USG) with a refractometer (available for less than $150) is less subjective than comparing urine color and also simple to use. Urine volume is another indicator of hydration status but inconvenient to collect and measure. For color analysis or specific gravity, use midstream urine collection for consistency and accuracy. Remember that body weight changes during exercise give the best indication of hydration status. Because of urine and body weight dynamics, measure urine before exercise and check body weight (percentage of body weight change) before, during, and after exercise sessions to estimate fluid balance.

5. To ensure proper pre-exercise hydration, the athlete should consume approximately 500 to 600 mL (17 to 20 fl oz) of water or a sports drink 2 to 3 hours before exercise and 200 to 300 mL (7 to 10 fl oz) of water or a sports drink 10 to 20 minutes before exercise.

6. Fluid replacement should approximate sweat and urine losses and at least maintain hydration at less than 2% body weight reduction. This generally requires 200 to 300 mL (7 to 10 fl oz) every 10 to 20 minutes. Specific individual recommendations are calculated based on sweat rates, sport dynamics, and individual tolerance. Maintaining hydration status in athletes with high sweat rates, in sports with limited fluid access, and during high-intensity exercise can be difficult, and special efforts should be made to minimize dehydration. Dangerous hyperhydration is also a risk if athletes drink based on published recommendations and not according to individual needs.

7. Postexercise hydration should aim to correct any fluid loss accumulated during the practice or event. Ideally completed within 2 hours, rehydration should contain water to restore hydration status, carbohydrates to replenish glycogen stores, and electrolytes to speed rehydration. The primary goal is the immediate return of physiologic function (especially if an exercise bout will follow). When rehydration must be rapid, the athlete should compensate for obligatory urine losses incurred during the rehydration process and drink about 25% to 50% more than sweat losses to assure optimal hydration 4 to 6 hours after the event.

8. Fluid temperature influences the amount consumed. While individual differences exist, a cool beverage of 10° to 15°C (50° to 59°F) is recommended.

9. The Wet Bulb Globe Temperature (WBGT) should be ascertained in hot environments. Very high relative humidity limits evaporative cooling; the air is nearly saturated with water vapor, and evaporation is minimized. Thus, dehydration associated with high sweat losses can induce a rapid core temperature increase due to the inability to dissipate heat. Measuring core temperature rectally allows the athlete's thermal status to be accurately determined. See the NATA position statement on heat illnesses for expanded information on this topic.

10. In many situations, athletes benefit from including carbohydrates (CHOs) in their rehydration protocols. Consuming CHOs during the pre-exercise hydration session (2 to 3 hours pre-exercise), as in item 5, along with a normal daily diet increases glycogen stores. If exercise is intense, then consuming CHOs about 30 minutes pre-exercise may also be beneficial. Include CHOs in the rehydration beverage during exercise if the session lasts longer than 45 to 50 minutes or is intense. An ingestion rate of about 1 g/min (0.04 oz/min) maintains optimal carbohydrate metabolism: for example, 1 L of a 6% CHO drink per hour of exercise. CHO concentrations greater than 8% increase the rate of CHO delivery to the body but compromise the rate of fluid emptying from the stomach and absorbed from the intestine. Fruit juices, CHO gels, sodas, and some sports drinks have CHO concentrations greater than 8% and are not recommended *during* an exercise session as the sole beverage. Athletes should consume CHOs at least 30 minutes before the normal onset of fatigue and earlier if the environmental conditions are unusually extreme, although this may not apply for very intense short-term exercise, which may require earlier intake of CHOs. Most CHO forms (ie, glucose, sucrose, glucose polymers) are suitable, and the absorption rate is maximized when multiple forms are consumed simultaneously. Substances to be limited include fructose (which may cause gastrointestinal distress); those to be avoided include caffeine, alcohol (which may increase urine output and reduce fluid retention), and carbonated beverages (which may reduce voluntary fluid intake due to stomach fullness).

11. Those supervising athletes should be able to recognize the basic signs and symptoms of dehydration: thirst, irritability, and general discomfort, followed by headache, weakness, dizziness, cramps, chills, vomiting, nausea, head or neck heat sensations, and decreased performance. Early diagnosis of dehydration decreases the occurrence and severity of heat illness. A conscious, cognizant, dehydrated athlete without gastrointestinal distress can aggressively rehydrate orally, while one with mental compromise from dehydration or gastrointestinal distress should be transported to a medical facility for intravenous rehydration. For a complete description of heat illnesses and issues

related to hyperthermia, see the NATA position statement on heat illnesses.

12. Inclusion of sodium chloride in fluid-replacement beverages should be considered under the following conditions: inadequate access to meals or meals not eaten; physical activity exceeding 4 hours in duration; or during the initial days of hot weather. Under these conditions, adding modest amounts of salt (0.3 to 0.7 g/L) can offset salt loss in sweat and minimize medical events associated with electrolyte imbalances (eg, muscle cramps, hyponatremia). Adding a modest amount of salt (0.3 to 0.7 g/L) to all hydration beverages would be acceptable to stimulate thirst, increase voluntary fluid intake, and decrease the risk of hyponatremia and should cause no harm.

13. Calculate each athlete's sweat rate (sweating rate = pre-exercise body weight − postexercise body weight + fluid intake − urine volume/exercise time in hours) for a representative range of environmental conditions, practices, and competitions (Table 3). This time-consuming task can be made easier by weighing a large number of athletes before an intense 1-hour practice session and then reweighing them at the end of the 1-hour practice. Sweat rate can now be easily calculated (do not allow rehydration or urination during this 1 hour when sweat rate is being determined to make the task even easier). This calculation is the most fundamental consideration when establishing a rehydration protocol. Average sweat rates from the scientific literature or other athletes can vary from 0.5 L/h to more than 2.5 L/h (0.50 to 2.50 kg/h) and are not ideal to use.

14. Heat acclimatization induces physiologic changes that may alter individual fluid-replacement considerations. First, sweat rate generally increases after 10 to 14 days of heat exposure, requiring a greater fluid intake for a similar bout of exercise. An athlete's sweat rate should be reassessed after acclimatization. Second, moving from a cool environment to a warm environment increases the overall sweat rate for a bout of exercise. The athlete's hydration status must be closely monitored for the first week of exercise in a warm environment. Third, increased sodium intake may be warranted during the first 3 to 5 days of heat exposure, since the increased thermal strain and associated increased sweat rate increase the sodium lost in sweat. Adequate sodium intake optimizes fluid palatability and absorption during the first few days and may decrease exercise-associated muscle cramping. After 5 to 10 days, the sodium concentration of sweat decreases, and normal sodium intake suffices.

15. All sports requiring weight classes (ie, wrestling, judo, rowing) should mandate a check of hydration status at weigh-in to ensure that the athlete is not dehydrated. A USG less than or equal to 1.020 or urine color less than or equal to 4 should be the upper range of acceptable on weigh-in. Any procedures used to induce dramatic dehydration (eg, diuretics, rubber suits, exercising in a sauna) are strictly prohibited.

16. Hyperhydration by ingesting a pre-exercise glycerol and water beverage has equivocal support from well-controlled studies. At this time, evidence is insufficient to endorse the practice of hyperhydration via glycerol. Also, a risk of side effects such as headaches and gastrointestinal distress exists when glycerol is consumed.

17. Consider modifications when working with prepubescent and adolescent athletes who exercise intensely in the heat and may not fully comprehend the medical and performance consequences of dehydration. Focus special attention on schedules and event modification to minimize environmental stress and maximize time for fluid replacement. Make available the most palatable beverage possible. Educate parents and coaches about rehydration and the signs of dehydration. Monitor and remove a child from activity promptly if signs or symptoms of dehydration occur.

18. Large-scale event management (eg, tournaments, camps) requires advance planning. Ample fluid and cups should be conveniently available. With successive practice sessions during a day or over multiple days (as in most summer sport camps), check hydration status daily before allowing continued participation. Be aware of unhealthy behaviors, such as eating disorders and dehydration in weight-class sports. Use extra caution with novice and unconditioned athletes, and remember, many athletes are not supervised on a daily basis. If the WBGT dictates, modify events (change game times or cancel) or change game dynamics (insert nonroutine water breaks, shorten game times). Recruit help from fellow athletic trainers in local schools, student athletic trainers, and athletes from other sports to ensure that hydration is maintained at all venues (ie, along a road race course, on different fields during a tournament). Be sure all assistants can communicate with the supervising athletic trainer at a central location. For successive-day events, provide educational materials on rehydration principles to inform athletes and parents of this critical component of athletic performance.

19. Implementing a hydration protocol for athletes will only succeed if athletes, coaches, athletic trainers, and team physicians realize the importance of maintaining proper hydration status and the steps required to accomplish this goal. Here are the most critical components of hydration education:

- Educate athletes on the effects of dehydration on physical performance.
- Inform athletes on how to monitor hydration status.
- Convince athletes to participate in their own hydration protocols based on sweat rate, drinking preferences, and personal responses to different fluid quantities.
- Encourage coaches to mandate rehydration during practices and competitions, just as they require other drills and conditioning activities.
- Have a scale accessible to assist athletes in monitoring weight before, during, and after activity.
- Provide the optimal oral rehydration solution (water, CHOs, electrolytes) before, during, and after exercise.
- Implement the hydration protocol during all practices and games, and adapt it as needed.
- Finally, encourage event scheduling and rule modifications to minimize the risks associated with exercise in the heat.

BACKGROUND AND LITERATURE REVIEW

Dehydration and Exercise

Physiologic Implications. All physiologic systems in the human body are influenced by dehydration.[1,2] The degree of

Table 1. Sample Hydration Protocol Worksheet

Parameter to Consider	Example A: College Soccer, Katie (60 kg)*	Example B: High School Basketball, Mike (80 kg)*
1) WBGT	28.3°C (83°F)	21.1°C (70°F)
2) Sweat rate†	1.7 L/h	1.2 L/h
3) Acclimatized	Yes	No
4) Length of activity	2 45-minute halves	4 10-minute quarters
5) Intensity	Game situation (maximal)	Game situation (maximal)
6) Properly prehydrated	No (began −2% body weight)	Yes
7) Individual container	Yes	No (just cups)
8) Type of beverage	5% to 7% CHO‡ solution	5% to 7% CHO solution
9) Assess hydration status	At halftime (with scale)	No
10) Available breaks	Halftime	Quarters, half, timeouts
11) Amount given	Maximal comfortable predetermined amount given at half time (about 700 to 1000 L)	200 mL at quarter breaks 400 mL at half time 100 mL at 1 timeout/half
12) End hydration status	−4.8% body weight	Normal hydration
13) Hydrated body weight	60 kg	80 kg
Pre-exercise body weight	58.8 kg	80 kg
Halftime body weight	57.5	No measure
Postexercise body weight	57.1	80.1 kg

*Assumptions: Both are starters and play a full game.
†Sweat rate determined under similar parameters described in example (ie, acclimatization state, WBGT, intensity, etc) under normal game conditions (ie, no injury timeouts, overtime, etc).
Note: Keep results on record for future reference.
‡CHO, carbohydrate.

Table 2. Indexes of Hydration Status

Condition	% Body Weight Change*	Urine Color	USG†
Well hydrated	+1 to −1	1 or 2	<1.010
Minimal dehydration	−1 to −3	3 or 4	1.010–1.020
Significant dehydration	−3 to −5	5 or 6	1.021–1.030
Serious dehydration	>5	>6	>1.030

*% Body weight change = [(pre-exercise body weight − postexercise body weight)/pre-exercise body weight] × 100.
†USG, urine specific gravity.
See Figure for urine color chart and references. Please note that obtaining a urine sample may not be possible if the athlete is seriously dehydrated. These are physiologically independent entities, and the numbers provided are only general guidelines.

dehydration dictates the extent of systemic compromise. Isolating the physiologic changes that contribute to decrements in performance is difficult, as any change in 1 system (ie, cardiovascular) influences the performance of other systems (ie, thermoregulatory, muscular).[3]

The body attempts to balance endogenous heat production and exogenous heat accumulation by heat dissipation via conduction, convection, evaporation, and radiation.[4] The relative contribution of each method depends on the ambient temperature, relative humidity, and exercise intensity. As ambient temperature rises, conduction and convection decrease markedly, and radiation becomes nearly insignificant.[4,5] Heat loss from evaporation is the predominant heat-dissipating mechanism for the exercising athlete. In warm, humid conditions, evaporation may account for more than 80% of heat loss. In hot, dry conditions, evaporation may account for as much as 98% of cooling.[5] If sufficient fluids are not consumed to offset the rate of water loss via sweating, progressive dehydration will occur. The sweating response is critical to body cooling during exercise in the heat. Therefore, any factor that limits evaporation (ie, high humidity, dehydration) will have pro-

found effects on physiologic function and athletic performance.

Water is the major component of the human body, accounting for approximately 73% of lean body mass.[6] Body water is distributed within and between cells and in the plasma. At rest, approximately 30% to 35% of total body mass is intracellular fluid, 20% to 25% is interstitial fluid, and 5% is plasma.[6,7] Water movement between compartments occurs due to hydrostatic pressure and osmotic-oncotic gradients.[6,7] Because sweat is hypotonic relative to body water, the elevation of extracellular tonicity results in water movement from intracellular to extracellular spaces.[6–9] As a consequence, all water compartments contribute to water deficit with dehydration.[6,10] Most of the resultant water deficits associated with dehydration, however, come from muscle and skin.[11] The resulting hypovolemic-hyperosmolality condition is thought to precipitate many of the physiologic consequences associated with dehydration.[12]

A major consequence of dehydration is an increase in core temperature during physical activity, with core temperature rising an additional 0.15 to 0.20°C for every 1% of body weight lost (due to sweating) during the activity.[13,14] The added thermal strain occurs due to both impaired skin blood flow and altered sweating responses,[15–21] which is best illustrated by the delayed onset of skin vasodilation and sweating when a dehydrated person begins to exercise.[6] These thermoregulatory changes may negate the physiologic advantages resulting from increased fitness[21,22] and heat acclimatization.[21,23] Additionally, heat tolerance is reduced and exercise time to exhaustion occurs at lower core temperatures with hypohydration.[24]

Accompanying the increase in thermal strain is greater cardiovascular strain, as characterized by decreased stroke volume, increased heart rate, increased systemic vascular resistance, and possibly lower cardiac output and mean arterial pressure.[25–31] Similar to body temperature changes, the magnitude of cardiovascular changes is proportional to the water

31

Table 3. Sample Sweat Rate Calculation*

A Name	B Date	C Before Exercise	D After Exercise	E ΔBW (C-D)	F Drink Volume	G Urine Volume†	H Sweat Loss (E+F−G)	I Exercise Time	J Sweat Rate (H/I)
		Body Weight							
		kg	kg	g	mL	mL	mL	min	mL/min
		(lb/2.2)	(lb/2.2)	(kg × 1000)	(oz × 30)	(oz × 30)	(oz × 30)	h	mL/h
		kg	kg	g	mL	mL	mL	min	mL/min
		(lb/2.2)	(lb/2.2)	(kg × 1000)	(oz × 30)	(oz × 30)	(oz × 30)	h	mL/h
		kg	kg	g	mL	mL	mL	min	mL/min
		(lb/2.2)	(lb/2.2)	(kg × 1000)	(oz × 30)	(oz × 30)	(oz × 30)	h	mL/h
		kg	kg	g	mL	mL	mL	min	mL/min
		(lb/2.2)	(lb/2.2)	(kg × 1000)	(oz × 30)	(oz × 30)	(oz × 30)	h	mL/h
Kelly K.‡	9/15	61.7 kg	60.3 kg	1400 g	420 mL	90 mL	1730 mL	90 min	19 mL/min
		(lb/2.2)	(lb/2.2)	(kg × 1000)	(oz × 30)	(oz × 30)	(oz × 30)	1.5 h	1153 mL/h

*Reprinted with permission from Murray R. Determining sweat rate. *Sports Sci Exch.* 1996;9(Suppl 63).

†Weight of urine should be subtracted *if urine was excreted prior to postexercise body weight.*

‡In the example, Kelly K. should drink about 1 L (32 oz) of fluid during each hour of activity to remain well hydrated.

deficit. For example, heart rate rises an additional 3 to 5 beats per minute for every 1% of body weight loss.[14] The stroke-volume reduction seen with dehydration appears to be due to reduced central venous pressure, resulting from reduced blood volume and the additional hyperthermia imposed by dehydration.[6,14,25,32–34]

Both hypovolemia[7,17,35,36] and hypertonicity[7,35,37–39] have been suggested as mechanisms for the altered thermoregulatory and cardiovascular responses during dehydration. Manipulation of each factor independently has resulted in decreased blood flow to the skin and sweating responses.[28,34] Some authors[17,35] have argued that hypovolemia is primarily responsible for the thermoregulatory changes by reducing cardiac preload and may alter the feedback to the hypothalamus via the atrial pressure receptors (baroreceptors). The hypothalamic thermoregulatory centers may induce a decrease in the blood volume perfusing the skin in order to reestablish a normal cardiac preload. Some studies[40,41] have provided support for this hypothesis, but it is clearly not the only variable influencing thermoregulation during hypohydration. Two hypotheses explain the role of hyperosmolality on the thermoregulatory system. Peripheral regulation may occur via the strong osmotic pressure influence of the interstitium, limiting the available fluid sources for the eccrine sweat glands.[42] However, while this peripheral influence is likely, it seems more feasible that central brain regulation plays the largest role.[7] The neurons surrounding the thermoregulatory control centers in the hypothalamus are sensitive to osmolality.[43,44] Changes in the plasma osmolality of the blood perfusing the hypothalamus affect body water regulation and the desire for fluid consumption.[28,32,45] It is likely that both hypovolemia and hypertonicity contribute to body fluid regulation.

Potential changes at the level of the muscle tissue include a possible increased rate of glycogen degradation,[18,46,47] elevated muscle temperature,[48] and increased lactate levels.[49] These changes may be caused by a decrease in blood perfusion of the muscle tissue during the recovery between contractions.[50]

The psychological changes associated with exercise in a dehydrated state should not be overlooked. Dehydration increases the rating of perceived exertion and impairs mental functioning.[14,51] Dehydration also decreases the motivation to exercise and decreases the time to exhaustion, even in instances when strength is not compromised.[52–54] These are important factors when considering the motivation required by high-level athletes to maintain maximal performance.

Performance Implications. Studies investigating the role of dehydration on muscle strength have generally shown decrements in performance at 5% or more dehydration.[15,33,55–58] The greater the degree of dehydration, the more negative the impact on physiologic systems and overall athletic performance.

Most studies[30,55,59–62] that address the influence of dehydration on muscle endurance show that dehydration of 3% to 4% elicits a performance decrement, but in 1 study,[33] this finding was not supported. Interestingly, hypohydrated wrestlers who were working at maximal or near-maximal muscle activity for more than 30 seconds had a decrease in performance.[63] The environmental conditions may also play an important role in muscle endurance.[33,48]

The research concerning maximal aerobic power and the physical work capacity for extended exercise is relatively consistent. Maximal aerobic power usually decreases with more than 3% hypohydration.[6] In the heat, aerobic power decrements are exaggerated.[33] Even at 1% to 2% hypohydration in a cool environment,[64,65] loss of aerobic power is demonstrated. Two important studies have noted a decrease in physical work capacity with less than 2% dehydration during intense exercise in the heat.[66,67] When the percentage of dehydration increased, physical work capacity decreased by as much as 35% to 48%,[68] and physical work capacity often decreased even when maximal aerobic power did not change.[46,64,65] Hypohydration of 2.5% of body weight results in significant performance decrements while exercising in the heat, regardless of fitness or heat acclimation status, although enhanced fitness and acclimation can lessen the effects of dehydration.[69] Partial rehydration will enhance performance during an ensuing exercise session in the heat, which is important when faced with the reality of sports situations.[49,70] The performance decrements noted with low to moderate levels of hypohydration may be due to an increased perception of fatigue.[50]

Rehydration and Exercise

Factors Influencing Rehydration. The degree of environmental stress is determined by temperature, humidity, wind speed, and radiant energy load, which induce physiologic changes that affect the rehydration process.[71–73] Fluid intake increases substantially when ambient temperature rises above 25°C; the rehydration stimulus can also be psychological.[74,75] An athlete exercising in the heat will voluntarily ingest more fluid if it is chilled.[76–78] Individual differences in learned behavior also play a role in the rehydration process.[71] An athlete who knows that rehydrating enhances subsequent performance is more apt to consume fluid before significant dehydration occurs, so appropriate education of athletes is essential.

The physical characteristics of the rehydration beverage can dramatically influence fluid replacement.[71,75,78] Salinity, color, sweetness, temperature, flavor, carbonation, and viscosity all affect how much an athlete drinks.[16,75,79–85] Since most fluid consumed by athletes is with meals, the presence of ample fluid during meals and adequate amount of time to eat are critical to rehydration.[79] When access to meals is limited, a CHO-electrolyte beverage will help maintain CHO and electrolyte intake along with hydration status.[86]

Other factors that contribute to fluid replacement include the individual's mood (calmness is associated with enhanced rehydration) and the degree of concentration required by the task.[71] For example, industrial laborers need frequent breaks to rehydrate because they must remain focused on a specific task. This need for concentration may explain why many elite mountain bikers use a convenient back-mounted hydration system instead of the typical rack-mounted water bottle. The back-mounted water reservoir may allow the cyclist to enhance rehydration while remaining focused on terrain, speed, gears, braking, and exertion.[87] Accessibility to a fluid and ease of drinking may explain why athletes consume more fluid while cycling compared with running in a simulated duathlon.[88]

Hydration before Exercise. An athlete should begin exercising well hydrated. Many athletes who perform repeated bouts of exercise on the same day or on consecutive days can become chronically dehydrated. When a hypohydrated athlete begins to exercise, physiologic mechanisms are compromised,[64,89,90] and the extent of the dysfunction is related to the degree of thermal stress experienced by the athlete.[91] Athletes may require substantial assistance in obtaining fluids as evidenced by the phenomena of voluntary (when individuals drink insufficient quantities to replace fluid losses) and involuntary dehydration.[92]

Athletes should ingest 500 mL of fluid 2 hours before the event (which allows ample time to urinate excess fluid) to ensure proper hydration and physiologic function at the onset of exercise.[79,93,94] Mandatory pre-exercise hydration is physiologically advantageous and more effective than hydration dictated by often insufficient personal preference.[95,96] Ingesting a nutritionally balanced diet and fluids during the 24 hours before an exercise session is also crucial. Increasing CHO intake before endurance activity may be beneficial for performance[97–99] and may even enhance performance for activities as short as 10 minutes,[100] but it may have a limited effect on resistance exercise.[101]

There has been recent interest in potential benefits of purposefully overhydrating before exercise to postpone the onset of water deficit.[33,102–108] While an enhanced hydration state is often reported with glycerol use, this does not always translate into a performance improvement.[109] A recent study[110] found increased exercise time and plasma volume during exercise to exhaustion in the heat when subjects were rehydrated with water and glycerol before exercise as compared with rehydration using an equal volume of water without

glycerol. However, another study[111] found no benefits of glycerol ingestion when the ensuing exercise took place in a thermoneutral environment. Hyperhydrating before exercise, even without glycerol, may enhance thermoregulatory function[112] and limit the performance decrements normally noted with dehydration[109] while exercising in the heat (WBGT > 25°C). A key point is that the benefits associated with glycerol use seem to be negated when proper hydration status is maintained during exercise.[113] However, many athletes are unable to maintain hydration, so hyperhydration may be beneficial in extreme conditions when fluid intake cannot match sweat loss.

Rehydration during Exercise. Proper hydration during exercise will influence cardiovascular function, thermoregulatory function, muscle functioning, fluid volume status, and exercise performance. This topic has been extensively reviewed through the years, but some recent compilations are especially notable.* Proper hydration during exercise enhances heat dissipation (increased skin blood flow and sweating rate), limits plasma hypertonicity, and helps sustain cardiac output.[79,119,120] The enhanced evaporative cooling that can occur (due to increased skin blood flow and maintained perfusion of working muscles) is the result of sustained cardiac filling pressure.[26] Rehydration during exercise conserves the centrally circulating fluid volume and allows maximal physiologic responses to intense exercise in the heat.

Two important purposes of rehydration are to decrease the rate of hyperthermia and to maintain athletic performance.[35,121] A classic study[122] showed that changes in rectal temperature during exercise depended on the degree of fluid intake. When water intake equaled sweat loss, rise in core temperature was slowest when compared with ad libidum water and no-water groups. This benefit of rehydration on thermoregulatory function is likely due to increased blood volume,[123] reduced hyperosmolality,[124] reduced cellular dehydration,[125] and improved maintenance of extravascular fluid volume.[126] Some studies[127,128] have not shown a physiologic or performance benefit when rehydration occurred during a 1-hour intense exercise session in mild environmental conditions. The likely reason for a lack of benefit in these studies was the fact that the exercise session did not elicit enough sweat loss to cross the physiologic threshold of percentage of body weight loss (eg, −2%) that would negatively influence performance and physiologic function. For example, in 1 of the studies,[127] the subjects had only lost 1.5% of body weight at the completion of the exercise session.

Athletes generally do not rehydrate to pre-exercise levels during exercise due to personal choice,[75,129] fluid availability,[129] the circumstances of competition,[79] or a combination of these factors. Athletes should aim to drink quantities equal to sweat and urine losses, and while they rarely meet this goal, athletes can readily handle these large volumes (>1 L/h).[130–132] Additionally, athletes may not need to exactly match fluid intake with sweat loss to maintain water balance given the small contribution of water from metabolic processes.[133]

Appealing to individual taste preferences may encourage athletes to drink more fluids. In addition, including CHOs and electrolytes (especially sodium and potassium) in the rehydration drink can maintain blood glucose, CHO oxidation, and electrolyte balance and can maintain performance

---

*References 6, 27, 71, 76, 79, 107, 108, 114–118.

if the exercise session exceeds about 50 minutes in duration.[79,118,130,134–152] Also, recent evidence[153,154] indicates that athletes performing extremely intense intermittent activity with total exercise times of less than 50 minutes may benefit from ingestion of CHOs in the rehydration beverage.

Rates of gastric emptying and intestinal absorption should also be considered.[118,155–160] Fluid volume,[161] fluid calorie content, fluid osmolality, exercise intensity,[162] environmental stress,[162] and fluid temperature[107] are some of the most important factors[28] in determining the rates of gastric emptying and small intestine absorption (the small intestine is the primary site of fluid absorption). The single most important variable may be the volume of fluid in the stomach.[163,164] Maintaining 400 to 600 mL of fluid in the stomach (or the maximum tolerated) will optimize gastric emptying.[79] If CHOs are included in the fluid, the concentration should be 4% to 8%. Concentrations higher than 8% slow the rate of fluid absorption.[165,166] Intense exercise (>80% of VO_2 max) may also decrease the rate of gastric emptying.[155] Frequent ingestion (every 15 to 20 minutes) of a moderate fluid volume (200 mL) may be ideal, but it is not feasible in sports with extended periods between breaks. The rates of gastric emptying and intestinal absorption likely influence the speed of movement of the ingested fluids into the plasma volume.[167] Since the gastric emptying and intestinal absorption rates are not compromised with the addition of a 6% carbohydrate solution as compared with water, fluid replacement and energy replenishment are equally achievable.[116,167–171] The rate of gastric emptying is slowed[163,172] by significant dehydration (>4%), which complicates rehydration and may increase gastrointestinal discomfort.[163,172] Regardless, rehydration will still benefit the athlete's hydration status.[172]

Rehydration during exercise is also influenced by the state of acclimatization of the athlete. Heat acclimatization is achieved after 5 to 10 days of training in a hot environment and will increase sweat rate, decrease electrolyte losses in the sweat, and allow athletes to better tolerate exercise in the heat.[173,174] Heat acclimatization modestly increases rehydration needs due to greater sweating. Fortunately, an athlete who is heat acclimatized has fewer deficits associated with dehydration[175] and tends to be a "better" voluntary drinker (ingests fluid earlier and more often).[1,34]

An athlete who exercises for more than 4 hours and hydrates excessively (well beyond sweat loss) only with water or low-solute beverages may be susceptible to a relatively rare condition known as symptomatic hyponatremia (also known as water intoxication).[76,108,176,177] Ultimately, the body cannot excrete the consumed fluid rapidly enough to prevent intracellular swelling, which is sufficient to produce neuropsychological manifestations. Patients present with serum sodium levels below 130 to 135 mmol/L, and the sequelae of hyponatremia can result in death if not treated.[177] The condition can most likely be avoided if sodium is consumed with the rehydration beverage and if fluid intake does not exceed sweat losses.[76,79,108]

Every athlete will benefit from attempting to match intake with sweating rate and urine losses. Individual differences exist for gastric emptying and availability of fluids during particular sports. Rehydration procedures should be tested in practice and individually modified to maximize performance in competition.[97,108,116,156]

Rehydration after Exercise. Replenishing fluid volume[178,179] and glycogen stores is critical in the recovery of many body processes, including the cardiovascular, thermoregulatory, and metabolic activities.[71,97,178,180,181]

Based on volume and osmolality, the best fluid to drink after exercise to replace the fluids that are lost via sweating may not be water.[71,182–184] Consuming water alone decreases osmolality, which limits the drive to drink and slightly increases urine output. Including sodium in the rehydration beverage (or diet) allows fluid volume to be better conserved and increases the drive to drink.[71,125,178,184–186] Including CHOs in the rehydration solution may improve the rate of intestinal absorption of sodium and water[118,178] and replenishes glycogen stores.[118,187,188] Replenishing glycogen stores can enhance performance in subsequent exercise sessions[189,190] and may enhance immune function.[191] While a normal diet commonly restores proper electrolyte concentrations,[192] many athletes are forced to rehydrate between exercise sessions in the absence of meals.[178] In addition, some athletes' meals are eaten as long as 6 hours after an exercise session, which may compromise electrolyte availability during rehydration after intense exercise in hot conditions.

While replenishing fluid to equal sweating losses is often recommended, this formula does not replace urine losses. Ingestion equal to 150% of weight loss resulted in optimal rehydration 6 hours after exercise.[185]

Assessment of Hydration Status. Body weight changes, urine color, subjective feelings, and thirst, among other indicators, offer cues to the need for rehydration.[193] When preparing for an event, an athlete should know the sweat rate, assess current hydration status, and develop a rehydration plan. Determinations of sweat rate can be made.[18,134] Hydration status can be assessed by measuring body weight before and after exercise sessions; monitoring urine color, USG, or urine volume; or using a combination of these factors.[194,195] A urine color chart is included in this manuscript (Figure).[196] The general indexes of hydration status are provided in Table 3. A refractometer offers a precise reading of USG and can be used as a general indicator of hydration state. A reading of less than 1.010 reflects a well-hydrated condition, while a reading of more than 1.020 reflects dehydration.[134] Urine osmolality and urine conductivity may also be useful tools in assessing hydration status.[197]

The hydration plan should take into account the length of the event, the individual's sweat rate, exercise intensity, the temperature and humidity, and the availability of fluids (is fluid constantly available, as in cycling, or is it consumed in a large bolus during a break?). Habits of the coach or athlete, or both, may need to be altered in order to maximize the hydration process. Any plan for rehydrating during competition should be instituted and perfected during practice sessions; it should also be individually implemented, given the large variation among people in what constitutes a "comfortable" amount of rehydration.[198,199] A sample hydration protocol for preparing an elite athlete for an event has been documented.[200]

Composition of Rehydration Fluid. During exercise, the body uses 30 to 60 g of CHOs per hour that need to be replaced to maintain CHO oxidation and delay the onset of glycogen depletion fatigue.[201–205] Thus, including 60 g of CHOs in 1 L of fluid will not hinder fluid absorption and provides an adequate supply of CHOs during or while recovering from an exercise bout. The CHO concentration in the ideal fluid-replacement solution should be in the range of to 6% to 8% (g/100 mL).[117] The simple sugars, glucose or sucrose in simple or polymer form, are the best additives to the replacement fluid. Absorption is maximized if multiple forms of CHO are ingested simultaneously (ie, fluid is absorbed more quickly from the intestine if both glucose and fructose are present than if only glucose is present).[107,116,206] The amount of fructose in the beverage should be limited to about 2% to 3% (2 to 3 g/100 mL of the beverage), since larger quantities may play a role in decreasing rates of absorption and oxidation and causing gastrointestinal distress.[107,207] Ultimately, CHO composition depends on the relative need to replace fluids or CHOs. During events, when a high rate of fluid intake is necessary to sustain hydration, the CHO composition should be kept low (eg, <7%) to optimize gastric emptying and fluid absorption. During conditions when high rates of fluid replacement are not as necessary (ie, during recovery from an exercise session, mild environmental conditions, etc), the carbohydrate concentration can be increased to optimize CHO delivery with minimal risk of jeopardizing the hydration status.

Small quantities of sodium may enhance palatability and retention, stimulate thirst, and prevent hyponatremia in a susceptible individual.* Sodium concentration should be approximately 0.3 to 0.7 g/L.[72,80,108,157,208] Other valuable sources of practical information concerning the composition of rehydration beverages and rehydration in general are available.†

Recognizing Dehydration in Athletes. The early signs and symptoms of dehydration include thirst and general discomfort and complaints. These are followed by flushed skin, weariness, cramps, and apathy. At greater water deficits, dizziness, headache, vomiting, nausea, heat sensations on the head or neck, chills, decreased performance, and dyspnea may be present.[5,79,211,212] The degree of dehydration, the mental status, and the general medical condition of the athlete will dictate the mode, amount, type, and rate of rehydration. Identifying the early signs of dehydration can limit the onset or degree of an exertional heat illnesses.[5,79,211,212] A comprehensive review of the prevention, identification, and treatment of the exertional heat illness can be found in the position stands by the NATA and the American College of Sports Medicine.[211,213]

Event Management. Some events are conducted under environmental conditions that are extreme and force the athlete to reduce intensity or risk a heat illness. These hazardous heat stresses can be avoided by scheduling athletic events during the coolest part of the day or a cooler time of the year.[211,214] The reality of sport administration is that many events take place regardless of the environmental conditions. Individuals supervising an event in a hot humid environment must ensure that athletes have ample access to fluids, are encouraged to match fluid intakes with sweat losses, and are monitored for dehydration and exertional heat illness. Whenever possible, minimize the exercise intensity of athletes in the extreme heat, since this is the largest contributor to dehydration and heat illness. When successive exercise sessions occur on the same day or on ensuing days, hydration status, sleep, meals, and other factors that maximize performance and enhance safety should be maintained. Given the variety of events an athletic trainer may supervise, we cannot formulate an event management recommendation for all sports. However, the general concepts are interchangeable across sports and venues. For example, game modifications such as decreasing the length of play or inserting

nontraditional water breaks (especially in youth sports and practice situations) will reduce the rate of heat illness. Closely monitoring environmental conditions via the WBGT or the heat index will allow an informed approach to hydration and sweat modification. Athletes who are educated on how to prevent and recognize dehydration are empowered to participate actively in implementing their own hydration protocols, thereby enhancing both performance and safety. The person responsible for the medical supervision of an event should have a detailed plan to address facilities, equipment, supplies, staffing, communication systems, education, and implementation of event policy.[213,215–220]

ACKNOWLEDGMENTS

This position statement was reviewed for the NATA by the Pronouncements Committee and reviewers Kristine L. Clark, PhD, RD, David Lamb, PhD, and Jack Ransone, PhD, ATC.

REFERENCES

1. Murray R. Nutrition for the marathon and other endurance sports: environmental stress and dehydration. *Med Sci Sports Exerc.* 1992; S319–S323.

2. Murray R. Fluid needs in hot and cold environments. *Int J Sports Nutr.* 1995;5:S62–S73.

3. Casa DJ. Exercise in the heat, I: fundamentals of thermal physiology, performance implications, and dehydration. *J Athl Train.* 1999;34:246–252.

4. Werner J. Temperature regulation during exercise: an overview. In: Gisolfi CV, Lamb DR, Nadel ER, eds. *Exercise, Heat, and Thermoregulation.* Dubuque, IA: Brown and Benchmark; 1993:49–77.

5. Armstrong LE, Maresh CM. The exertional heat illnesses: a risk of athletic participation. *Med Exerc Nutr Health.* 1993;2:125–134.

6. Sawka MN, Coyle EF. Influence of body water and blood volume on thermoregulation and exercise performance in the heat. *Exerc Sport Sci Rev.* 1999;27:167–218.

7. Morimoto T, Itoh T, Takamata A. Thermoregulation and body fluid in hot environment. *Progress Brain Res.* 1998;115:499–508.

8. Costill DL, Cote R, Fink W. Muscle water and electrolytes following varied levels of dehydration in man. *J Appl Physiol.* 1976;40:6–11.

9. Durkot MJ, Martinez O, McQuade D, Francesconi R. Simultaneous determination of fluid shifts during thermal stress in a small-animal model. *J Appl Physiol.* 1986;61:1031–1034.

10. Nose H, Mack GW, Shi X, Nadel ER. Shift in body fluid compartments after dehydration in humans. *J Appl Physiol.* 1988;65:318–324.

11. Nose H, Morimoto T, Ogura K. Distribution of water losses among fluid compartments of tissues under thermal dehydration in the rat. *Jpn J Physiol.* 1983;33:1019–1029.

12. Szlyk-Modrow PC, Francesconi RP, Hubbard RW. Integrated control of body fluid balance during exercise. In: Buskirk ER, Puhl SM, eds. *Body Fluid Balance: Exercise and Sport.* New York, NY: CRC Press; 1996:117–136.

13. Sawka MN, Young AJ, Francesconi RP, Muza SR, Pandolf KB. Thermoregulatory and blood responses during exercise at graded hypohydration levels. *J Appl Physiol.* 1985;59:1394–1401.

14. Montain SJ, Coyle EF. Influence of graded dehydration on hyperthermia and cardiovascular drift during exercise. *J Appl Physiol.* 1992;73:1340–1350.

15. Adolph EF, ed. *Physiology of Man in the Desert.* New York, NY: Interscience; 1947.

16. Claremont AD, Costill DL, Fink W, Van Handel P. Heat tolerance following diuretic induced dehydration. *Med Sci Sports Exerc.* 1976;8:239–243.

17. Fortney SM, Nadel ER, Wenger CB, Bove JR. Effect of blood volume on sweating rate and body fluids in exercising humans. *J Appl Physiol.* 1981;51:1594–1600.

---

*References 38, 80, 108, 131, 157, 185, 208.
†References 18, 76, 107, 118, 156, 159, 160, 168, 178, 205, 209, 210.

18. Murray R. Dehydration, hyperthermia, and athletes: science and practice. *J Athl Train*. 1996;31:248–252.

19. Nadel ER, Fortney SM, Wenger CB. Effect of hydration state on circulatory and thermal regulations. *J Appl Physiol*. 1980;49:715–721.

20. Sawka MN, Gonzalez RR, Young AJ, Dennis RC, Valeri CR, Pandolf KB. Control of thermoregulatory sweating during exercise in the heat. *Am J Physiol*. 1989;257:R311–R316.

21. Buskirk ER, Iampietro PF, Bass DE. Work performance after dehydration: effects of physical conditioning and heat acclimatization. *J Appl Physiol*. 1958;12:189–194.

22. Cadarette BS, Sawka MN, Toner MM, Pandolf KB. Aerobic fitness and the hypohydration response to exercise heat-stress. *Aviat Space Environ Med*. 1984;55:507–512.

23. Sawka MN, Hubbard RW, Francesconi RP, Horstman DH. Effects of acute plasma volume expansion on altering exercise-heat performance. *Eur J Appl Physiol*. 1983;51:303–312.

24. Sawka MN, Young AJ, Latzka WA, Neufer PD, Quigley MD, Pandolf KB. Human tolerance to heat strain during exercise: influence of hydration. *J Appl Physiol*. 1992;73:368–375.

25. Gonzalez-Alonso J, Mora-Rodriguez R, Below PR, Coyle EF. Dehydration markedly impairs cardiovascular function in hyperthermic endurance athletes during exercise. *J Appl Physiol*. 1997;82:1229–1236.

26. Rowell LB. *Human Circulation Regulation During Physiological Stress*. New York, NY: Oxford University Press; 1986.

27. Coyle EF, Montain SJ. Thermal and cardiovascular responses to fluid replacement during exercise. In: Gisolfi CV, Lamb DR, Nadel ER, eds. *Exercise, Heat, and Thermoregulation*. Dubuque, IA: Brown and Benchmark; 1993:179–212.

28. Sawka MN. Physiological consequences of hypohydration: exercise performance thermoregulation. *Med Sci Sports Exerc*. 1992;24:657–670.

29. Gonzalez-Alonso J, Mora-Rodriguez R, Below PR, Coyle EF. Dehydration reduces cardiac output and increases systemic and cutaneous vascular resistance during exercise. *J Appl Physiol*. 1995;79:1487–1496.

30. Saltin B. Circulatory response to submaximal and maximal exercise after thermal dehydration. *J Appl Physiol*. 1964;19:1125–1132.

31. Sproles CB, Smith DP, Byrd RJ, Allen TE. Circulatory responses to submaximal exercise after dehydration and rehydration. *J Sports Med*. 1976;16:98–105.

32. Armstrong LE, Maresh CM, Gabaree CV, et al. Thermal and circulatory responses during exercise: effects of hypohydration, dehydration, and water intake. *J Appl Physiol*. 1997;82:2028–2035.

33. Sawka MN, Montain SJ, Latzka WA. Body fluid balance during exercise-heat exposure. In: Buskirk EW, Puhl SM, eds. *Body Fluid Balance: Exercise and Sport*. New York, NY: CRC Press; 1996:139–157.

34. Sawka MN, Pandolf KB. Effect of body water loss on physiological function and exercise performance. In: Gisolfi CV, Lamb DR, eds. *Fluid Homeostasis During Exercise*. Carmel, IN: Brown and Benchmark; 1990:1–30.

35. Nose H, Takamata A. Integrative regulations of body temperature and body fluid in humans exercising in a hot environment. *Int J Biometeorol*. 1997;40:42–49.

36. Fortney SM, Vroman NB, Beckett WS, Permutt S, LaFrance ND. Effect of exercise hemoconcentration and hyperosmolality on exercise responses. *J Appl Physiol*. 1988;65:519–524.

37. Candas V, Libert JP, Brandenberger G, Sagot JC, Amoros C, Kahn JM. Hydration during exercise: effects on thermal and cardiovascular adjustments. *Eur J Appl Physiol*. 1986;55:113–122.

38. Harrison MH, Edwards RJ, Fennessy PA. Intravascular volume and tonicity as factors in the regulation of body temperature. *J Appl Physiol*. 1978;44:69–75.

39. Senay LC. Temperature regulation and hypohydration: a singular view. *J Appl Physiol*. 1979;47:1–7.

40. Gaddis GM, Elizondo RS. Effect of central blood volume decrease upon thermoregulation responses to exercise in the heat. *Fed Proc*. 1984;43:627.

41. Mack G, Nose H, Nadel ER. Role of cardiopulmonary baroreflexes during dynamic exercise. *J Appl Physiol*. 1988;65:1827–1832.

42. Nielsen B, Hansen G, Jorgensen SO, Nielsen E. Thermoregulation in exercising man during dehydration and hyperhydration with water and saline. *Int J Biometeorol*. 1971;15:195–200.

43. Nakashima T, Hori T, Kiyohara T, Shibata M. Effects of local osmolality changes on medial preoptic thermosensitive neurons in hypothalamic slices. *In Vitro Thermal Physiol*. 1984;9:133–137.

44. Silva NL, Boulant JA. Effects of osmotic pressure, glucose and temperature on neurons in preoptic tissue slices. *Am J Physiol*. 1984;247:R335–R345.

45. Takamata A, Mack GW, Stachenfeld NS, Nadel ER. Body temperature modification of osmotically induced vasopressin secretion and thirst in humans. *Am J Physiol*. 1995;269:R874–R880.

46. Burge CM, Carey MF, Payne WR. Rowing performance, fluid balance, and metabolic function, following dehydration and rehydration. *Med Sci Sports Exerc*. 1993;25:1358–1364.

47. Hargeaves M, Dillo P, Angus D, Febbraio M. Effect of fluid ingestion on muscle metabolism during prolonged exercise. *J Appl Physiol*. 1996;80:363–366.

48. Edwards RHT, Harris RC, Hultman E, Kaizer L, Koh D, Nordesjo L. Effect of temperature on muscle energy metabolism and endurance during successive isometric contractions, sustained to fatigue, of the quadriceps muscle in man. *J Physiol*. 1972;220:335–352.

49. Casa DJ, Maresh CM, Armstrong LE, et al. Intravenous versus oral rehydration during a brief period: responses to subsequent exercise in the heat. *Med Sci Sports Exerc*. 2000;32:124–133.

50. Buskirk ER, Puhl SM. Effects of acute body weight loss in weight-controlling athletes. In: Buskirk ER, Puhl SM, eds. *Body Fluid Balance: Exercise and Sport*. New York, NY: CRC Press; 1996:283–296.

51. Gopinthan PM, Pichan G, Sharma VM. Role of dehydration in heat stress-induced variations in mental performance. *Arch Environ Health*. 1988;43:15–17.

52. Montain SJ, Smith SA, Mattot RP, Zientara GP, Jolesz FA, Sawka MN. Hypohydration effects on skeletal muscle performance and metabolism: a 31P-MRS study. *J Appl Physiol*. 1998;84:1889–1994.

53. Lidell WSS. The effects of water and salt intake upon the performance of men working in hot and humid environments. *J Physiol*. 1955;127:11–46.

54. Strydom NB, Wyndham CH, van Graan CH, Holdsworth LD, Morrison JF. The influence of water restriction on the performance of men during a road march. *S Afr Med J*. 1966;40:539–544.

55. Bosco JS, Greenleaf JE, Bernauer EM, Card DH. Effects of acute dehydration and starvation on muscular strength and endurance. *Acta Physiol Pol*. 1974;25:411–421.

56. Bosco JS, Terjung RL, Greenleaf JE. Effects of progressive hypohydration on maximal isometric muscular strength. *J Sports Med Phys Fitness*. 1968;8:81–86.

57. Houston ME, Marrin DA, Green HJ, Thomson JA. The effect of rapid weight loss on physiological function in wrestlers. *Physician Sportsmed*. 1981;9(11):73–78.

58. Webster S, Rutt R, Weltman A. Physiological effects of a weight loss regimen practiced by college wrestlers. *Med Sci Sports Exerc*. 1990;22:229–234.

59. Bijlani RL, Sharma KN. Effect of dehydration and a few regimes of rehydration on human performance. *Ind J Physiol Pharmacol*. 1980;24:255–266.

60. Mnatzakian PA, Vaccaro P. Effects of 4% dehydration and rehydration on hematological profiles and muscular endurance of college wrestlers. *Med Sci Sports Exerc*. 1982;14:117s.

61. Serfass RC, Stull GA, Alexander JF, Ewing JL. The effects of rapid weight loss and attempted rehydration on strength and endurance of the handgripping muscles in college wrestlers. *Res Q Exerc Sport*. 1968;55:46–52.

62. Torranin C, Smith DP, Byrd RJ. The effect of acute thermal dehydration and rapid rehydration on isometric and isotonic endurance. *J Sports Med Phys Fitness*. 1979;19:1–9.

63. Horswill CA. Applied physiology of amateur wrestling. *Sports Med*. 1992;14:114–143.

64. Armstrong LE, Costill DL, Fink WJ. Influence of diuretic-induced dehydration on competitive running performance. *Med Sci Sports Exerc*. 1985;17:456–461.

65. Caldwell JE, Ahonen E, Nousianen U. Differential effects of sauna-,

diuretic- and exercise-induced hypohydration. *J Appl Physiol*. 1984;57: 1018–1023.

66. Pinchan G, Gauttam RK, Tomar OS, Bajaj AC. Effects of primary hypohydration on physical work capacity. *Int J Biometeorol*. 1988;32: 176–180.

67. Walsh RM, Noakes TD, Hawley JA, Dennis SC. Impaired high-intensity cycling performance time at low levels of dehydration. *Int J Sports Med*. 1994;15:392–398.

68. Craig FN, Cummings EG. Dehydration and muscular work. *J Appl Physiol*. 1966;21:670–674.

69. Cheung SS, McClellan TM. Heat acclimation, aerobic fitness, and hydration effects on tolerance during uncompensable heat stress. *J Appl Physiol*. 1998;84:1731–1739.

70. Castellani JW, Maresh CM, Armstrong LE, et al. Intravenous versus oral rehydration: effects on subsequent exercise heat stress. *J Appl Physiol*. 1997;82:799–806.

71. Armstrong LE, Maresh CM. Fluid replacement during exercise and recovery from exercise. In: Buskirk ER, Puhl SM, eds. *Body Fluid Balance: Exercise and Sport*. New York, NY: CRC Press; 1996:259–281.

72. Greenleaf JE. Environmental issues that influence intake of replacement beverages. In: Marriott BM, ed. *Fluid Replacement and Heat Stress*. Washington, DC: National Academy Press; 1994:195–214.

73. Meyer F, Bar-Or O, Salsberg A, Passe D. Hypohydration during exercise in children: effect on thirst, drink preferences, and rehydration. *Int J Sports Nutr*. 1994;4:22–35.

74. Welch BE, Buskirk ER, Iampietro PF. Relation of climate and temperature to food and water intake. *Metabolism*. 1958;7:141.

75. Greenleaf JE. Problem: thirst, drinking behavior, and involuntary dehydration. *Med Sci Sports Exerc*. 1992;24:645–656.

76. Epstein Y, Armstrong LE. Fluid-electrolyte balance during labor and exercise: concepts and misconceptions. *Int J Sports Nutr*. 1999;9:1–12.

77. Herrera JA, Maresh CM, Armstrong LE, et al. Perceptual responses to exercise in the heat following rapid oral and intravenous rehydration. *Med Sci Sports Exerc*. 1998;30(5s):6.

78. Hubbard RW, Sandick BL, Matthew WT, et al. Voluntary dehydration and allesthesia for water. *J Appl Physiol*. 1984;57:868.

79. American College of Sports Medicine. Position stand: Exercise and fluid replacement. *Med Sci Sports Exerc*. 1996;28(1):i–vii.

80. Meyer F, Bar-Or O. Fluid and electrolyte loss during exercise. *Sports Med*. 1994;18:4–9.

81. Passe DH, Horn M, Murray R. The effects of beverage carbonation on sensory responses and voluntary fluid intake following exercise. *Int J Sports Nutr*. 1997;7:286–297.

82. Wilk B, Bar-Or O. Effect of drink flavor and NaCl on voluntary drinking and hydration in boys exercising in the heat. *J Appl Physiol*. 1996;80: 1112–1117.

83. Wilk B, Kriemler S, Keller H, Bar-Or O. Consistency in preventing voluntary dehydration in boys who drink a flavored carbohydrate-NaCl beverage during exercise in the heat. *Int J Sports Nutr*. 1998;8:1–9.

84. Wilmore JH, Morton AR, Gilbey HJ, Wood RJ. Role of taste preference on fluid intake during and after 90 min of running at 60% of VO_{2max} in the heat. *Med Sci Sports Exerc*. 1998;30:587–595.

85. Booth DA. Influences on human fluid consumption. In: Ramsay DJ, Booth DA, eds. *Thirst: Physiological and Psychological Aspects*. London, UK: Springer-Verlag; 1991:53.

86. Montain SJ, Shippee RL, Tharion WJ. Carbohydrate-electrolyte solution effects on physical performance of military tasks. *Aviat Space Environ Med*. 1997;68:384–391.

87. McClung JM, Casa DJ, Berger EM, Dellis WO, Knight JC, Wingo JE. Fluid replacement during mountain bike races in the heat: rack mounted vs. back mounted rehydration. *Med Sci Sports Exerc*. 1999;31(5s):322.

88. Iuliano S, Naughton G, Collier G, Carlson J. Examination of the self-selected fluid intake practices by junior athletes during a simulated duathlon event. *Int J Sports Nutr*. 1998;8:10–23.

89. Rothstein A, Towbin EJ. Blood circulation of temperature of men dehydrating in the heat. In: Adolph EF, ed. *Physiology of Man in the Desert*. New York, NY: Interscience; 1947:172–196.

90. Brown AH, Towbin EJ. Relative influence of heat, work, and dehydration on blood circulation. In: Adolph EF, ed. *Physiology of Man in the Desert*. New York, NY: Interscience; 1947:197–207.

91. Sawka MN, Francesconi RP, Young AJ, Pandolf KB. Influence of hydration level and body fluids on exercise performance in the heat. *JAMA*. 1984;252:1165–1169.

92. Greenleaf JE, Sargent F II. Voluntary dehydration in man. *J Appl Physiol*. 1965;20:719–724.

93. Greenleaf JE, Castle BL. Exercise temperature regulation in man during hypohydration and hyperhydration. *J Appl Physiol*. 1971;30:847–853.

94. Moroff SV, Bass DB. Effects of overhydration on man's physiological responses to work in the heat. *J Appl Physiol*. 1965;20:267–270.

95. Rico-Sanz J, Fronera WR, Rivera MA, Rivera-Brown A, Mole PA, Meredith CN. Effects of hyperhydration on total body water, temperature regulation and performance of elite young soccer players in a warm climate. *Int J Sports Med*. 1995;17:85–91.

96. Rothstein A, Adolph EF, Wills JH. In: Adolph EF, ed. *Physiology of Man in the Desert*. New York, NY: Interscience; 1947:254–270.

97. Hawley JA, Dennis SC, Noakes TD. Carbohydrate, fluid, and electrolyte requirements of the soccer player: a review. *Int J Sports Nutr*. 1994;4: 221–236.

98. Hawley JA, Schabort EJ, Noakes TD, Dennis SC. Carbohydrate loading and exercise performance and update. *Sports Med*. 1997;24:73–81.

99. Schabort EJ, Bosch AN, Weltan SM, Noakes TD. The effect of a preexercise meal on time to fatigue during prolonged cycling exercise. *Med Sci Sports Exerc*. 1999;31:464–471.

100. Ventura JL, Estruch A, Rodas G, Segura R. Effect of prior ingestion of glucose or fructose on the performance of exercise of intermediate duration. *Eur J Appl Physiol*. 1994;68:345–349.

101. Mitchell JB, DiLauro PC, Pizza FX, Cavender DL. The effect of preexercise carbohydrate status on resistance exercise performance. *Int J Sports Nutr*. 1997;7:185–196.

102. Montner P, Stark DM, Riedesel ML, et al. Pre-exercise glycerol hydration improves cycling endurance time. *Int J Sports Med*. 1996;17: 27–33.

103. Freund BJ, Montain SJ, Young AJ, et al. Glycerol hyperhydration: hormonal, renal, and vascular fluid responses. *J Appl Physiol*. 1995;79: 2069–2077.

104. Lyons TP, Riedesel ML, Meuli LE, Chick TW. Effects of glycerol-induced hyperhydration prior to exercise in the heat on sweating and core temperature. *Med Sci Sports Exerc*. 1990;22:477–483.

105. Riedesel ML, Allen DY, Peake GT, Al-Qattan K. Hyperhydration with glycerol solutions. *J Appl Physiol*. 1987;63:2262–2268.

106. Leutkeimer MJ, Thomas EL. Hypervolemia and cycling time trial performance. *Med Sci Sports Exerc*. 1994;26:503–509.

107. Hoswill CA. Effective Fluid Replacement. *Int J Sports Nutr*. 1998;8: 175–195.

108. Maughan RJ. Optimizing hydration for competitive sport. In: Lamb DR, Murray R, eds. *Optimizing Sport Performance*. Carmel, IN: Cooper Publishing; 1997:139–183.

109. Casa DJ, Wingo JE, Knight JC, Dellis WO, Berger EM, McClung JM. Influence of a pre-exercise glycerol hydration beverage on performance and physiological function during mountain bike races in the heat. *J Athl Train*. 1999;34:S25.

110. Kavouras SA, Casa DJ, Herrera JA, et al. Rehydration with glycerol: endocrine, cardiovascular, and thermoregulatory effects during exercise in 37°C. *Med Sci Sports Exerc*. 1998;30(5s):332.

111. Inder WJ, Swanney MP, Donald RA, Prickett TCR, Hellemans J. The effect of glycerol and desmopressin on exercise performance and hydration in triathletes. *Med Sci Sports Exerc*. 1998;30:1263–1269.

112. Rico-Sanz J, Frontera WR, Rivera MA, Rivera-Brown A, Mole PA, Meredith CN. Effects of hyperhydration on total body water, temperature regulation and performance of elite young soccer players in a warm climate. *Int J Sports Med*. 1996;17:85–91.

113. Latzka WA, Sawka MN, Montain SJ, et al. Hyperhydration: thermoregulatory effects during compensable exercise-heat stress. *J Appl Physiol*. 1997;83:860–866.

114. Coyle EF, Hamilton M. Fluid replacement during exercise: effects on physiological homeostasis and performance. In: Gisolfi CV, Lamb DR,

eds. *Fluid Homeostasis During Exercise*. Carmel, IN: Cooper Publishing; 1990:281–303.

115. Bar-Or O, Wilk B. Water and electrolyte replenishment in the exercising child. *Int J Sports Nutr*. 1996;6:93–99.

116. Gisolfi CV. Fluid balance for optimal performance. *Nutr Reviews*. 1996;54:S159–S168.

117. Hargreaves M. Physiological benefits of fluid and energy replacement during exercise. *Aust J Nutr Diet*. 1996;53:S3–S7.

118. Murray R. The effects of consuming carbohydrate-electrolyte beverages on gastric emptying and fluid absorption during and following exercise. *Sports Med*. 1987;4:322–351.

119. Montain SJ, Coyle EF. Influence of graded dehydration on hyperthermia and cardiovascular drift during exercise. *J Appl Physiol*. 1992;73:1340–1350.

120. Raven PB, Stevens GHJ. Cardiovascular function and prolonged exercise. In: Lamb DR, Murray R, eds. *Prolonged Exercise*. Indianapolis, IN: Benchmark Press; 1988:43–74.

121. Febbraio MA, Murton P, Selig SE et al. Effect of CHO ingestion on exercise metabolism and performance in different ambient temperatures. *Med Sci Sports Exerc*. 1996;28:1380–1387.

122. Pitts GC, Johnson RC, Consolazio FC. Work in the heat as affected by intake of water, salt, and glucose. *Am J Physiol*. 1944;142:253–259.

123. Fortney SM, Wenger CB, Bove JR, Nadel ER. Effect of blood volume on forearm venous volume and cardiac stroke volume during exercise. *J Appl Physiol*. 1983;55:884–890.

124. Greenleaf JE, Kozlowski S, Nazar K, Kaciuba-Ucilko H, Brzezinska Z, Ziemba A. Ion-osmotic hyperthermia during exercise in dogs. *Am J Physiol*. 1976;230:74–78.

125. Nadel ER, Mack GW, Nose H. Influence of fluid replacement beverages on body fluid homeostasis during exercise and recovery. In: Gisolfi CV, Lamb DR, eds. *Fluid Homeostasis During Exercise*. Carmel, IN: Cooper Publishing; 1990:181–198.

126. Gonzalez-Alonso JR, Mora-Rodriquez R, Below PR, Coyle EF. Reductions in cardiac output, mean blood pressure, and skin vascular conductance with dehydration are reversed when venous return is increased. *Med Sci Sports Exerc*. 1994;26(5s):163.

127. McConell GK, Stephens TJ, Canny BJ. Fluid ingestion does not influence intense 1-h exercise performance in a mild environment. *Med Sci Sports Exerc*. 1999;31:386–392.

128. Robinson TA, Hawley JA, Palmer GS, et al. Water ingestion does not improve 1-h cycling performance in moderate ambient temperatures. *Eur J Appl Physiol*. 1995;71:153–160.

129. Broad EM, Burke LM, Cox GR, Heeley P, Riley M. Body weight changes and voluntary fluid intakes during training and competition in team sports. *Int J Sport Nutr*. 1996;6:307–320.

130. Below PR, Mora-Rodriguez R, Gonzalez-Alonso J, Coyle EF. Fluid and carbohydrate ingestion independently improve performance during 1 h of intense exercise. *Med Sci Sports Exerc*. 1995;27:200–210.

131. Lambert GP, Chang RT, Joensen D, et al. Simultaneous determination of gastric emptying and intestinal absorption during cycle exercise in humans. *Int J Sports Med*. 1996;17:48–55.

132. Mitchell JB, Voss KW. The influence of volume on gastric emptying and fluid balance during prolonged exercise. *Med Sci Sports Exerc*. 1991;23:314–319.

133. Rogers G, Goodman C, Rosen C. Water budget during ultra-endurance exercise. *Med Sci Sports Exerc*. 1997;29:1477–1481.

134. Armstrong LE. *Keeping Your Cool in Barcelona: The Effects of Heat, Humidity, and Dehydration on Athletic Performance, Strength, and Endurance*. Colorado Springs, CO: United States Olympic Committee; 1992:1–29.

135. Ball TC, Headley SA, Vanderburgh PM, Smith JC. Periodic carbohydrate replacement during 50 min of high-intensity cycling improves subsequent sprint performance. *Int J Sports Nutr*. 1995;5:151–158.

136. Burke ER, Ekblom B. Influence of fluid ingestion and dehydration on precision and endurance performance in tennis. In: Bachl N, Prokop L, Suckert R, eds. *Current Topics in Sports Medicine: Proceedings of the World Congress of Sports Medicine*. Wien, Austria: Urban and Schwarzeberg; 1984:379–388.

137. Davis JM, Lamb DR, Pate RR, Slentz CA, Burgess WA, Bartoli WP. Carbohydrate-electrolyte drinks: effects on endurance cycling in the heat. *Am J Clin Nutr*. 1988;48:1023–1030.

138. El-Sayed MS, Balmer J, Rattu AJM. Carbohydrate ingestion improves endurance performance during a 1 h simulated cycling time trial. *J Sports Sci*. 1997;15:223–230.

139. El-Sayed MS, Rattu AJM, Roberts I. Effects of carbohydrate feeding before and during prolonged exercise on subsequent maximal exercise performance capacity. *Int J Sports Nutr*. 1995;5:215–224.

140. Hawley JA, Dennis SC, Noakes TD. Oxidation of carbohydrate ingested during prolonged exercise. *Sports Med*. 1992;14:27–42.

141. Jeukendrop A, Brouns F, Wagenmakers AJM, Saris WHM. Carbohydrate-electrolyte feedings improve 1h time trial cycling performance. *Int J Sports Med*. 1997;18:125–129.

142. Kirkendall D, Foster C, Dean J, Grogan J, Thompson N. Effect of glucose polymer supplementation on performance of soccer players. In: Reilly T, Lees A, David K, Murphy W, Spon E, Spon FN, eds. *Science and Football: Proceedings of the First World Congress of Science and Football*. London, UK: 1988:33–41.

143. Leatt PB, Jacobs I. Effect of glucose polymer ingestion on glycogen depletion during a soccer match. *Can J Sports Sci*. 1989;14:112–116.

144. Nicholas CM, Williams C, Lakomy HKA, Phillips G, Nowitz A. Influence of ingesting a carbohydrate-electrolyte solution on endurance capacity during intermittent, high-intensity shuttle running. *J Sports Sci*. 1995;13:283–290.

145. Sugiura K, Kobayashi K. Effect of carbohydrate ingestion on sprint performance following continuous and intermittent exercise. *Med Sci Sports Exerc*. 1998;30:1624–1630.

146. Simard C, Tremblay A, Jobin M. Effects of carbohydrate intake before and during an ice hockey game on blood and muscle energy substrates. *Res Q Exerc Sport*. 1988;59:144–147.

147. Smith K, Smith N, Wishart C, Green S. Effect of a carbohydrate-electrolyte beverage on fatigue during a soccer-related running test. *J Sports Sci*. 1998;16:502–503.

148. Tsintzas K, Williams C. Human muscle glycogen metabolism during exercise: effect of carbohydrate supplementation. *Sports Med*. 1998;25:7–23.

149. Tsintzas OK, Williams C, Singh R, Wilson W, Burrin J. Influence of carbohydrate-electrolyte drinks on marathon running performance. *Eur J Appl Physiol*. 1995;70:154–160.

150. Tsintzas OK, Williams C, Wilson W, Burrin J. Influence of carbohydrate supplementation early in exercise on endurance running capacity. *Med Sci Sports Exerc*. 1996;28:1373–1379.

151. Utter A, Kang J, Nieman D, Warren B. Effect of carbohydrate substrate availability on rating of perceived exertion during prolonged running. *Int J Sports Nutr*. 1997;7:274–285.

152. Wilber RL, Moffatt RJ. Influence of carbohydrate ingestion on blood glucose and performance in runners. *Int J Sports Nutr*. 1992;2:317–327.

153. Davis JM, Jackson DA, Broadwell MS, Queary JL, Lambert CL. Carbohydrate drinks delay fatigue during intermittent, high-intensity cycling in active men and women. *Int J Sports Nutr*. 1997;7:261–273.

154. Lambert CP, Flynn MG, Boone JB, Michaud TJ, Rodriguez-Zayas J. Effects of carbohydrate feeding on multiple-bout resistance exercise. *J Sports Sci*. 1991;5:192–197.

155. Costill DL. Gastric emptying of fluid during exercise. In: Gisolfi CV, Lamb DR, eds. *Fluid Homeostasis During Exercise*. Carmel, IN: Cooper Publishing; 1990:97–121.

156. Gisolfi CV, Duchman SM. Guidelines for optimal replacement beverages for different athletic events. *Med Sci Sports Exerc*. 1992;24:679–687.

157. Gisolfi CV, Summers R, Schedl H. Intestinal absorption of fluids during rest and exercise. In: Gisolfi CV, Lamb DR, eds. *Fluid Homeostasis During Exercise*. Carmel, IN: Cooper Publishing; 1990:129–175.

158. Maughan RJ, Rehrer NJ. Gastric emptying during exercise. *Sports Sci Exch*. 1993;6:5.

159. Schedl HP, Maughan RJ, Gisolfi CV. Intestinal absorption during rest and exercise: implications for formulating an oral rehydration solution. *Med Sci Sports Exerc*. 1994;3:267–280.

160. Shi X, Gisolfi CV. Fluid and carbohydrate replacement during intermittent exercise. *Sports Med*. 1998;25:157–172.

161. Mitchell JB, Grandjean PW, Pizza FX, Starling RD, Holtz RW. The

effect of volume on rehydration and gastric emptying following exercise-induced dehydration. *Med Sci Sports Exerc.* 1994;26:1135–1143.

162. Neufer PD, Young AJ, Sawka MN. Gastric emptying during exercise: effects of heat stress and hypohydration. *Eur J Appl Physiol.* 1989;58: 433–439.

163. Neufer PD, Young AJ, Sawka MN. Gastric emptying during running and walking: effects of varied exercise intensity. *Eur J Appl Physiol.* 1989;58:440–445.

164. Noakes TD, Rehrer NJ, Maughan RJ. The importance in volume in regulating gastric emptying. *Med Sci Sports Exerc.* 1991;23:307–313.

165. Costill DL, Saltin B. Factors limiting gastric emptying during rest and exercise. *J Appl Physiol.* 1974;37:679–683.

166. Ryan AJ, Lambert GP, Shi X, Chang RT, Summers RW, Gisolfi CV. Effect of hypohydration on gastric emptying and intestinal absorption during exercise. *J Appl Physiol.* 1998;84:1581–1588.

167. Murray R, Bartoli WP, Eddy DE, Horn MK. Gastric emptying and plasma deuterium accumulation following ingestion of water and two carbohydrate-electrolyte beverages. *Int J Sports Nutr.* 1997;7:144–153.

168. Costill DL. Carbohydrates for exercise: dietary demands for optimal performance. *Int J Sports Med.* 1988;9:1–18.

169. Davis JM, Burgess WA, Slentz CA, Bartoli WP, Pate RR. Effects of ingesting 6% and 12% glucose/electrolyte beverages during prolonged intermittent cycling in the heat. *Eur J Appl Physiol.* 1988;57:563–569.

170. Gisolfi CV, Spranger KJ, Summers RW, Schedl HP, Bleiler TL. Effects of cycle exercise on intestinal absorption in humans. *J Appl Physiol.* 1991;71:2518–2527.

171. Houmard JA, Egan PC, Johns RA, Neufer PD, Chenier TC, Israel RG. Gastric emptying during 1h of cycling and running at 75% VO$_{2max}$. *Med Sci Sports Exerc.* 1991;23:320–325.

172. Rehrer NJ, Beckers EJ, Brouns F, Hoor FT, Saris WH. Effects of dehydration on gastric emptying and gastrointestinal distress while running. *Med Sci Sports Exerc.* 1990;22:790–795.

173. Armstrong LE, Maresh CM. The induction and decay of heat acclimatization in trained athletes. *Sports Med.* 1991;12:302–312.

174. Montain SJ, Maughan RJ, Sawka MN. Fluid replacement strategies for exercise in hot weather. *Athl Ther Today.* 1996;July:24–27.

175. Sawka MN, Toner MM, Francesconi RP, Pandolf KB. Hypohydration and exercise: effects of heat acclimation, gender, and environment. *J Appl Physiol.* 1983;55:1147–1153.

176. Armstrong LE, Curtis WC, Hubbard RW, Francesconi RP, Moore R, Askew W. Symptomatic hyponatremia during prolonged exercise in the heat. *Med Sci Sports Exerc.* 1993;25:543–549.

177. Garigan T, Ristedt DE. Death from hyponatremia as a result of acute water intoxication in an army basic trainee. *Mil Med.* 1999;164:234.

178. Maughan RJ, Leiper JB, Shirreffs SM. Rehydration and recovery after exercise. *Sports Sci Exch.* 1996;9:3.

179. Murray R. Fluid replacement: the American College of Sports Medicine position stand. *Sports Sci Exch.* 1996;9(4s):63.

180. Maughan RJ, Leiper JB, Shirreffs SM. Factors influencing the restoration of fluid and electrolyte balance after exercise in the heat. *Br J Sports Med.* 1997;31:175–182.

181. Maughan RJ, Shirreffs SM. Recovery from prolonged exercise: restoration of water and electrolyte balance. *J Sports Sci.* 1997;15:297–303.

182. Costill DL, Sparks KE. Rapid fluid replacement following thermal dehydration. *J Appl Physiol.* 1973;34:299–303.

183. Gonzalez-Alonso J, Heaps CL, Coyle EF. Rehydration after exercise with common beverages and water. *Int J Sports Med.* 1992;13:399–406.

184. Nose H, Mack GW, Shi X, Nadel ER. Role of osmolality and plasma volume during rehydration in humans. *J Appl Physiol.* 1988;65:325–331.

185. Shirreffs SM, Taylor AJ, Leiper JB, Maughan RJ. Post-exercise rehydration in man: effects of volume consumed and drink sodium content. *Med Sci Sports Exerc.* 1996;28:1260–1271.

186. Wemple RD, Morocco TS, Mack GW. Influence of sodium replacement on fluid ingestion following exercise-induced dehydration. *Int J Sports Nutr.* 1997;7:104–116.

187. Fallowfield JL, Williams C. Carbohydrate intake and recovery from prolonged exercise. *Int J Sports Nutr.* 1993;3:150–164.

188. Ivy JL. Carbohydrate supplements during and immediately post exercise. In: Marriott BM, ed. *Fluid Replacement and Heat Stress.* Washington, DC: National Academy Press; 1994:55–68.

189. Murray R, Eddy DE, Murray TW, Seifert JG, Paul GL, Halaby GA. The effect of fluid and carbohydrate feedings during intermittent cycling exercise. *Med Sci Sports Exerc.* 1987;19:597–604.

190. Nicholas CW, Green PA, Hawkins RD, Williams C. Carbohydrate intake and recovery of intermittent running capacity. *Int J Sports Nutr.* 1997;7:251–260.

191. Nieman DC. Influence of carbohydrate on the immune response to intensive, prolonged exercise. *Exerc Immunol Rev.* 1998;4:64–76.

192. Armstrong LE. Considerations for replacement beverages: fluid electrolyte balance and heat illness. In: Marriott BM, ed. *Fluid Replacement and Heat Stress.* Washington, DC: National Academy Press; 1994:37–54.

193. Nadel ER, Mack GW, Nose H. Thermoregulation, exercise, and thirst: interrelationships in humans. In: Gisolfi CV, Lamb DR, Nadel ER, eds. *Exercise, Heat, and Thermoregulation.* Dubuque, IA: Brown and Benchmark; 1993:225–251.

194. Armstrong LE, Maresh CM, Castellani JW, et al. Urinary indices of hydration status. *Int J Sports Nutr.* 1994;4:265–279.

195. Armstrong LE, Herrera Soto JA, Hacker FT, Casa DJ, Kavouras SA, Maresh CM. Urinary indices during dehydration, exercise, and rehydration. *Int J Sports Nutr.* 1998;8:345–355.

196. Armstrong LE. *Performing in Extreme Environments.* Champaign, IL: Human Kinetics; 2000.

197. Shirreffs SM, Maughan RJ. Urine osmolality and conductivity as indices of hydration status in athletes in the heat. *Med Sci Sports Exerc.* 1998;30:1598–1602.

198. Fallon KE, Broad E, Thompson MW, Reull PA. Nutritional and fluid intake in a 100-km ultramarathon. *Int J Sports Nutr.* 1998;8:24–35.

199. Maughan R, Goodburn R, Griffin J, et al. Fluid replacement in sport and exercise—a consensus statement. *Br J Sports Med.* 1993;27:34–35.

200. Armstrong LE, Hubbard RW, Jones BH, Jones JT. Preparing Alberto Salazar for the heat of the 1984 Olympic Marathon. *Physician Sportsmed.* 1986;14(3):73–81.

201. Burgess WA, Davis JM, Bartoli WP, Woods JA. Failure of low dose carbohydrate feeding to attenuate glucoregulatory hormone responses and improve endurance performance. *Int J Sports Nutr.* 1991;1:338–352.

202. Coggan AR, Coyle EF. Reversal of fatigue during prolonged exercise by carbohydrate infusion or ingestion. *J Appl Physiol.* 1987;63:2388–2395.

203. Coyle EF, Coggan AR, Hemmert MK, Ivy JL. Muscle glycogen utilization during prolonged strenuous exercise when fed carbohydrate. *J Appl Physiol.* 1986;61:165–172.

204. Coyle EF, Hagberg JM, Hurley BF, Martin WH, Ehsani AA, Holloszy JO. Carbohydrate feeding during prolonged strenuous exercise can delay fatigue. *J Appl Physiol.* 1983;55:230–235.

205. Coyle EF, Montain SJ. Carbohydrate and fluid ingestion during exercise: are there trade-offs? *Med Sci Sports Exerc.* 1992;24:671–678.

206. Shi X, Summers RW, Schedl HP, Flanagan SW, Chang R, Gisolfi G. Effects of carbohydrate type and concentration and solution osmolality on water absorption. *Med Sci Sports Exerc.* 1995;27:1607–1615.

207. Murray R, Paul GL, Seifert JG, Eddy DE, Halaby GA. The effects of glucose, fructose, and sucrose ingestion during exercise. *Med Sci Sports Exerc.* 1989;21:275–282.

208. Leutkeimer MJ, Coles MG, Askew EW. Dietary sodium and plasma volume levels with exercise. *Sports Med.* 1997;23:279–286.

209. Coyle EF. Fluid and carbohydrate replacement during exercise: how much and why? *Sports Sci Exch.* 1994;7:3.

210. Casa DJ. Exercise in heat, II: critical concepts in rehydrations, exertional heat illness, and maximizing athletic performance. *J Athl Train.* 1999; 34:253–262.

211. American College of Sports Medicine. Position stand: heat and cold illnesses during distance running. *Med Sci Sports Exerc.* 1996;28(12):i–x.

212. Armstrong LE, Hubbard RW, Kraemer WJ, Deluca JP, Christensen EL. Signs and symptoms of heat exhaustion during strenuous exercise. *Ann Sports Med.* 1987;3:182–189.

213. Binkley HM, Beckett J, Casa DJ, Eubank TK, Kleiner DM, Plummer P.

National Athletic Trainers' Association position statement: heat illnesses in athletes. *J Athl Train*. In press.

214. Nielsen B. Olympics in Atlanta: a fight against physics. *Med Sci Sports Exerc*. 1996;28:665–668.

215. Adner MM, Scarlet JJ, Casey J, Robison W, Jones BH. The Boston Marathon medical care team: ten years of experience. *Physician Sportsmed*. 1988;16(7):98–106.

216. Roberts WO. Medical management and administration manual for long distance road racing. In Brown CH, Gudjonsson B, eds. *IAAF Medical Manual for Athletics and Road Racing Competitions A Practical Guide*.

Monaco: International Amateur Athletic Federation Publications; 1998: 39–75.

217. Earle MV, ed. *1998–1999 NCAA Sports Medicine Handbook*. Overland Park, KS: National Collegiate Athletic Association; 1998.

218. Elias SR, Roberts WO, Thorson DC. Team sports in hot weather: guidelines for modifying youth soccer. *Physician Sportsmed*. 1991;19(5):67–78.

219. Kleiner DM, Glickman SE. Medical considerations and planning for short distance road races. *J Athl Train*. 1994;29:145–151.

220. Roberts WO. Exercise-associated collapse in endurance events: a classification system. *Physician Sportsmed*. 1989;17(5):49–55.

Fluid Replacement Review Questions:

1. What are the advantages and disadvantages of the various ways to assess hydration status?

2. From a physiological perspective, why does substantial dehydration compromise performance and physiological function?

3. What components should be part of a rehydration beverage and how much of each?

4. What is an individualized rehydration plan? How do you figure out the sweat rate of your athlete?

5. Why use percent dehydration? What advantage does that calculation have over just reporting weight lost?

NATA Position Statement:
Head Down Contact and
Spearing in Tackle Football

In This Section: Football players are at a higher risk for spinal injuries than other athletes because of head-down tackling techniques. Athletic trainers should educate their athletes to help reduce the risk of cervical spine injury. This position statement explains how football injuries are caused by spearing and details a proper tackling technique.

National Athletic Trainers' Association Position Statement: Head-Down Contact and Spearing in Tackle Football

Jonathan F. Heck*; Kenneth S. Clarke†; Thomas R. Peterson‡;
Joseph S. Torg§; Michael P. Weis‖

*Richard Stockton College, Pomona, NJ; † SLE Worldwide, Inc, Fort Wayne, IN (Retired); ‡University of Michigan, Ann Arbor, MI (Retired); §Temple University, Philadelphia, PA; ‖MCRC Physical Therapy, West Orange, NJ

Jonathan F. Heck, MS, ATC, Kenneth S. Clarke, PhD, Thomas R. Peterson, MD, Joseph S. Torg, MD, and Michael P. Weis, PT, ATC, contributed to conception and design; acquisition and analysis and interpretation of the data; and drafting, critical revision, and final approval of the article.
Address correspondence to National Athletic Trainers' Association, Communications Department, 2952 Stemmons Freeway, Dallas, TX 75247.

Objective: To present recommendations that decrease the risk of cervical spine fractures and dislocations in football players.

Background: Axial loading of the cervical spine resulting from head-down contact is the primary cause of spinal cord injuries. Keeping the head up and initiating contact with the shoulder or chest decreases the risk of these injuries. The 1976 rule changes resulted in a dramatic decrease in catastrophic cervical spine injuries. However, the helmet-contact rules are rarely enforced and head-down contact still occurs frequently.

Our recommendations are directed toward decreasing the incidence of head-down contact.

Recommendations: Educate players, coaches, and officials that unintentional and intentional head-down contact can result in catastrophic injuries. Increase the time tacklers, ball carriers, and blockers spend practicing correct contact techniques. Improve the enforcement and understanding of the existing helmet-contact penalties.

Key Words: catastrophic injuries, cervical spine, head injuries, injury prevention, neck injuries, paralysis, quadriplegia

Catastrophic cervical spine injuries (CSIs) resulting in quadriplegia (paralysis of all 4 extremities) are among the most devastating injuries in all of sport. In football, the primary mechanism for these injuries is axial loading that occurs, whether intentional or unintentional, as a result of head-down contact and spearing. Head-first contact also increases the risk of concussion and closed head injury. In 1976, the National Collegiate Athletic Association (NCAA) and the National Federation of State High School Associations (NFSHSA) changed their football rules to broaden the concept of spearing to include any deliberate use of the helmet as the initial point of contact against an opponent. They did this in an effort to reduce the incidence of catastrophic CSIs.

Subsequent data on the occurrence of quadriplegia in organized football dramatically demonstrated that the NCAA and NFSHSA rule changes were successful. The incidence has remained at a relatively low level, with a mild increase at the end of the 1980s (Figure 1). However, in spite of this accomplishment, head-down contact still occurs frequently. The helmet-contact penalties also are not enforced adequately. Clearly, a reduction in the incidence of head-down contact and increased enforcement of the existing rules will further reduce the risk of both paralytic and nonparalytic injuries.

The purpose of this position statement is to (1) provide scientifically proven concepts and recommendations to minimize the risk of catastrophic CSIs in football; (2) clarify that head-down contact and spearing pose a risk to all positional players regardless of intent; (3) establish the value and necessity of ongoing educational practices for players, coaches, and officials regarding dangerous and proper playing techniques; and (4) emphasize that increasing safety depends on the participation of sports medicine professionals, coaches, players, officials, administrators, and governing bodies.

RECOMMENDATIONS

The National Athletic Trainers' Association (NATA) recommends the following regarding head-down contact and spearing in football. These recommendations should be considered by sports medicine professionals, coaches, players, officials, administrators, and governing bodies who work with athletes at risk for cervical spine injuries.

Practices and Concepts

1. Axial loading is the primary mechanism for catastrophic CSI. Head-down contact, defined as initiating contact with the top or crown of the helmet, is the only technique that results in axial loading.

2. Spearing is the intentional use of a head-down contact technique. Unintentional head-down contact is the inadvertent dropping of the head just before contact. Both head-down

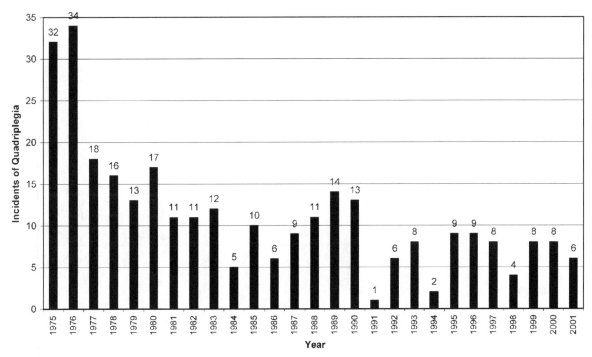

Figure 1. Incidence of quadriplegia in high school and college athletes. Data from the National Football Head and Neck Injury Registry (1976–1991) and the National Center for Catastrophic Sports Injury Research (1992–present).[1–4]

techniques are dangerous and may result in axial loading of the cervical spine and catastrophic injury (Figure 2).

3. Catastrophic CSI resulting from axial loading is neither caused nor prevented by players' standard equipment.

4. Injuries that occur as a result of head-down contact are technique related and are preventable to the extent that head-down contact is preventable.

5. Attempts to determine a player's intent regarding intentional or unintentional head-down contact are subjective. Therefore, coaching, officiating, and playing techniques must focus on decreasing all head-down contact, regardless of intent.

6. Catastrophic CSI occurs most often to defensive players. However, all players are at risk. Ball carriers and blockers

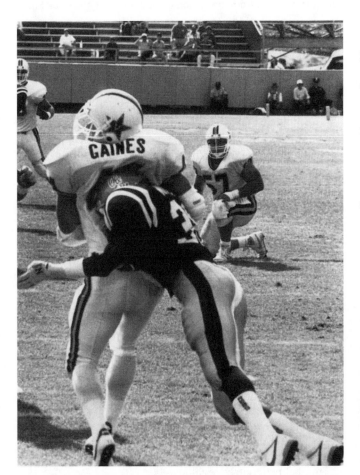

Figure 2. Head-down contact poses significant risks of catastrophic cervical spine injury. This defensive back (dark jersey) sustained fractures of his 4th, 5th, and 6th cervical vertebrae. The hit resulted in quadriplegia.

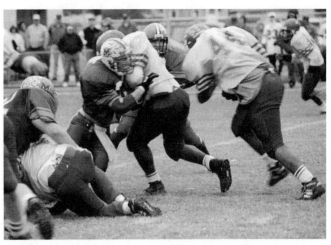

Figure 3. Initiating contact with the shoulder while keeping the head up reduces the risk of catastrophic injury, as demonstrated by the blocker and potential tackler.

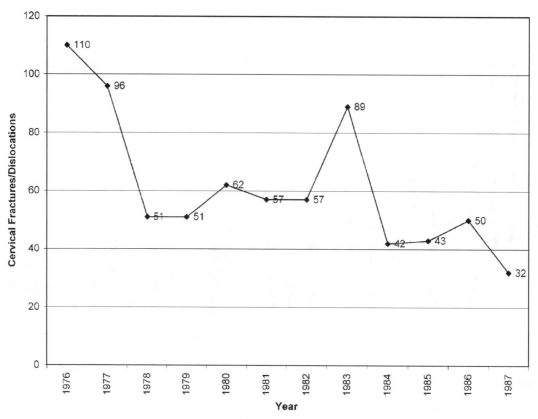

Figure 4. Incidence of cervical fractures and dislocations in high school athletes. Data from the National Football Head and Neck Injury Registry.

have also become quadriplegics by lowering their heads at contact. Expanding the concept of head-down contact beyond tackler spearing and the "intentional attempt to punish an opponent" will decrease the risk of serious injury to players in other positions.

7. As emphasized in the college and high school rule books, making contact with the shoulder or chest while keeping the head up greatly reduces the risk of serious head and neck injury. With the head up, the player can see when and how impact is about to occur and can prepare the neck musculature for impact. Even if inadvertent head-first contact is made, then the force is absorbed by the neck musculature, the intervertebral discs, and the cervical facet joints. This is the safest contact technique.

8. Each time a player initiates contact with his head down, he risks paralysis. Therefore, increased attention to the frequency of head-down contact occurring in games and practices is needed. It is a reasonable conclusion that a reduction in the cause (head-down contact) will further reduce the effect (catastrophic CSI).

9. Data collection on all catastrophic CSIs is important. Attention to the number of nonparalytic cervical spine fractures and dislocations is needed, as each incident has the potential for paralysis. These data are less reliable and harder to obtain than data for paralytic injuries. Both injury types require diligent reporting to the National Center for Catastrophic Sports Injury Research (mailing address: CB 8700, 204 Fetzer Gymnasium, University of North Carolina, Chapel Hill, NC 27599-8700, e-mail: mueller@email.unc.edu).

Rules and Officiating

10. Officials should enforce the existing rules to further reduce the incidence of head-down contact. A clear discrepancy exists between the incidence of head-down/head-first contact and the level of enforcement of the helmet-contact penalties. Stricter officiating would bring more awareness to coaches and players about the effects of head-down contact.

11. The current annual education programs for all officials should emphasize the purpose of the helmet-contact rules and the dangers associated with head-down/head-first contact. Emphasis should be on the fact that the primary purpose of the helmet-contact penalties is to protect the athlete who leads with his head. Although the technique is dangerous to both players, it is the athlete who initiates head-down contact who risks permanent quadriplegia.

12. Not all head-first contacts that result in serious injury are intentional. A major area of concern for officials remains application of the penalties to athletes who unintentionally initiate contact with their helmets. Athletic governing bodies should address this issue in order to improve penalty enforcement.

13. Athletic governing bodies should coordinate a protocol to document and quantify all penalties called through their organizations. This will identify the enforcement level of the helmet-contact penalties.

14. Athletic governing bodies should periodically survey their football officials regarding their interpretations and perceptions of the helmet-contact rules. Existing rules and

Table 1. Available Videos

Title	Available From
Prevent Paralysis: Don't Hit With Your Head[5]	Dick Lester, Riddell Inc E-Mail: dlester@riddellsports.com Cost: Free
See What You Hit[6]	The Spine in Sports Foundation www.spineinsports.org Cost: Free
Spine Injury Management[7]	Human Kinetics www.humankinetics.com Cost: $39.95

comments need to specifically include the ball carrier in the application of these penalties.

15. Those preparing the football rule books should consider revising the wording "blocking and tackling techniques" with "contact techniques" (or similar). This revised wording would then include all position players and all types of contact.

16. A task force of athletic trainers, coaches, team physicians, officials, and league administrators should be developed at all levels of play to monitor rule enforcement and the frequency of head-down contact by an annual, random review of game films.

Education and Coaching

17. The athlete should know, understand, and appreciate the risk of making head-down contact, regardless of intent. Formal team educational sessions (conducted by the athletic trainer or team physician or both with the support of the coaching staff) should be held at least twice per season. One session should be conducted before contact begins and the other at the midpoint of the season. Parents should be invited to the first educational session at the high school level. Recommended topics are mechanisms of head and neck injuries, related rules and penalties, the incidence of catastrophic injury, the severity and prognosis of these injuries, and the safest contact positions. The use of videos such as *Prevent Paralysis: Don't Hit With Your Head*,[5] *See What You Hit*,[6] or the prevention portion of *Spine Injury Management*[7] should be mandatory (Table 1). The use of supplemental media and materials are strongly recommended.

18. Correct contact technique should be taught at the earliest organized level. Pop Warner, Midget, and Pee Wee football leagues should perpetually emphasize the importance of coaching and teaching heads-up football.

19. It is crucial that educational programs extend to the television, radio, and print media for both local and national affiliates regarding the dangers of head-down contact and the reasons for the helmet-contact rules. This will promote awareness of these issues and provide extended education to viewers, listeners, and readers.

20. Initiating contact with the shoulder/chest while keeping the head up is the safest way to play football. The game can be played aggressively with this technique with much less risk of serious injury (Figure 3). However, it is a technique that must be learned. To be learned, it must be practiced extensively. Athletes who still drop their head just before contact require additional practice time. It is imperative for coaches to teach, demonstrate, and practice this technique throughout the year for all position players. Specific emphasis should be placed on contact techniques at least 4 times spread over the entire season. Tacklers, ball carriers, and blockers must receive practice time until it is instinctive to keep the head up.

21. Initiating contact with the face mask is a rules violation and must not be taught. If the athlete uses poor technique by lowering his head, he places himself in the head-down position and at risk of serious injury.

22. Every coaching staff must display and implement a clear philosophy regarding the reduction of head-down contact. The head coach should clearly convey this philosophy to the assistant coaches and the entire team and pursue an enforcement policy during practice. A player's technique must be corrected anytime he is observed lowering his head at contact. Coaches should also use weekly game film reviews to provide players with feedback about their head positions.

23. Athletes should have a year-round supervised neck-strengthening program with appropriate equipment and techniques. Although the role of strength training is secondary to correcting contact technique in axial-loading injury prevention, it provides the strength and endurance required to maintain the neck in extension. It also provides protection against cervical nerve root neurapraxia (burners).

24. Schools, responsible administrators, and the sports medicine team should recognize cyclic turnover in coaches and establish programs that educate new and re-educate existing coaches to appropriate teaching and practicing methods. This will provide a documented and consistent approach to the prevention of these injuries.

HISTORY AND BACKGROUND

In 1931, the American Football Coaches Association compiled the first Football Fatality Report.[8] By 1962, its findings caused the American Medical Association Committee on Medical Aspects of Sports to host a national conference on head protection for athletes.[8] The conference convened the principal authorities of that era in what was emerging as "sports medicine" to discuss the current issues involving changes in the football helmet and the advent of the football face mask. The focus was the rapidly rising fatality rate among high school and college football players suffering from closed head injuries. Football authorities were divided as to whether the new protective headgear was good for the sport.

Into the 1970s, opinion was more prevalent than scientific data in addressing these problems. The American Medical Association Committee arrived at a collective expert opinion and encouraged pragmatic scholarly attention to the health and safety issues within sport. Among the recommendations resulting from the 1962 conference were condemning the practice of spearing and the need for research to develop standards for football helmets.[9] Initially, spearing was defined by rule as "intentionally and maliciously striking the opponent with one's helmet after the opponent had been downed."

After the 1962 conference, Blyth from the University of North Carolina assumed the data collection for the Fatality Report of the America Football Coaches Association.[10] Helmet manufacturers began to sponsor research on impact standards for helmets, and high school and college rules committees confirmed that spearing was an illegal form of football contact after the whistle.

American Medical Association Position Statement

The practice of teaching "face into the numbers" was growing in the 1960s as the helmets evolved and coaches felt that players could therefore better withstand the use of the helmeted head.[8,11,12] "Face into the numbers" was increasingly popular, because it allowed the blocker or tackler to keep his eyes forward and neck "bulled" and to move with the opponent, without having the intent to spear.[8] In essence, coaches considered using the helmet as the primary point of contact a superior technique.

In 1967, however, the American Medical Association Committee on Medical Aspects of Sports declared, in a groundbreaking position statement, its opinion that most spearing was unintentional and non-malicious, ie, "inadvertent."[11] It identified the flaw with teaching "face-into-the-numbers" contact. Athletes do not always execute with precision, and the tendency to duck the head at contact is natural. This position statement was adopted by the NFSHSA as a joint statement in 1968.

Football Helmet Standards

In spite of this timely recognition of unsafe head position, the annual football fatality data reports revealed a continued rise in frequency during the 1960s.[10] Although it was reported that the risk of death from football did not exceed the actuarial risk of death among males of that age in non-football activities,[13] the need for helmet design standards became more and more evident.

Consequently, the helmet manufacturers agreed in 1969 to pool their resources through a newly devised interdisciplinary National Operating Committee for Safety in Athletic Equipment (NOCSAE).[8] This committee was charged with the development of consensus standards for helmets in football by an independent investigator. Hodgson, from Wayne State University, was selected as the investigator because of his extensive research in this area.[14] A safety standard was achieved in 1973, and the first helmets were tested on the NOCSAE standard in 1974.[12] The NOCSAE standards went into effect for colleges in 1978 and for high schools in 1980.[15] It was commonly understood that the helmets being produced and used by the mid-1970s met the NOCSAE standards, and all helmets being worn were, in fact, associated with the same low rates of clinical concussions.[16]

The increase in head injury fatalities throughout the 1960s and early 1970s was attributed to the introduction of hardshell helmets and face masks in the early 1960s, which resulted in playing techniques that increased exposure of the head to contact.[1,8] Helmet standards and head injuries received football's priority attention during this time.[8] Similar attention to serious neck injuries in the 1960s was lacking because the incidence of nonfatal quadriplegia was not being tracked and therefore was unknown.

Catastrophic Injury Data

The Annual Football Fatality Report was the only ongoing source of data into the 1970s. Schneider[17] included serious neck injuries in his landmark survey of catastrophic injuries in football in the early 1960s. But it was not until the mid-1970s that 2 concurrent and independent studies by Clarke[18] and Torg et al[19,20] again examined quadriplegia. These data revealed the increased incidence of paralyzed football players.

The total number of head and neck injuries from 1971 to 1975[19,20] was calculated and retrospectively compared with the data from 1959 to 1963 compiled by Schneider.[17] The number of intracranial hemorrhages and deaths had decreased by 66% and 42%, respectively. This suggested that the new helmet standards had been effective in minimizing serious head injuries. However, the number of cervical spine fractures, subluxations, and dislocations had increased by 204%, and the number of athletes with cervical quadriplegia had increased by 116%.

Clarke and Torg led the proponents of the spearing rule changes that were implemented by the NFSHSA and NCAA in 1976. These rule changes preceded the publication of their data.[18–20] The purpose of the rule changes was to protect the spearer, whether inadvertent or intentional, from neurotrauma.[5,8,11,12,15,21–25] On the basis of these data, it was concluded that the improved protective capabilities of the polycarbonate helmets accounted for a decrease in head injuries but encouraged playing techniques that used the top or crown of the helmet as the initial point of contact and put the cervical spine at risk.[1]

The results of the 1976 rule change are an example of one of the most successful injury interventions in sport (Figures 1 and 4). In the first year after the rule change, the number of injuries resulting in quadriplegia in high school and college players decreased by 53%.[1] By 1984, the number dropped by 87%. Other than increases in 1988, 1989, and 1990 to the low teens, these cases have remained in the single digits through the most recent years of available data. This decrease is attributed to the rule change and to improved coaching techniques at the high school and college levels.[8,12,15,19,23,24,26–34]

In order to track nonfatal catastrophic injuries, Torg et al[1] established the National Football Head and Neck Injury Registry in 1975, which collected data on CSIs through the early 1990s. In 1977, the NCAA initiated funding for a National Survey of Catastrophic Injuries directed by Mueller and Blyth.[2–4] In 1982, this project was expanded to include all sports and renamed the National Center for Catastrophic Sports Injury Research. Both projects used similar methods of collecting data. These sources included coaches, school administrators, medical personnel, athletic organizations, a national newspaper-clipping service, and professional associates. The collection of these data was crucial in preventing catastrophic injuries.[12]

In 1987, a joint endeavor was initiated between the National Center for Catastrophic Sports Injury Research and the section on Sports Medicine of the American Association of Neurological Surgeons. As a result, Cantu became responsible for monitoring the collected medical data.[2] This project continues to collect data on these injuries.

Mechanism of Injury

In the early 1970s, several theories existed regarding the mechanisms of CSIs and quadriplegia. The theories of hyperflexion and hyperextension, based on postinjury radiographs, were considered 2 primary causes.[1] Forced hyperflexion was considered a primary cause of severe CSI in football and other sports.[1,35–57] Hyperextension and the concept of the posterior

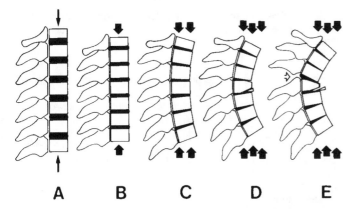

Figure 5. (A) Axial loading of the cervical spine (B) first results in compressive deformation of the intervertebral discs. As the energy input continues and maximum compressive deformation is reached, angular deformation and buckling occur (C). The spine fails in a flexion mode, with resulting fracture, dislocation, or subluxation (D and E).

Table 2. Percentage of Plays Involving at Least 1 Head-Down Contact Between Tacklers and Ball Carriers During a 1990 High School Season[103]

Play	%
All plays	25
Running plays	37
Kick returns	38
Pass plays	7

Table 3. Percentage of Plays Involving Head-Down Contact by High School and College Tacklers or Ball Carriers

Position	%
Tacklers, film (1990)[103]	26
Tacklers, live (1993)[101]	6
College tacklers, live (1993)[101]	8
Ball carriers, film (1990)[103]	16
Ball carriers, film (1989)[19]	20

rim of the helmet acting as a guillotine also received attention as an injury mechanism.[58–62] Both of these injury mechanisms received acceptance throughout the 1970s.

In contrast to these early theories, Torg et al[19,20] determined that most cases of permanent quadriplegia occurring between 1971 and 1975 were due to head-down contact or direct compression to the cervical spine. This resulted from the player initiating contact with the top of his helmet. The direct-compression or axial-loading concept eventually replaced the numerous other inaccurate, theoretic mechanisms of CSI. The identification of an accurate mechanism of injury was vitally important to the prevention of these injuries.[12,30] This allowed the development of a precise plan to reduce the incidence of quadriplegia.[8] Axial loading is now accepted as the primary cause of cervical-spine fracture and dislocation in football. Numerous studies have supported the role of axial loading[20,63–97] in catastrophic CSI and refuted the role of hyperflexion and hyperextension in these injuries.[1,19,23,24,30–32,63–65,68,72,94,98,99]

Axial Loading. In the course of contact activity, such as football, the cervical spine is repeatedly exposed to dangerous energy inputs.[93] Fortunately, most forces are dissipated by controlled spinal motion through the cervical paravertebral muscles, eccentric contractions, and intervertebral discs.[19] However, the vertebrae, intervertebral discs, and supporting ligamentous structures can be injured when contact occurs on the top or crown of the helmet with the head, neck, and trunk positioned in such a way that forces are transmitted along the vertical axis of the cervical spine. In this situation, the cervical spine can assume the characteristics of a segmented column. With the neck in the neutral position, the cervical spine is extended as a result of normal cervical lordosis (Figure 5). When the neck is flexed to 30°, the cervical spine becomes straight. When a force is applied to the vertex, the energy is transmitted along the longitudinal axis of the cervical spine and is no longer dissipated by the paravertebral muscles. This results in the cervical spine being compressed between the abruptly decelerated head and the force of the oncoming trunk.[65] Essentially, the head is stopped, the trunk keeps moving, and the spine is crushed between the two. When maximum vertical compression is reached, the cervical spine fails in a flexion mode, with a fracture, subluxation, or facet dislocation resulting.[63] In the laboratory, fracture or dis-

location has occurred with less than 150 ft-lb of kinetic energy.[28] A running football player can possess 1500 ft-lb of kinetic energy.[28]

Distribution of Serious Injuries

Defensive football players receive the majority of fatalities and catastrophic CSIs, accounting for approximately 4 times those of offensive players.[2–4,12,15,19,20,23] Tackling is the leading cause, followed by being tackled and then blocking.[2–4,12,15] By position, defensive backs and special teams players are at the greatest risk[2,3,12,15,16,19,23] with ball-carrier positions, linebackers, and defensive linemen having the next highest incidences of serious injury.[2,12,15]

Each time a player initiates contact with his head down, he risks quadriplegia.[2,15,19,22–25,27–33,97,100–106] Each time an athlete initiates contact head first, he increases the risk of concussion.[22,29,101–103,107,108] Although catastrophic injuries have occurred to position players at various rates, mechanism of injury does not discriminate by position or intent.[103,105,107,109] Head-down contact poses a risk to every player who employs this technique.[22,103–105]

Incidence of Head-Down Contact

According to Hodgson and Thomas,[28] the number of paralyzed players does not accurately identify the risk of hitting with the head down. Because of the decrease in catastrophic injuries since the 1976 rule changes, it is often assumed that head-down contact rarely occurs. Two authors have examined the incidence of head-down contact in the 1990s:[22,101,103] twice on film in slow motion and once in live situations. Selected data appear in Tables 2 and 3.

One study compared the incidence of head-down contact between tacklers and ball carriers before and after the rule change on the high school level.[103] No significant change was seen in the incidence of head-down contact between the seasons. Approximately 20 head-down contacts occurred per team in a single game. There was 1 head-down contact for every 1.8 kick returns. Special teams' players have been among the leading position players associated with catastrophic injuries. Considering that kicking plays account for only about 7% of

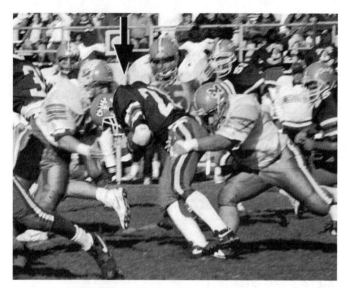

Figure 6. Ball-carrier head-down contact, an often overlooked danger, increases the risk of head and neck injuries.

the plays involving a ball carrier, this play is probably the most dangerous play in football.

Ball-carrier spearing (Figure 6) is interesting in that defensive players were 4 times more likely to hit with their head down when tackling a head-down ball carrier. It is possible that a head-down ball carrier influences a tackler to "get lower" and use a similar technique.[22,103] This coincides well with Drake's[101,102] finding that tacklers were 3 times more likely to make head-down contact when tackling below the waist.

During the 1990 season, 200 head-down contacts occurred during one team's season, and an estimated 2.8 million head-down contacts took place nationally between tacklers and ball carriers on the high school level. This translated into approximately 1 case of quadriplegia for every 251 000 head-down contacts. Based upon these numbers, a high school should have 1 case of quadriplegia for every 11 000 games.[103] Although these numbers are rough estimates at best, they demonstrate the room for additional improvement in decreasing the incidence of spearing and head-down contact.

Rules and Officiating

The current helmet-contact rules for high school and college are shown in Tables 4 and 5, respectively. In 1976, the high school rule change defined butt blocking and face tackling and made them illegal. It was also a "point of emphasis" that coaches could no longer teach "face in the numbers" as a contact technique.[112] On the collegiate level, the rules were adapted to make "deliberate" use of the helmet illegal. Also, the rule book included a "Coaching Ethics" statement from the American Football Coaches Association that the helmet cannot be used as a primary point of contact in the teaching of blocking and tackling.[113] Since 1976, 2 significant changes to the helmet-contact rules have been made. First, in the mid-1980s, the spearing penalty was lessened from an automatic ejection to a 15-yard penalty. Second, in the early 1990s, the NCAA made the face mask an official part of the helmet.

Although the rule change is credited with reducing catastrophic injuries, the role officials have played by enforcing these rules is questionable (Table 6). To illustrate this, in 2001, college officials called 1 spearing penalty in every 73 games

Table 4. Helmet-Contact Rules and Selected Comments from the 2002 National Federation of State High School Associations' *Official Football Rules*[110]

Rules

1. Spearing is the intentional use of the helmet in an attempt to punish an opponent.
2. Face tackling is driving the face mask, frontal area, or top of the helmet directly into the runner.
3. Butt blocking is a technique involving a blow driven directly into an opponent with the face mask, frontal area, or top of the helmet as the primary point of contact either in close line play or in the open field.
4. Illegal personal contact occurs when a player intentionally uses his helmet to butt or ram an opponent.

Points of Emphasis

1. Illegal acts such as spearing, face tackling, and butt blocking should always be penalized.
2. Coaches have the responsibility to teach the proper technique of blocking and tackling. Officials have the responsibility to penalize all illegal contact.

Shared Responsibility and Football-Helmet Warning Statement

1. The rules against butting, ramming, or spearing the opponent with the helmeted head are there to protect the helmeted person as well the opponent being hit. The athlete who does not comply with these rules is a candidate for catastrophic injury.
2. The teaching of the blocking/tackling techniques which keep the helmeted head from receiving the brunt of the impact is now required by rule and coaching ethics.

Table 5. Helmet-Contact Rules and Comments in the National Collegiate Athletic Association's *2001 Football Rules and Interpretations*[111]

Rules

1. Spearing is the deliberate use of the helmet (including the face mask) in an attempt to punish an opponent.
2. No player intentionally shall strike a runner with the crown or top of the helmet.
3. No player intentionally shall use his helmet (including the face mask) to butt or ram an opponent.

Points of Emphasis

1. The NCAA Rules Committee is strongly opposed to tackling and blocking techniques that are potentially dangerous for both the tackler/blocker and the opponent.
2. Coaches are reminded to instruct their players not to initiate contact with any part of their helmets, including the face mask.

Coaching Ethics

The following are unethical practices:

1. Using the football helmet as a weapon. The helmet is for the protection of the players.
2. Spearing. Players, coaches, and officials should emphasize the elimination of spearing.

Table 6. Selected 2001 National Collegiate Athletic Association Penalty-Enforcement Data from Major Division 1 Conferences[114]

Penalty Type	No. Called
Total penalties	20 837
Holding	3347
Face mask	945
Spearing	17
Butting or ramming	8

and 1 butting or ramming penalty in every 156 games. No spearing penalties were called in 12 of the 20 major Division 1 conferences.[114] During the 1992 NCAA season, officials called 55 spearing penalties (1 in every 21 games) and 16 related to butting or ramming.[115]

On the high school level, officials called an estimated 1 spearing penalty in every 20 games.[116] During one team's high school season, no spearing penalties were called.[20] This appears to be the norm rather than the exception. These data contradict the NFSHSA recommendation that infractions involving a safety issue should always be enforced.[110,117] At this level of enforcement, it is doubtful whether actual penalties have decreased the incidence of head-down contact or the mechanism of injury.[116] If illegal helmet contact is not penalized, the message is sent that the technique is acceptable.[118] Adequate enforcement of the rules will clearly further reduce the risk of catastrophic injuries.[4,12,15,21–23,29–31,101,102,106,115]

Surveys of football officials have revealed many inconsistencies with regard to the helmet-contact penalties. Football officials may not have a uniform understanding of these rules. Fifty percent of New Jersey officials felt that all head-first contact was illegal.[116] Thirty-two percent felt that the rules were difficult to interpret.[116] Another 38% were unsure whether the rules were written in a way that allowed easy enforcement.[116] A survey of college officials found similar results regarding the wording of the rules.[115] A large number of high school and college officials believed that determining an athlete's intent made the rules difficult to enforce.

The helmet-contact penalties are unique in football because they are the only action penalties that penalize a player for his own protection.[105,109] However, many officials and coaches erroneously perceive the primary purpose of the penalties as protecting the athlete who gets hit.[105,109,115,116] This is reflected by one group's findings that nearly one third of high school players did not know that it was illegal to tackle with the top of the helmet or run over an opponent head first.[119]

Despite the intent of the 1976 rule change to address unintentional or inadvertent spearing, the primary rule still has an association with the "intentional attempt to punish." The wording of the helmet-contact rules does imply the need for intent.[116] On the college level, the rules do not address unintentional head-down contact at all. High school rules do address head-down contact through the penalties for face tackling and butt blocking; however, these rules exclude mention of the ball carrier. Although rules do exist at the high school level, officials may enforce them even less than they enforce the spearing penalty.[116,120] Football's objective should be to alter athlete behavior to eliminate head-down contact, not merely to discourage it.[121]

An appropriate inquiry, which cannot be answered, is, "How many of the approximately 200+ hits resulting in paralysis were flagged at the time of contact?" Although a penalty flag on a play that involves a head or neck injury cannot prevent that injury, it may prevent one later on.[120] In reviewing the video *Prevent Paralysis: Don't Hit With Your Head*, football officials did not feel that the rules allowed them to penalize the majority of the hits demonstrated on this film that resulted in quadriplegia.[122] A "litmus test" for the enforcement of the helmet-contact rules is their application to actual hits that have resulted in paralysis. There is no better definition of the type of contact that we must eliminate.

Safest Contact Position

Initiating contact with the shoulder while keeping the head up is the safest contact position.[2–4,11,12,15,22,28,49,103,110,123] With the head up, the athlete can see when and how impact is about to occur and can prepare the neck musculature. This information applies to all position players, including ball carriers. The game can be played just as aggressively with this technique with much less risk of serious injury. Tacklers can still "unload" a big hit, and ball carriers can still break tackles.[105,109]

Conversely, with the head down, the athlete does not have the advantage of good vision and preparation for the instant of contact. He is likely to receive the full force of the impact on the head instead of the shoulders, chest, or arm. He is more apt to hit low on the opponent's body (including the opponent's hard-driving knees), and exposes his cervical spine to impact in its most vulnerable position.[11] Albright et al[124] found that college and high school players had sufficient nonfatal CSIs to warrant concern over the teaching of head-butting techniques.

Coaches have expressed that they have taught players to tackle correctly, but the players still have a tendency to lower their heads just before contact.[15,28] It seems that players have learned to approach contact with their head up, but they need to maintain this position during contact.[103–105,109] It is instinctive for players to protect their eyes and face from injury by lowering their heads at impact.[22,103–105,109] Coaches must spend enough practice time to overcome this instinct. Players who drop their heads at the last instant are demonstrating that they need additional practice time with correct contact techniques in game-like situations. In addition to teaching correct contact in the beginning of the season, coaches should put specific emphasis on this 3 more times throughout the season.[21,22,104]

The "See What You Hit" concept has gained popularity in recent years. It is intended to teach athletes to keep their heads up and can be an effective tool. However, caution is required to ensure that coaches and athletes do not misinterpret this slogan as support for initiating contact with the face mask.

Strengthening the neck musculature is an accepted part of neck-injury prevention.[15,29,49,97,100] Although such strengthening cannot prevent axial loading in the head-down position, it can help athletes keep the head up during contact. Athletes should have access to some type of neck-strengthening equipment, and, ideally, the program should be year round. If this is not possible, then adequate time (4 to 6 weeks before the season begins) should be allowed for strength gains. During the season, athletes should continue to lift at least 1 day per week to maintain their strength levels.[125]

Litigation

The occurrence of a catastrophic head or neck injury is characteristically accompanied by litigation.[126–140] The proliferation of litigation for these injuries began in the 1980s. Multimillion-dollar verdicts are now common. Of the $45.8 million awarded in verdicts between 1970 and 1985, $38.7 million was awarded between 1980 and 1985.[126,127] Ironically, the litigation in football is inversely proportional to the injury statistics. During the time when there was a drastic decrease in catastrophic injuries, litigation increased.[126] Any allegation of fault can have devastating financial consequences for school districts, coaches, medical personnel, and equipment manufacturers.

The increase in litigation had serious effects on the football helmet industry. Between 1975 and 1985, 11 of 14 football helmet manufacturers left the marketplace.[126] This exit from the marketplace was due to the cost of defending product liability claims[126] and not to shortcomings regarding the NOCSAE helmet standards. Dramatic increases in liability insurance premiums followed the increase in litigation. At that point, many helmet manufacturers became self-insured or accepted the risk of being underinsured. Approximately 40% of the helmet price was set aside for product liability.[126] Litigation will continue, and medical practitioners will have to determine, as the helmet manufacturers did, if they can afford to work in athletics.[126] For these individuals and others, the implications of the increase in the number of athletic-injury lawsuits are obvious. The chance of being named in a lawsuit is significantly increased, regardless of fault or their role in the injury.[126,127,139]

Many steps can be taken to decrease the risk of catastrophic injuries and being found at fault for these injuries.[104,123,127,140] A top priority is to ensure players know, understand, and appreciate the risks of making head-first contact in football.[8,104,140] The videos *Prevent Paralysis: Don't Hit with Your Head*"[5] and *See What You Hit*[6] and the prevention section of *Spine Injury Management*[7] are excellent education tools. Parents of high school players should also be given the opportunity to view at least one of these videos. Coaches have a responsibility to spend adequate time teaching and practicing correct contact techniques with all position players. Everyone associated with football has a moral and legal responsibility to do all in their power to attempt to eliminate head-down contact from the sport.[104,105,109,140]

ACKNOWLEDGMENTS

We gratefully acknowledge the efforts of Douglas M. Kleiner, PhD, ATC/L, CSCS, FACSM; Frederick O. Mueller, PhD; Robert G. Watkins, MD; and the Pronouncements Committee in the preparation of this document.

DISCLAIMER

NATA publishes its position statements as a service to promote the awareness of certain issues to its members. The information contained in the position statements is neither exhaustive nor exclusive to all circumstances or individuals. Variables such as institutional human resource guidelines, state or federal statutes, rules, or regulations, as well as regional environmental conditions, may impact the efficacy and/or reliability of these statements. NATA advises individuals to carefully and independently investigate each of its position statements (including the applicability of same to any particular circumstance or individual) and states that such position statements should not be relied upon as an independent basis for treatment but rather as a resource available to its members. Moreover, no opinion is expressed herein regarding the quality of treatment that adheres to or differs from NATA's position statements. NATA reserves the right to rescind or modify its position statements at any time.

REFERENCES

1. Torg JS, Guille JT, Jaffe S. Injuries to the cervical spine in American football players. *J Bone Joint Surg Am*. 2002;84:112–122.

2. Mueller FO, Cantu RC. Annual survey of catastrophic football injuries: 1977–1992. In: Hoerner EF, ed. *Head and Neck Injuries in Sports ASTM STP 1229*. Philadelphia, PA: American Society for Testing and Materials; 1994:20–27.

3. Mueller FO, Cantu RC. The annual survey of catastrophic football injuries: 1977–1988. *Exerc Sport Sci Rev*. 1991;19:261–312.

4. Cantu RC, Mueller FO. Catastrophic football injuries: 1977–1998. *Neurosurgery*. 2000;47:673–675.

5. Torg JS. *Prevent Paralysis: Don't Hit With Your Head* [videotape]. Philadelphia, PA: Penn Sports Medicine; 1992.

6. *See What You Hit* [videotape]. Atlanta, GA: Kestrel Communications Inc; 2000.

7. *Spine Injury Management* [videotape]. Champaign, IL: Human Kinetics; 2001.

8. Clarke KS. Cornerstones for future directions in head/neck injury prevention in sports. In: Hoerner EF, ed. *Head and Neck Injuries in Sports ASTM STP 1229*. Philadelphia, PA: American Society for Testing and Materials; 1994:3–9.

9. Hard-shelled helmets for athletes, experts say. *JAMA*. 1962;180:23–24.

10. Blyth C, Arnold D. *The Thirty-Ninth Annual Survey of Football Fatalities,1931–1970*. Chicago, IL: American Football Coaches Association, National Collegiate Athletic Association, and National Federation of State High School Associations; 1978.

11. American Medical Association Committee on Medical Aspects of Sports. *Spearing in Football: Tips on Athletic Training*. Chicago, IL: American Medical Association, National Federation of State High School Athletic Associations; 1968:6–7.

12. Mueller FO, Blyth CS. Fatalities from head and cervical spine injuries occurring in tackle football: 40 years' experience. *Clin Sports Med*. 1987;6:185–196.

13. Clarke KS. Calculated risk of sports fatalities. *JAMA*. 1966;197:894–896.

14. Hodgson V. National Operating Committee on Standards for Athletic Equipment Football Certification Program. Available at: http://www.nocsae.org/nocsae/RESEARCH/Hodgson.htm. Accessed September 23, 2002.

15. Mueller FO, Blyth CS, Cantu RC. Catastrophic spine injuries in football. *Physician Sportsmed*. 1989;17(10):51–53.

16. Clarke KS, Powell, JW. Football helmets and neurotrauma: an epidemiological overview of three seasons. *Med Sci Sports*. 1979;11:138–145.

17. Schneider RC. Serious and fatal neurosurgical football injuries. *Clin Neurosurg*. 1964;12:226–236.

18. Clarke KS. A survey of sport-related spinal cord injuries in schools and colleges, 1973–1975. *J Safety Res*. 1977;9:140–146.

19. Torg JS, Quedenfeld TC, Moyer RA, Truex R, Spealman AD, Nichols CE. Severe and catastrophic neck injuries resulting from tackle football. *J Am Coll Health Assoc*. 1977;25:224–226.

20. Torg JS, Truex R Jr, Quedenfeld TC, Burstein A, Spealman A, Nichols CE III. The National Football Head and Neck Injury Registry: report and conclusions, 1978. *JAMA*. 1979;241:1477–1479.

21. Heck JF. An analysis of football's spearing rules. *Sideliner J Athl Train Soc N J*. 1993;9:8,9,15.

22. Heck JF. The incidence of spearing by high school football ball carriers and their tacklers. *J Athl Train*. 1992;27:120–124.

23. Torg JS, Vegso JJ, Sennett B. The National Football Head And Neck Injury Registry: 14-year report on cervical quadriplegia. *Clin Sports Med*. 1987;6:61–72.

24. Torg JS, Sennett B, Vegso JJ. Spinal injury at the third and fourth cervical vertebrae resulting from the axial loading mechanism: an analysis and classification. *Clin Sports Med*. 1987;6:159–183.

25. Wilberger JE, Maroon JC. Cervical spine injuries in athletes. *Physician Sportsmed*. 1990;18(3):57–70.

26. Albright JP, Mcauley E, Martin RK, Crowley ET, Foster DT. Head and neck injuries in college football: an eight-year analysis. *Am J Sports Med*. 1985;13:147–152.

27. Anderson C. Neck injuries: backboard, bench or return to play. *Physician Sportsmed*. 1993;21(8):23–34.

28. Hodgson VR, Thomas LM. Play head-up football. *Natl Fed News*. 1985;2:24–27.

29. Saal JA, Sontag MJ. Head injuries in contact sports: sideline decision making. *Phys Med Rehabil.* 1987;1:649–658.

30. Torg JS. Epidemiology, pathomechanics, and prevention of athletic injuries to the cervical spine. *Med Sci Sports Exerc.* 1985;17:295–303.

31. Torg JS. Epidemiology, pathomechanics, and prevention of football-induced cervical spinal cord trauma. *Exerc Sport Sci Rev.* 1992;20:321–338.

32. Torg JS. Epidemiology, biomechanical and cinematographic analysis of football induced cervical spine trauma. *Athl Train J Natl Athl Train Assoc.* 1990;25:147–159.

33. Torg JS, Sennett B, Vegso JJ, Pavlov H. Axial loading injuries to the middle cervical spine segment: an analysis and classification of twenty-five cases. *Am J Sports Med.* 1991;19:6–20.

34. Diehl J. The National Federation: how rules are written. Paper presented at: National Athletic Trainers' Association 53rd Annual Meeting and Clinical Symposia; June 14–18, 2002; Dallas, TX.

35. Schneider RC. *Head and Neck Injuries in Football: Mechanisms, Treatment, and Prevention.* Baltimore, MD: Williams & Wilkins; 1973.

36. Dolan KD, Feldick HG, Albright JP, Moses JM. Neck injuries in football players. *Am Fam Physician.* 1975;12:86–91.

37. Funk FJ, Wells RE. Injuries of the cervical spine in football. *Clin Orthop.* 1975;109:50–58.

38. Silver JR. Injuries of the spine sustained in rugby. *Br Med J (Clin Res Ed).* 1984;288:37–43.

39. Melvin WJ, Dunlop HW, Hetherington RF, Kerr JW. The role of the faceguard in the production of flexion injuries to the cervical spine in football. *Can Med Assoc J.* 1965;93:1110–1117.

40. Ciccone R, Richman RM. The mechanism of injury and the distribution of three thousand fractures and dislocations caused by parachute jumping. *J Bone Joint Surg Am.* 1948;30:77–97.

41. Ellis WG, Green D, Holzaepfel NR, Sahs AL. The trampoline and serious neurologic injuries: a report of five cases. *JAMA.* 1960;174:1673–1676.

42. Hage P. Trampolines: an "attractive nuisance." *Physician Sportsmed.* 1982;10(12):118–122.

43. Kravitz H. Problems with the trampoline, I: too many cases of permanent paralysis. *Pediatr Ann.* 1978;7:728–729.

44. Tator CH, Edmonds VE. National survey of spinal injuries in hockey players. *Can Med Assoc J.* 1984;130:875–880.

45. Tator CH, Ekong CE, Rowed DW, Schwartz ML, Edmonds VE, Cooper PW. Spinal injuries due to hockey. *Can J Neurol Sci.* 1984;11:34–41.

46. Torg JS, Das M. Trampoline-related quadriplegia: review of the literature and reflections on the American Academy of Pediatrics' position statement. *Pediatrics.* 1984;74:804–812.

47. Carvell JE, Fuller DJ, Duthie RB, Cockin J. Rugby football injuries to the cervical spine. *Br Med J (Clin Res Ed).* 1983;286:49–50.

48. Gehweiler JA Jr, Clark WM, Schaaf RE, Powers B, Miller MD. Cervical spine trauma: the common combined conditions. *Radiology.* 1979;130:77–86.

49. Leidholt JD. Spinal injuries in athletes: be prepared. *Orthop Clin North Am.* 1973;4:691–707.

50. Macnab I. Acceleration injuries of the cervical spine. *J Bone Joint Surg Am.* 1964;46:1797–1799.

51. McCoy GF, Piggot J, Macafee AL, Adair IV. Injuries of the cervical spine in schoolboy rugby football. *J Bone Joint Surg Br.* 1984;66:500–503.

52. Paley D, Gillespie R. Chronic repetitive unrecognized flexion injury of the cervical spine (high jumper's neck). *Am J Sports Med.* 1986;14:92–95.

53. Piggot J, Gordon DS. Rugby injuries to the cervical cord. *Br Med J.* 1979;1:192–193.

54. Williams JP, McKibbin B. Cervical spine injuries in rugby union football. *Br Med J.* 1978;2:1747.

55. Wu WQ, Lewis RC. Injuries of the cervical spine in high school wrestling. *Surg Neurol.* 1985;23:143–147.

56. O'Carroll PF, Sheehan JM, Gregg TM. Cervical spine injuries in rugby football. *Ir Med J.* 1981;74:377–379.

57. Scher AT. "Crashing" the rugby scrum: an avoidable cause of cervical spinal injury: case reports. *S Afr Med J.* 1982;61:919–920.

58. Burke DC. Hyperextension injuries of the spine. *J Bone Joint Surg Br.* 1971;53:3–12.

59. Edilken-Monroe B, Wagner LK, Harris JH Jr. Hyperextension dislocation of the cervical spine. *AJR Am J Roentgenol.* 1986;146:803–808.

60. Forsyth HF. Extension injuries of the cervical spine. *J Bone Joint Surg Am.* 1964;46:1792–1797.

61. Marar BC. Hyperextension injuries of the cervical spine: the pathogenesis of damage to the spinal cord. *J Bone Joint Surg Am.* 1974;56:1655–1662.

62. Alexander E Jr, Davis CH Jr, Field CH. Hyperextension injuries of the cervical spine. *AMA Arch Neurol Psychiatry.* 1958;19:146–150.

63. Torg JS, Quedenfeld TC, Burstein A, Spealman AD, Nichols CE III. National Football Head and Neck Injury Registry: report on cervical quadriplegia, 1971 to 1975. *Am J Sports Med.* 1979;7:127–32.

64. Torg JS, Vegso JJ, O'Neill MJ, Sennett B. The epidemiologic, pathologic, biomechanical, and cinematographic analysis of football-induced cervical spine trauma. *Am J Sports Med.* 1990;18:50–7.

65. Torg JS. Epidemiology, pathomechanics, and prevention of athletic injuries to the cervical spine. *Med Sci Sports Exerc.* 1985;17:295–303.

66. Yoganandan N, Sances A Jr, Maiman DJ, Myklebust JB, Pech P, Larson SJ. Experimental spinal injuries with vertical impact. *Spine.* 1986;11:855–60.

67. Mertz HJ, Hodgson VR, Thomas LM, Nyquist GW. An assessment of compressive neck loads under injury-producing conditions. *Physician Sportsmed.* 1978;6(11):95–106.

68. Hodgson VR, Thomas LM. Mechanism of cervical spine injury during impact to the protected head. In: *Proceedings of the Twenty-Fourth Staap Car Crash Conference.* Warrendale, PA: Society of Automotive Engineers; 1980: 17–42.

69. Sances A Jr, Myklebust JB, Maiman DJ, Larson SJ, Cusick JF, Jodat RW. The biomechanics of spinal injuries. *Crit Rev Biomed Eng.* 1984;11:1–76.

70. Gosch HH, Gooding E, Schneider RC. An experimental study of cervical spine and cord injuries. *J Trauma.* 1972;12:570–576.

71. Maiman DJ, Sances A Jr, Myklebust JB, et al. Compression injuries of the cervical spine: a biomechanical analysis. *Neurosurgery.* 1983;13:254–260.

72. Roaf R. A study of the mechanics of the spinal injuries. *J Bone Joint Surg Br.* 1960;42:810–823.

73. White AA III, Punjabi MM. *Clinical Biomechanics of the Spine.* Philadelphia, PA: Lippincott; 1978.

74. Bauze RJ, Ardran GM. Experimental production of forward dislocation in the human cervical spine. *J Bone Joint Surg Br.* 1978;60:239–245.

75. Nightingale RW, McElhaney JH, Richardson WJ, Best TM, Myers BS. Experimental impact injury to the cervical spine: relating motion of the head and the mechanism of injury. *J Bone Joint Surg Am.* 1996;78:412–421.

76. Kazarian L. Injuries to the human spinal column: biomechanics and injury classification. *Exerc Sport Sci Rev.* 1981;9:297–352.

77. Kewalramani LS, Orth MS, Taylor RG. Injuries to the cervical spine from diving accidents. *J Trauma.* 1975;15:130–142.

78. Albrand OW, Corkill G. Broken necks from diving accidents: a summer epidemic in young men. *Am J Sports Med.* 1976;4:107–110.

79. Albrand OW, Walter J. Underwater deceleration curves in relation to injuries from diving. *Surg Neurol.* 1975;4:461–465.

80. Maroon JC, Steele PB, Berlin R. Football head and neck injuries: an update. *Clin Neurosurg.* 1980;27:414–429.

81. Mennen U. Survey of spinal injuries from diving: a study of patients in Pretoria and Cape Town. *S Afr Med J.* 1981;59:788–790.

82. Rogers WA. Fractures and dislocations of the cervical spine: an end-result study. *J Bone Joint Surg Am.* 1957;39:341–376.

83. Scher AT. Diving injuries to the cervical spinal cord. *S Afr Med J.* 1981;59:603–605.

84. Scher AT. Injuries to the cervical spine sustained while carrying loads on the head. *Paraplegia.* 1978;16:94–101.

85. Scher AT. "Tear-drop" fractures of the cervical spine: radiological features. *S Afr Med J.* 1982;61:355–356.

86. Scher AT. The high rugby tackle: an avoidable cause of cervical spinal injury? *S Afr Med J.* 1978;53:1015–1018.

87. Scher AT. Vertex impact and cervical dislocation in rugby players. *S Afr Med J*. 1981;59:227–228.

88. Bishop PJ. Impact postures and neck loading in head first collisions: a review. In: Hoerner EF, ed. *Head and Neck Injuries in Sports ASTM STP 1229*. Philadelphia, PA: American Society for Testing and Materials; 1994:127–141.

89. Burstein AH, Otis JC. The response of the cervical spine to axial loading: feasibility for intervention. In: Hoerner EF, ed. *Head and Neck Injuries in Sports ASTM STP 1229*. Philadelphia, PA: American Society for Testing and Materials; 1994:142–153.

90. Pintar FA, Yoganandan N, Sances A JF, Cusick JF. Experimental production of head-neck injuries under dynamic forces. In: Hoerner EF, ed. *Head and Neck Injuries in Sports ASTM STP 1229*. Philadelphia, PA: American Society for Testing and Materials; 1994:203–211.

91. Yoganandan N, Pintar FA, Sances A Jr, Reinartz J, Larson SJ. Strength and kinematic response of dynamic cervical spine injuries. *Spine*. 1991; 16(10 suppl):S511–S517.

92. Yoganandan N, Sances A Jr, Maiman DJ, Myklebust JB, Pech P, Larson SJ. Experiemical spinal injuries with vertical impact. *Spine*. 1986;11: 855–859.

93. Burstein AH, Otis JC, Torg JS. Mechanisms and pathomechanics of athletic injuries to the cervical spine. In: Torg JS, ed. *Athletic Injuries to the Head, Neck, and Face*. Philadelphia, PA: Lea & Febiger; 1982: 139–154.

94. Torg JS, Truex RC Jr, Marshall J, et al. Spinal injury at the level of the third and fourth cervical vertebrae from football. *J Bone Joint Surg Am*. 1977;59:1015–1019.

95. Allen BL Jr, Ferguson RL, Lehmann TR, O'Brien RP. A mechanistic classification of closed, indirect fractures and dislocations of the lower cervical spine. *Spine*. 1982;7:1–27.

96. Jackson DW, Lohr FT. Cervical spine injuries. *Clin Sports Med*. 1986; 5:373–386.

97. Watkins RG. Neck injuries in football players. *Clin Sports Med*. 1986; 5:215–246.

98. Carter DR, Frankel VH. Biomechanics of hyperextension injuries to the cervical spine in football. *Am J Sports Med*. 1980;8:302–309.

99. Virgin H. Cineradiographic study of football helmets and the cervical spine. *Am J Sports Med*. 1980;8:310–317.

100. Cantu RC. Head and spine injuries in the young athlete. *Clin Sports Med*. 1988;7:459–472.

101. Drake GA. Research provides more suggestions to reduce serious football injuries. *Natl Fed News*. November/December 1994;18–21.

102. Drake GA. Catastrophic football injuries and tackling techniques. In: Hoerner EF, ed. *Safety in American Football, ASTM STP 1305*. Philadelphia, PA: American Society for Testing and Materials; 1996:42–49.

103. Heck JF. The incidence of spearing during a high school's 1975 and 1990 football seasons. *J Athl Train*. 1996;31:31–37.

104. Heck JF. Preventing catastrophic head and neck injuries in football. *From Gym Jury*. 1998;10(1):7.

105. Heck JF. Re-examining spearing: the incidence of cervical spine injury hides the risks. *Am Football Coach*. 1999;5(8):52–54.

106. Football-related spinal cord injuries among high school players: Louisiana, 1989. *MMWR Morb Mortal Wkly Rep*. 1990;39:586–587.

107. Buckley WE. Concussions in college football: a multivariate analysis. *Am J Sports Med*. 1988;16:51–56.

108. Cantu RC. Guidelines for return to contact sports after a cerebral concussion. *Physician Sportsmed*. 1986;14(10):75–83.

109. Heck JF. The state of spearing in football: incidence of cervical spine injuries doesn't indicate the risks. *Sports Med Update*. 1998;13(2):4–7.

110. National Federation of State High School Associations. *Official Football Rules*. Indianapolis, IN: National Federation of State High School Associations; 2002.

111. National Collegiate Athletic Association. *2001 Football Rules and Interpretations*. Indianapolis, IN: National Collegiate Athletic Association; 2001.

112. National Federation of State High School Associations. *Official Football Rules*. Elgin, IL: National Federation of State High School Associations; 1976.

113. National Collegiate Athletic Association. *Football Rules Changes and/or Modifications*. Kansas City, MO: National Collegiate Athletic Association; January 23, 1976.

114. National Collegiate Athletic Association. *2001 Consolidated NCAA Foul Report*. Indianapolis, IN: National Collegiate Athletic Association; 2002.

115. Peterson TR. Roundtable: head and neck injuries in football. Paper presented at: American Society for Testing and Materials' International Symposium on Head and Neck Injuries in Sports; May 1993; Atlanta, GA.

116. Heck JF. A survey of New Jersey high school football officials regarding spearing rules. *J Athl Train*. 1995;30:63–68.

117. Lutz R. Good judgment critical in making call. Available at: http://www.mcoa.org/articles/fb_003.html. Accessed July 9, 2002.

118. National Federation of State High School Associations. *Official Football Rules*. Indianapolis, IN: National Federation of State High School Associations; 1988.

119. Lawrence DS, Stewart GW, Christy DM, Gibbs, LI, Ouellette M. High school football-related cervical spinal cord injuries in Louisiana: the athlete's perspective. Available at: http://www.injuryprevention.org/states/la/football/football.htm. Accessed July 15, 2002.

120. National Federation of State High School Associations. *Official Football Rules*. Indianapolis, IN: National Federation of State High School Associations; 1994.

121. Bishop PJ. Factors related to quadriplegia in football and the implications for intervention strategies. *Am J Sports Med*. 1996;24:235–239.

122. Heck JF. The football official's role in the prevention of catastrophic neck injuries. Presented at: Southern New Jersey Football Officiating Association Meeting; September 1994; Audubon, NJ.

123. Kleiner DM, Almquist JL, Bailes J, et al. *Prehospital Care of the Spine-Injured Athlete*. Dallas, TX: Inter-Association Task Force for Appropriate Care of the Spine-Injured Athlete; 2001.

124. Albright JP, Moses JM, Feldick HD, Dolan KD, Burmeister LF. Nonfatal cervical spine injuries in interscholastic football. *JAMA*. 1976;236:1243–1245.

125. Graves JE, Pollock ML, Leggett SH, et al. Effect of reduced training frequency on muscular strength. *Int J Sports Med*. 1988;9:316–319.

126. Patterson D. Legal aspects of athletic injuries to the head and cervical spine. In: Torg JS, ed. *Athletic Injuries to the Head, Neck, and Face*. 2nd ed. St. Louis, MO: Mosey Year Book; 1991:198–209.

127. Patterson D. Legal aspects of athletic injuries to the head and cervical spine. *Clin Sports Med*. 1987;6:197–210.

128. *Boulet v Brunswick Corporation*, 126 Mich App 240 (1982).

129. *Dibortolo v Metropolitan School District*, 440 NE2d 506 Ind Ct App (1982).

130. *Gerrity v Beatty*, 71 Ill 2d 47 (1978).

131. *Green v Orleans Parish School Board*, 365 So2d 834, 836 La Ct App (1978).

132. *Jackson v Board of Education 109*, Ill App 3d 716, 441 NE2d 120 (1982).

133. *Landers v School District #203*, 66 Ill App 3d 78, 383 NE2d 645 (1978).

134. *Low v Texas Tech University*, 540 SW2d 297 Tex Supreme Ct (1976).

135. *Peterson v Multnomah County School District*, 669 P2d 387, 393 (1983).

136. *Stehn v Bernarr Macfadden Foundations, Inc*, 434 F2d811 6th Cir (1970).

137. *Vendrell v School District No 26C*, 233 Ore 1 (1962).

138. *Wissel v Ohio High School Athletic Association*, 78 Ohio App 3d 529 (1992).

139. Black J. Legal implications for the secondary school athlete. Paper presented at: National Athletic Trainers' Association 53rd Annual Meeting and Clinical Symposia; June 14–18, 2002: Dallas, TX.

140. Heck JF, Weis MP, Gartland JM, Weis CR. Minimizing liability risks of head and neck injuries in football. *J Athl Train*. 1994;29:128–139.

Head-Down Contact & Spearing Review Questions:

1. Explain the anatomical scenario in which head-down contact and spearing in tackle football oftentimes result in catastrophic cervical spine injury.

2. This position statement recommends that players, coaches and officials be educated that unintentional and intentional head-down contact can result in catastrophic injury. As an athletic trainer, what actions can you take to help educate players, coaches and officials about the risk of head-down contact?

3. The NCAA and NFSHSA rule changes aimed at reducing the incidence of catastrophic cervical spine injuries have been successful. However, head-down contact still occurs frequently. Explain why head-down contact still occurs on football fields today and detail ways in which you, as an athletic trainer, can minimize the number of head-down contacts occurring to the athletes for which you are responsible.

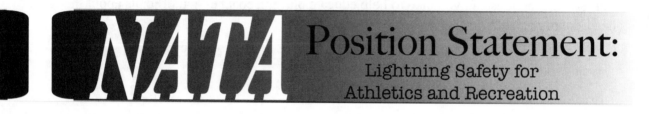

NATA Position Statement:
Lightning Safety for Athletics and Recreation

In This Section: Lightning casualities and injuries during sports and recreational activities have increased at an alarming rate in recent decades. This position statement provides specific recommendations for the implementation of a lightning safety plan and the treatment of lightning-strike victims.

National Athletic Trainers' Association Position Statement: Lightning Safety for Athletics and Recreation

Katie M. Walsh, EdD, ATC-L*; Brian Bennett, MEd, ATC†;
Mary Ann Cooper, MD‡; Ronald L. Holle, MS§; Richard Kithil, MBA¶;
Raul E. López, PhD§

*East Carolina University, Greenville, NC; †The College of William and Mary, Williamsburg, VA; ‡The University of Illinois at Chicago, Chicago, IL; §National Severe Storms Laboratory, Norman, OK; ¶The National Lightning Safety Institute, Louisville, CO

Objective: To educate athletic trainers and others about the dangers of lightning, provide lightning-safety guidelines, define safe structures and locations, and advocate prehospital care for lightning-strike victims.

Background: Lightning may be the most frequently encountered severe-storm hazard endangering physically active people each year. Millions of lightning flashes strike the ground annually in the United States, causing nearly 100 deaths and 400 injuries. Three quarters of all lightning casualties occur between May and September, and nearly four fifths occur between 10:00 AM and 7:00 PM, which coincides with the hours for most athletic or recreational activities. Additionally, lightning casualties from sports and recreational activities have risen alarmingly in recent decades.

Recommendations: The National Athletic Trainers' Association recommends a proactive approach to lightning safety, including the implementation of a lightning-safety policy that identifies safe locations for shelter from the lightning hazard. Further components of this policy are monitoring local weather forecasts, designating a weather watcher, and establishing a chain of command. Additionally, a flash-to-bang count of 30 seconds or less should be used as a minimal determinant of when to suspend activities. Waiting 30 minutes or longer after the last flash of lightning or sound of thunder is recommended before athletic or recreational activities are resumed. Lightning-safety strategies include avoiding shelter under trees, avoiding open fields and spaces, and suspending the use of land-line telephones during thunderstorms. Also outlined in this document are the prehospital care guidelines for triaging and treating lightning-strike victims. It is important to evaluate victims quickly for apnea, asystole, hypothermia, shock, fractures, and burns. Cardiopulmonary resuscitation is effective in resuscitating pulseless victims of lightning strike. Maintenance of cardiopulmonary resuscitation and first-aid certification should be required of all persons involved in sports and recreational activities.

Key Words: lightning, policies and procedures, lightning casualties, severe-storm hazards, environmental hazards, emergency action plan, thunderstorms, lightning-safety policy, athletics, recreation

O ver the past century, lightning has consistently been 1 of the top 3 causes of weather-related deaths in this country.[1,2] It kills approximately 100 people and injures hundreds more each year.[2–5] Lightning is an enormous and widespread danger to the physically active population, due in part to the prevalence of thunderstorms in the afternoon to early evening during the late spring to early fall and a societal trend toward outdoor physical activities.[2,3,6] Certain areas of the United States have higher propensities for thunderstorm activity, and thus, higher casualty rates: the Atlantic seaboard, southwest, southern Rocky Mountains, and southern plains states.[2,7]

Worldwide, approximately 2000 thunderstorms and 50 to 100 lightning flashes occur every second.[8] In 1997, the National Lightning Detection Network recorded nearly 27 000 000 cloud-to-ground lightning strikes in the United States (Christoph Zimmerman, Global Atmospherics, Inc, Tucson, AZ, unpublished data). Many of these strikes caused fires, power outages, property damage, loss of life, and disabling injuries. Property damage from lightning is estimated to cost $5 000 000 000 to $6 000 000 000 annually in this country.[9] While print and television news reports of lightning-strike incidents to recreational athletes are frequent during the thunderstorm season, many people are unsure about what to do and where to go to improve their safety during thunderstorms. It is incumbent on all individuals, particularly those who are leaders in athletics and recreation, to appreciate the lightning hazard, learn the published lightning-safety guidelines, and act prudently, wisely, and in a spirit that will encourage safe behavior in others.

The guidelines presented in this article govern all outdoor activities, as well as indoor swimming-pool activities. The purpose of this position statement is to recommend lightning-safety policy guidelines and strategies and to educate athletic trainers and others involved with athletic or recreation activities about the hazards of lightning.

Address correspondence to National Athletic Trainers' Association, Communications Department, 2952 Stemmons Freeway, Dallas, TX 75247.

RECOMMENDATIONS

1. Formalize and implement a comprehensive, proactive lightning-safety policy or emergency action plan specific to lightning safety.[1,7,10–14] The components of this policy should include the following:
   A. An established chain of command that identifies who is to make the call to remove individuals from the field or an activity.
   B. A designated weather watcher (ie, a person who actively looks for the signs of threatening weather and notifies the chain of command if severe weather becomes dangerous).
   C. A means of monitoring local weather forecasts and warnings.
   D. A listing of specific safe locations (for each field or site) from the lightning hazard.
   E. The use of specific criteria for suspension and resumption of activities (refer to recommendations 4, 5, and 6).
   F. The use of the recommended lightning-safety strategies (refer to recommendations 7, 8, and 9).
2. The primary choice for a safe location from the lightning hazard is any substantial, frequently inhabited building. The electric and telephone wiring and plumbing pathways aid in grounding a building, which is why buildings are safer than remaining outdoors during thunderstorms. It is important not to be connected to these pathways while inside the structure during ongoing thunderstorms.
3. The secondary choice for a safer location from the lightning hazard is a fully enclosed vehicle with a metal roof and the windows closed.[1,7,10,11,13,14] Convertible cars and golf carts do not provide protection from lightning danger. It is important not to touch any part of the metal framework of the vehicle while inside it during ongoing thunderstorms.
4. Seeking a safe structure or location at the first sign of lightning or thunder activity is highly recommended. By the time the flash-to-bang count approaches 30 seconds (or is less than 30 seconds), all individuals should already be inside or should immediately seek a safe structure or location.[1,13–15] To use the flash-to-bang method, the observer begins counting when a lightning flash is sighted. Counting is stopped when the associated bang (thunder) is heard. Divide this count by 5 to determine the distance to the lightning flash (in miles). For example, a flash-to-bang count of 30 seconds equates to a distance of 6 miles (9.66 km).
5. Postpone or suspend activity if a thunderstorm appears imminent before or during an activity or contest (regardless of whether lightning is seen or thunder heard) until the hazard has passed. Signs of imminent thunderstorm activity are darkening clouds, high winds, and thunder or lightning activity.
6. Once activities have been suspended, wait at least 30 minutes after the last sound of thunder or lightning flash before resuming an activity or returning outdoors.[1,13–15] A message should be read over the public address system and lightning-safety tips should be placed in game programs alerting spectators and competitors about what to do and where to go to find a safer location during thunderstorm activity.[13,15]
7. Extremely large athletic events are of particular concern with regard to lightning safety. Consider using a multidisciplinary approach to lessen lightning danger, such as integrating weather forecasts, real-time thunderstorm data, a weather watcher, and the flash-to-bang count to aid in decision making.
8. Avoid being in contact with, or in proximity to, the highest point of an open field or on the open water. Do not take shelter under or near trees, flag poles, or light poles.[1,8,10,13–15]
9. Avoid taking showers and using plumbing facilities (including indoor and outdoor pools) and land-line telephones during thunderstorm activity.[1,8,10,13–15] Cordless or cellular telephones are safer to use when emergency help is needed.
10. Individuals who feel their hair stand on end or skin tingle or hear crackling noises should assume the lightning-safe position (ie, crouched on the ground, weight on the balls of the feet, feet together, head lowered, and ears covered). Do not lie flat on the ground.[1,8,10,13–15]
11. Observe the following basic first-aid procedures, in order, to manage victims of lightning strike[16]:
    A. Survey the scene for safety. Ongoing thunderstorms may still pose a threat to emergency personnel responding to the situation.
    B. Activate the local emergency management system.
    C. Move the victim carefully to a safer location, if needed.
    D. Evaluate and treat for apnea and asystole.
    E. Evaluate and treat for hypothermia and shock.
    F. Evaluate and treat for fractures.
    G. Evaluate and treat for burns.
12. All persons should maintain current cardiopulmonary resuscitation (CPR) and first-aid certification.
13. All individuals should have the right to leave an athletic site or activity, without fear of repercussion or penalty, in order to seek a safe structure or location if they feel they are in danger from impending lightning activity.[13,15]

BACKGROUND

Lightning-Flash Development

Within a developing thunderstorm cloud, updrafts promote the collision of rising and descending ice and water particles, and the positive and negative charges are separated into distinct layers. Positive charges are taken via updrafts to the top of the cloud, while negative charges accumulate in the bottom of the cloud, creating the equivalent of a giant atmospheric battery.[8]

A cloud-to-ground lightning flash is the product of the buildup and discharge of static electric energy between the charged regions of the cloud and the earth. The negatively charged lower region of the cloud induces a positive charge on the ground below. The tremendous electric forces between these 2 opposite charges initiate the lightning flash, which begins as a barely visible step leader moving in a series of steps downward from the cloud. Various objects on the ground (trees, chimneys, people, etc) can produce positively charged, upward streamers. The connection of the step leader with an upward streamer determines the connection point on the ground. After contact, a bright return stroke propagates upward from the ground, while electrons move downward toward the earth.[8] This entire phenomenon happens in less than a fraction of a second,[8] but a large amount of charge is transferred to the earth from the cloud.

Most lightning flashes have several return strokes, separated by only 0.004 to 0.005 seconds.[8] The human eye can barely resolve the intervals between the strokes that cause the lightning flash to appear to flicker. A lightning flash is essentially a brief spark, similar to that received from touching a doorknob after walking across a carpeted room. The lightning channel is approximately 2.54 cm (1 inch) in diameter and averages 4.83 to 8.05 km (3 to 5 miles) in vertical height but can be 9.66 km (6 miles) or higher.[8] Cloud-to-ground lightning flashes typically have peak currents ranging from 10 000 to 200 000 Å, and the electric potential between the cloud and ground can be 10 000 000 to 100 000 000 V.[8]

Thunder is created when lightning quickly heats the air around it, sometimes to temperatures greater than approximately 27 800°C (50 000°F), which is about 5 times hotter than the surface of the sun.[8] The rapidly heated air around a lightning channel explodes, which in turn creates the sound we hear as a clap of thunder.[8] The audible range of thunder is about 16.09 km (10 miles) but can be more or less depending on local conditions.[1] Heat lightning is intracloud or intercloud lightning that is too distant for the accompanying thunder to be heard.[8] Although it is possible to have lightning without thunder, thunder never occurs in the absence of lightning.

Lightning Casualty Demographics

On average, lightning kills approximately 100 people each year in this country, while many hundreds more are injured.[2–5] The death toll from lightning for 1940 to 1973 was greater than that from tornadoes and hurricanes combined.[17] Ninety-two percent of lightning casualties occur between May and September, while July has the greatest number of casualties.[2,3,7,18] Furthermore, 45% of the deaths and 80% of the casualties occurred in these months between 10:00 AM and 7:00 PM,[2,3,7,8] which coincides with the most likely time period for athletic or recreational events. For these reasons, it is accurate to say that lightning is the most dangerous and frequently encountered severe-storm hazard that most people experience each year.[10,11]

The statistics on lightning casualty demographics compiled from the National Oceanographic and Atmospheric Administration publication *Storm Data* for the state of Colorado over the last few decades demonstrate an increase in the number of lightning casualties in persons involved in sports and outdoor recreation.[7,10,18,19] Fifty-two percent of lightning casualties were people involved in outdoor recreation.[7,18] In addition, these authors noted that the highest number of casualties from lightning was recorded in recreational and sports activities for each year of the study.[18] During the 1960s, more than 30% of lightning casualties occurred during outdoor recreation activities; during the 1970s, that figure rose to 47%.[17] Furthermore, the rate of increase of lightning casualties during sports was higher than the general United States population rate of increase during the same time period.[7,18]

Lightning casualty statistics from Colorado demonstrate that the most common sites for fatalities were open fields (27%), near trees (16%), and close to water (13%).[7,8,18] Statistics from the country as a whole mimic the numbers from Colorado. Open fields, ballparks, and playgrounds accounted for nearly 27% of casualties, and under trees (14%), water-related (8%), and golf-related (5%) deaths associated with lightning followed.[19] All these fatalities had 1 common denominator: being near the highest object or being the tallest object in the immediate area. This single factor accounted for 56% of all fatalities from Colorado. Thus, it is imperative to

avoid high ridges and high points on the terrain, and conversely, it is important to seek low-lying points on the terrain.[1,3,8,13–15]

The height above ground has been demonstrated to play a prominent role in determining the strike probability. Therefore, it is important to understand why minimizing vertical height is critical in decreasing the chances of becoming a victim of lightning. Warning signs of a high electromagnetic field and imminent lightning strike include hair standing on end and sounds similar to bacon sizzling or cloth tearing.[8] If these conditions occur, a cloud-to-ground lightning flash could strike in the immediate area. Therefore, one should immediately crouch in the lightning-safe position: feet together, weight on the balls of the feet, head lowered, and ears covered.[1] This position is intended to minimize the probability of a direct strike by both lowering the person's height and minimizing the area in contact with the surface of the ground. Taller objects are more likely to be struck (but not always) because their upward streamer occurs first, so that it is closer in proximity to the step leader coming downward from the cloud.

The ultimate message is that individuals in dangerous lightning situations should never wait to seek a safe location and pursue safety measures. It is important to be proactive by having all individuals inside a safe structure or location long before the lightning is close enough to be threatening.

Mechanisms of Lightning Injury

Injury from lightning can occur via 5 mechanisms.[16] A direct strike most commonly occurs to the head, and lightning current enters the orifices. This mechanism explains why eye and ear injuries in lightning-strike victims are abundantly reported in the literature.[16] The shock wave created by the lightning channel can also produce injuries, such as rupture of the tympanic membrane, a common clinical presentation in the lightning-strike victim.[16,23,24] Recommending that individuals cover their ears while in the lightning-safe position may help to mitigate this type of injury.

The second mechanism, contact injury, occurs when the lightning victim is touching an object that is in the pathway of a lightning current.[16] Side flash, the third mechanism, occurs when lightning strikes an object near the victim and then jumps from that object to the victim. This is the main danger to a person who is sheltered under an isolated, tall tree.[6] An upward streamer is triggered by the tree but when this connects with the step leader, the resulting stroke jumps to the victim, who represents an additional pathway to ground.

The fourth mechanism, a step voltage or ground current, occurs when the lightning current flowing in the ground radiates outward in waves from the strike point. If 1 of the individual's feet is closer to the strike than the other, a step voltage is created.[6,16] Humans are primarily salt minerals in an aqueous solution, and a lightning current preferentially travels up from the earth through this solution (that is, the person) rather than through the ground. The greater the differential step voltage (ie, the greater the distance between the 2 feet), the greater the likelihood of injury. Placing one's feet close together while in the crouched position and not lying flat on the ground are crucial in reducing the likelihood of injury from a step voltage or ground current.

Blunt injury is the fifth mechanism for lightning-strike injuries. Lightning current can cause violent muscular contractions that throw its victims many meters from the strike point.

Explosive and implosive forces created by the rapid heating and cooling by the lightning current are also enough to produce traumatic injuries.[16]

Common Effects of Lightning Injury

While lightning kills nearly 100 people annually in this country, the protracted suffering of the survivors should not be underestimated. Although the only acute cause of death from lightning injury is cardiac arrest,[20] the anoxic brain damage that can occur if the person is not rapidly resuscitated can be devastating. In addition, even for the survivor who did not sustain a cardiac arrest, permanent sequelae can include common brain-injury symptoms such as deficits in short-term memory and processing of new information, as well as severe and ongoing headaches, hyperirritability, sleep disturbances, and distractibility.[21,22] Others may develop chronic pain syndromes or absence-type seizures. Frequently, survivors are unable to return to their previous level of function. They may not be able to continue in their jobs or in their educational pursuits and may be permanently disabled.

Components of a Lightning-Safety Policy

The purpose of formalizing a policy on lightning safety is to provide written guidelines for safety during lightning storms. Ninety-two percent of National Collegiate Athletic Association Division I athletics departments responding to a survey did not have a formal, written lightning-safety policy.[12] The best means of reducing the lightning hazard to people is to be proactive. Athletic and recreational personnel should formalize and implement an emergency action plan specific to lightning safety before the thunderstorm season.[1,11,13–15] Dissemination of the plan is paramount, so that all persons will know what to do and where to go to improve their own safety during thunderstorms. The 6 components of a lightning-safety policy or emergency action plan for lightning are discussed in the following paragraphs.

The first component in an emergency action plan or policy for lightning safety is the establishment of a specific chain of command that identifies the person who has the authority to remove participants from athletic venues or activities. The second is to appoint a weather watcher who actively looks for signs of developing local thunderstorms, such as high winds, darkening clouds, and any lightning or thunder.

The third element of a lightning-safety policy is the stipulation for monitoring local weather forecasts. One method is to use weather radios that broadcast information on daily forecasts and approaching storm systems. Weather radios are an excellent informational tool for general storm movement and strength. While this information is extremely important in decision making, the National Weather Service does not broadcast information on specific storm cells or lightning. Therefore, in addition to monitoring weather radios, it is essential that the weather watcher be on constant lookout for conditions in the immediate vicinity of the athletic event and compare these conditions with the weather radio information.

When a local area is placed under a severe-storm watch or warning by the National Weather Service, weather radios can be programmed to give audible alert tones. A watch indicates conditions are favorable for severe weather; a warning means severe weather has been detected in the locale, and all persons should take the necessary precautions to preserve their own safety. If severe storms are in the vicinity, all individuals should more intently monitor thunderstorm activity, such as severity and direction of movement of the storm. It may also mean that steps should be taken to remove athletes from the field or perhaps to postpone or suspend athletic or recreational activities during the event or before the storm begins.

Safe Locations

The fourth aspect of a lightning-safety policy, defining and listing safe structures or locations to evacuate to in the event of lightning, is of utmost importance. While there are reports of people being injured by lightning inside buildings,[8] evacuating to a substantial building can considerably lower the risks of lightning injury compared with those of remaining outside during the thunderstorm. The lightning-safety policy should identify the safe structure or location specific to each venue. This information will enable individuals to know where to go in advance of any thunderstorm situation and appreciate how long it takes to get to the specific safe location from each field or event site.

The primary choice for a safe structure is any fully enclosed, substantial building.[1,3,8,13–15] Ideally, the building should have plumbing, electric wiring, and telephone service. The lightning current is more likely to follow these pathways to ground, which aids in electrically grounding the structure.[8] If a substantial building is not available, a fully enclosed vehicle with a metal roof and the windows completely closed is a reasonable alternative.[1,3,13–15] It is not the rubber tires that make the vehicle safe but the metal enclosure that guides the lightning current around the passengers, rather than through them. Do not touch any part of the metal framework while inside the vehicle.[8] Convertible vehicles and golf carts do not provide a high level of protection and cannot be considered safe from lightning.

Unsafe Locations

Unfortunately, those properties that serve to define a safe structure and improve the safety of its inhabitants also present a potential risk. Lightning current can enter a building via the electric or telephone wiring. It can also enter via a ground current through the incoming plumbing pipelines. This condition makes locker-room shower areas, swimming pools (indoor and outdoor), telephones, and electric appliances unsafe during thunderstorms because of the possible contact with current-carrying conduction. While such reports are rare, people have been killed or injured by lightning in their homes while talking on the telephone, taking a shower, or standing near household appliances such as dishwashers, stoves, or refrigerators.[1,3,8,13–15]

From 1959 through 1965, lightning killed 4 people and injured 36 others while they were talking on the telephone. These numbers comprised 0.42% (n = 960) of deaths and 2.1% (n = 1736) of injuries for the period.[5] Studying reports from *Storm Data*, researchers found that between 1959 and 1994, 2.4% of lightning casualties were telephone related.[2] Because they are not connected directly to a land-line phone, cellular and cordless telephones are reasonably safe alternatives for summoning help during a thunderstorm. It should be noted that injury from acoustic damage can occur via explosive static from the earpiece caused by a nearby lightning strike.

Even though a swimming pool may be indoors and apparently safe, it can be a dangerous location during thunderstorms.[25] The current can be propagated through plumbing and electric connections via the underwater lights and drains of most swimming pools. Lightning current can also enter the building, either into the electric wiring inside the building or through underground plumbing pipelines that enter the building.[8] If lightning strikes the building or ground nearby, the current will most likely follow these pathways to the swimmers through the water. Thus, indoor-pool activities are potentially dangerous and should be avoided during thunderstorms.[25]

Small structures, such as rain or picnic shelters or athletic storage sheds, are generally not properly protected and should be avoided during thunderstorms. These locations may actually increase the risk of lightning strike via a side flash and cause injury to the occupants.

Criteria for Postponement and Resumption of Activities

The fifth component of any lightning-safety policy is to clearly describe criteria for both the suspension and resumption of athletic or recreational activities. Various technologies currently on the market propose to assist in determining when lightning is in the immediate area. Within the developing area of this lightning technology, data-based research is insufficient to either support or dispute companies' claims regarding establishing when one is in danger of a lightning strike. Therefore the National Athletic Trainers' Association promotes the flash-to-bang standard to warn people of imminent lightning danger. The flash-to-bang method is the easiest and most convenient means for determining the distance to a lightning flash and can also be used to determine when to suspend or postpone activities. The flash-to-bang method is based on the fact that light travels faster than sound, which travels at a speed of approximately 1.61 km (1 mile) every 5 seconds.[1,8,13,14] To use the flash-to-bang method, begin counting on the lightning flash, and stop counting when the associated clap of thunder is heard. When storms have a high flash rate, it is important to correlate a specific flash with the thunder it produced. Divide the time to thunder (in seconds) by 5 to determine the distance (in miles) to the lightning flash.[1,8,13,14] For example, an observer obtains a count of 30 seconds from the time he or she spots the flash to when the thunder is heard. Thirty divided by 5 equals 6; therefore, that lightning flash was 6 miles (9.66 km) from the observer.

The 30-second rule is not an arbitrary guideline. López and Holle[26] studied storms in Oklahoma, Colorado, and Florida and found that in larger thunderstorms, the distance between successive flashes can be up to 6 miles (9.66 km) (ie, a flash-to-bang count of 30 seconds) in approximately 80% of the flash pairs. The authors also found the distance between successive flashes may be as great as 9 miles (14.48 km) or more, depending on local geography and atmospheric conditions. If a flash-to-bang count of 30 seconds is observed, the next flash could conceivably be at the observer's location.

Another important factor to consider when using the flash-to-bang method is that, although a relatively rare occurrence, lightning has been reported to strike 16.09 km (10 miles) or more from where it is raining.[1] Therefore, a flash-to-bang count of at least 30 seconds is strongly recommended as a determinant of when to suspend or postpone athletic or recreational activities.[13–15] As the flash-to-bang count approaches 30 seconds, all persons should be seeking, or already inside, a safe structure or location. This is the minimal guideline when using the flash-to-bang method to halt athletic or recreational activities. Seeking a safe location at the first sign of thunder or lightning activity is also highly recommended.

Another facet of the lightning-safety policy is embodied in the "30–30 rule" (Table 1), which relies on the flash-to-bang method. If a game, practice, or other activity is suspended or postponed due to lightning activity, it is important to establish strict criteria in the lightning-safety policy for resumption of activities. Waiting at least 30 minutes after the last lightning flash or sound of thunder is recommended.[13–15] When storm reports and flash data at the time of death or injury were compared, researchers found that the end of the storm, when the flash-rate frequency began to decline, was as deadly as the middle of the storm, when the lightning flash rate was at its peak. The authors postulated that once the flash rate begins to decline, people do not perceive the thunderstorm as dangerous and are struck by lightning when they return outdoors prematurely.[1] An important adage for athletic trainers, coaches, and officials to remember is, "if you see it (lightning) flee it, if you hear it (thunder), clear it."

The 30-minute rule can also be explained in another way. A typical thunderstorm moves at a rate of approximately 40.23 km (25 miles) per hour. Experts believe that 30 minutes allow the thunderstorm to be about 16.09 to 19.31 km (10 to 12 miles) from the area, minimizing the probability of a nearby, and therefore dangerous, lightning strike.[15] Blue sky in the local area or a lack of rainfall are not adequate reasons to breach the 30-minute return-to-play rule. Lightning can strike far from where it is raining, even when the clouds begin to clear and show evidence of blue sky.[1] This situation is often referred to as a "bolt out of the blue." Each time lightning is observed or thunder is heard, the 30-minute clock should be reset.

Obligation to Warn

The recommendation for reading lightning-safety messages over public address systems and placing placards conspicuously around each venue resulted from a fatal lightning strike in Washington, DC, in May 1991.[27] During a high school lacrosse game, a dangerous thunderstorm swept into the local area, and the game was suspended. Lightning killed 1 young person and injured 10 others who sought refuge under a tree. Many people stated that they did not know what to do or where to go to protect themselves from the dangers of lightning.

According to the basic principles of tort law, an individual has a duty to warn others of dangers that may not be obvious to a guest or subordinate of that person.[28] Black et al[29] defined the legal principle of "foreseeability" as "the ability to see or

Table 1. The 30-30 Rule[15]

Criteria for suspension of activities	By the time the flash-to-bang count approaches 30 seconds, all individuals should already be inside a safe shelter.
Criteria for resumption of activities	Wait at least 30 minutes after the last sound (thunder) or observation of lightning before leaving the safe shelter to resume activities.

know in advance, eg, reasonable anticipation, that harm or injury is a likely result from certain acts or omissions." With regard to dangerous lightning situations, it could be argued that an institution (or athletic department) has the duty to warn spectators, invited guests, and participants if conditions are such that lightning activity may be an imminent danger in the immediate area. Whereas lightning is understood by all to be a dangerous phenomenon, the importance of seeking safe shelter and the specific time that one should vacate to safety are generally not known. Based on research presented in this article regarding the number of lightning casualties resulting from the erroneous tendency of people to seek shelter under trees, it would be wise for an organization to promote lightning safety to its clientele and participants, including a list of specific safe locations or structures.

Warnings should be commensurate with the age and understanding of those involved. Announcements should be repeated over the public address system and colorful notices and safety instructions both placed in the event programs and posted in visible, high-traffic areas. Safety instructions should include the location of the nearest safe shelter, similar to airline pocket diagrams of nearest emergency exits. Being proactive with regard to the lightning threat demands not putting individuals at risk if a hazardous situation could have been prevented. If thunderstorm activity looks menacing before or during an event, consider canceling or postponing the event until the complete weather situation can be ascertained and determined to no longer be a threat. The first lightning flash from the thunderstorm cloud and storms that produce only a few flashes still pose a potential threat and should be treated as such. Every cloud-to-ground lightning flash is dangerous and potentially deadly and should not be taken lightly or viewed complacently. Therefore, it is the recommendation of the National Athletic Trainers' Association to postpone or suspend athletic and recreational activities before their onset, if thunderstorm activity appears imminent.

Prehospital Care of Victims

If a lightning-strike victim presents in asystole or respiratory arrest, it is critical to initiate CPR as soon as safely possible.[23] Because lightning-strike victims do not remain connected to a power source, they do not carry an electric charge and are safe to assess.[30] However, during an ongoing thunderstorm, lightning activity in the local area still poses a deadly hazard for the medical team responding to the incident. The athletic trainer or other medical personnel should consider his or her own personal safety before venturing into a dangerous situation to render care.

If medical personnel assume the risk of entering a dangerous lightning situation to render care, the first priority should be to move the victim to a safe location. In this way, a hazardous situation can be neutralized for the athletic trainer, as well as the victim. It is unlikely that moving a victim to an area of greater safety for resuscitation will cause any serious injury to the victim.[16] The primary and secondary survey of the victim's condition can then be conducted once safety is reached.

It is not uncommon to find a lightning-strike victim unconscious, with fixed and dilated pupils and cold extremities and in cardiopulmonary arrest. Case studies of individuals with prolonged apnea and asystole after a lightning strike have demonstrated successful resuscitations using CPR.[23,24,31] Once stopped, the heart will most likely spontaneously restart, but

Table 2. Recommended Prehospital Care for Treating Lightning-Strike Victims[16]

Perform the following steps in order:
1. Survey the scene for safety.
2. Activate the local emergency management system.
3. Carefully move the victim to a safe area, if needed.
4. Evaluate and treat for apnea and asystole.
5. Evaluate and treat for hypothermia and shock.
6. Evaluate and treat for fractures.
7. Evaluate and treat for burns.

breathing centers in the brain may be damaged. Respiratory arrest lasts longer than cardiac arrest, leading to secondary asystole from hypoxia.[16] Therefore, the basic principle of triage, "treat the living first," should be reversed in cases involving casualties from a lightning strike. It is imperative to treat those persons who are "apparently dead" first by promptly initiating CPR. See Table 2 for quick-reference guidelines in evaluating and treating victims of lightning strike.

CONCLUSIONS

Due to its pervasiveness during the times that most athletic events occur, lightning is a significant hazard to the physically active population. Lightning-casualty statistics show an alarming rise in the number of lightning casualties in recreational and sports settings in recent decades.[2,3,9] Each person must take responsibility for his or her own personal safety during thunderstorms.[10] However, because people are often under the direction of others, whether they are children or adults participating in organized athletics, athletic trainers, coaches, teachers, and game officials must receive education about the hazards of lightning and become familiar with proved lightning-safety strategies. A policy is only as good as its compliance and unwavering, broad-based enforcement.

It is important to be much more wary of the lightning threat than the rain. Lightning can strike in the absence of rain, as well as from apparently clear blue skies overhead, even though a thunderstorm may be nearby. The presence of lightning or thunder should be the determining factor in postponing or suspending games and activities, not the amount of rainfall on the playing field. Lightning should be the only critical factor in decision making for athletic trainers, umpires, officials, referees, and coaches.

Athletic trainers, umpires, officials, referees, coaches, teachers, and parents can make a difference in reducing the number of lightning casualties if they (1) formalize and implement a lightning-safety policy or emergency action plan specific to lightning safety; (2) understand the qualifications of safe structures or locations, in addition to knowing where they are in relation to each athletic field or activity site; (3) understand the 30–30 rule as a minimal determinant of when to suspend activities and follow it; being conservative and suspending activities at the first sign of lightning or thunder activity is also prudent and wise; (4) practice and follow the published lightning-safety guidelines and strategies; (5) and maintain CPR and standard first-aid certification.

ACKNOWLEDGMENTS

This position statement was reviewed for the National Athletic Trainers' Association by the Pronouncements Committee, Richard Ray, PhD, ATC, and Philip Krider, PhD.

REFERENCES

1. Holle RL, López RE, Howard KW, Vavrek J, Allsopp J. Safety in the presence of lightning. *Semin Neurol.* 1995;15:375–380.
2. López RE, Holle RL, Heitkamp TA, Boyson M, Cherington M, Langford K. The underreporting of lightning injuries and deaths in Colorado. *Bull Am Meteorol Soc.* 1993;74:2171–2178.
3. Duclos PJ, Sanderson LM. An epidemiological description of lightning-related deaths in the United States. *Int J Epidemiol.* 1990;19:673–679.
4. Craig SR. When lightning strikes: pathophysiology and treatment of lightning injuries. *Postgrad Med.* 1986;79:109–112,121–123.
5. Zegel FH. Lightning deaths in the United States: a seven-year survey from 1959 to 1965. *Weatherwise.* 1967;20:169.
6. Andrews CJ, Cooper MA, Darveniza M. *Lightning Injuries: Electrical, Medical, and Legal Aspects.* Boca Raton, FL: CRC Press; 1992.
7. López RE, Holle RL. Demographics of lightning casualties. *Semin Neurol.* 1995;15:286–295.
8. Uman MA. *All About Lightning.* New York, NY: Dover Publications; 1986.
9. Kithil R. Annual USA lightning costs and losses. National Lightning Safety Institute. Available at: www.lightningsafety.com/nlsi_lls/nlsi_annual_usa_losses.htm. Accessed January 19, 1999.
10. Holle RL, López RE. Lightning: impacts and safety. *World Meterol Bull.* 1998;47:148–155.
11. Holle RL, López RE, Vavrek J, Howard KW. Educating individuals about lightning. In: *Preprints of the American Meteorological Society 7th Symposium on Education*; January 11–16, 1998; Phoenix, AZ.
12. Walsh KM, Hanley MJ, Graner SJ, Beam D, Bazluki J. A survey of lightning policy in selected Division I colleges. *J Athl Train.* 1997;32:206–210.
13. Bennett BL. A model lightning safety policy for athletics. *J Athl Train.* 1997;32:251–253.
14. Bennett BL, Holle RL, López RE. Lightning safety guideline 1D. *1997–98 National Collegiate Athletic Association Sports Medicine Handbook.* Overland Park, KS: National Collegiate Athletic Association; 1997–1998:12–14.
15. Vavrek JR, Holle RL, López RE. Updated lightning safety recommendations. In: *Preprints of the American Meteorological Society 8th Symposium on Education*; January 10–15, 1999; Dallas, TX.
16. Cooper MA. Emergent care of lightning and electrical injuries. *Semin Neurol.* 1995;15:268–278.
17. Weigel EP. Lightning: the underrated killer. *NOAA [National Oceanographic and Atmospheric Administration].* 1976;6:4–11.
18. López RE, Holle RL, Heitkamp TA. Lightning casualties and property damage in Colorado from 1950 to 1991 based on storm data. *Weather Forecast.* 1995;10:114–126.
19. Curran EB, Holle RL, López RE. *Lightning Fatalities, Injuries, and Damage Reports in the United States: 1959–1994.* Washington, DC: National Oceanic and Atmospheric Administration; 1997. Technical Memorandum NWS SR-193.
20. Cooper MA. Lightning: prognostic signs for death. *Ann Emerg Med.* 1980;9:134–138.
21. Primeau M, Engelstatter GH, Bares KK. Behavioral consequences of lightning and electrical injury. *Semin Neurol.* 1995;15:279–285.
22. Andrews CJ, Darveniza M. Telephone-mediated lightning injury: an Australian survey. *J Trauma.* 1989;29:665–671.
23. Fontanarosa PB. Electrical shock and lightning strike. *Ann Emerg Med.* 1993;22(Pt 2):378–387.
24. Steinbaum S, Harviel JD, Jaffin JH, Jordan MH. Lightning strike to the head: case report. *J Trauma.* 1994;36:113–115.
25. Wiley S. Shocking news about lightning and pools. *USA Swimming Safety Q.* 1998;4:1–2.
26. López RE, Holle RL. The distance between subsequent lightning flashes. In: *Preprints of the International Lightning Detection Conference*; November 17–18, 1998; Tucson, AZ.
27. Sanchez R, Wheeler L. Lightning strike at St. Albans game kills Bethesda student, injures 10. *Washington Post.* May 18, 1991;A1.
28. Keeton WP, Dobbs DB, Keeton RE, Owen DG. *Prosser and Keeton on Torts.* 5th ed. St. Paul, MN: West Publishing; 1984.
29. Black HC, Nolan JR, Nolan-Haley JM. *Black's Law Dictionary.* 6th ed. St. Paul, MN: West Publishing; 1990.
30. Cooper MA. Myths, miracles, and mirages. *Semin Neurol.* 1995;15:358–361.
31. Jepsen DL. How to manage a patient with lightning injury. *Am J Nurs.* 1992;92:38–42.

Lightning Safety Review Questions:

1. What are the essential components of a comprehensive lightning safety policy? Review the lightning safety policy at your athletic training site. Based on this position statement, where is your policy falling short? What changes can you make to adopt more or all of the recommendations in this statement?

2. What is the best choice for a safe location during a lightning storm? Look at your outdoor practice/game locations. Which of the recommended safe locations are available for your athletes? What additions or alterations can you make to increase the number of safe locations?

3. What are the five mechanisms of a lightning injury? How can you minimize an athlete's risk of sustaining each of these types of lightning injury? How will you manage an athlete who is a victim of a lightning strike?

4. During a late afternoon soccer practice you see a lightning flash. When you see the next flash you begin counting and stop when the associated bang (thunder) is heard. You have counted to 40. A few minutes later you see a second lightning flash and again count until you hear the associated thunder. This time you count to 30. As the athletic trainer responsible for the health, safety and well-being of the athletes on this soccer field, what actions will you now take? What criteria will you use to determine when it is safe for these players to return to the field?

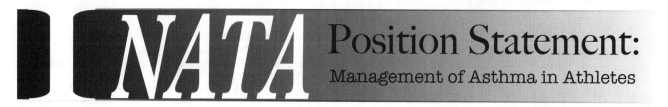

NATA Position Statement:
Management of Asthma in Athletes

In This Section: Breathing difficulties during athletic events and practices are commonly caused by undiagnosed or uncontrolled asthma. The following position statement describes a thorough approach to the diagnosis and management of asthma in athletes.

National Athletic Trainers' Association Position Statement: Management of Asthma in Athletes

Michael G. Miller*; John M. Weiler†; Robert Baker‡; James Collins§; Gilbert D'Alonzo‖

*Western Michigan University, Kalamazoo, MI; †University of Iowa and CompleWare, Iowa City, IA; ‡Michigan State University Kalamazoo Center for Medical Studies, Kalamazoo, MI; §San Diego Chargers, San Diego, CA; ‖Temple University School of Medicine, Philadelphia, PA

Michael G. Miller, EdD, ATC, CSCS; John M. Weiler, MD; Robert Baker, MD, PhD, ATC; James Collins, ATC; and Gilbert D'Alonzo, DO, contributed to conception and design; acquisition and analysis and interpretation of the data; and drafting, critical revision, and final approval of the article.

Address correspondence to National Athletic Trainers' Association, Communications Department, 2952 Stemmons Freeway, Dallas, TX 75247.

Objective: To present guidelines for the recognition, prophylaxis, and management of asthma that lead to improvement in the quality of care certified athletic trainers and other health care providers can offer to athletes with asthma, especially exercise-induced asthma.

Background: Many athletes have difficulty breathing during or after athletic events and practices. Although a wide variety of conditions can predispose an athlete to breathing difficulties, the most common cause is undiagnosed or uncontrolled asthma. At least 15% to 25% of athletes may have signs and symptoms suggestive of asthma, including exercise-induced asthma. Athletic trainers are in a unique position to recognize breathing difficulties caused by undiagnosed or uncontrolled asthma, particularly when asthma follows exercise. Once the diagnosis of asthma is made, the athletic trainer should play a pivotal role in supervising therapies to prevent and control asthma symptoms. It is also important for the athletic trainer to recognize when asthma is not the underlying cause for respiratory difficulties, so that the athlete can be evaluated and treated properly.

Recommendations: The recommendations contained in this position statement describe a structured approach for the diagnosis and management of asthma in an exercising population. Athletic trainers should be educated to recognize asthma symptoms in order to identify patients who might benefit from better management and should understand the management of asthma, especially exercise-induced asthma, to participate as active members of the asthma care team.

Key Words: airway hyperresponsiveness, airway obstruction, exercise-induced asthma, exercise-induced bronchospasm, pulmonary function tests, certified athletic trainer

INTRODUCTION

Asthma is defined as a chronic inflammatory disorder of the airways characterized by variable airway obstruction and bronchial hyperresponsiveness.[1] Airway obstruction can lead to recurrent episodes of wheezing, breathlessness, chest tightness, and coughing, particularly at night or in the early morning.[1] Asthma can be triggered by many stimuli, including allergens (eg, pollen, dust mites, animal dander), pollutants (eg, carbon dioxide, smoke, ozone), respiratory infections, aspirin, nonsteroidal anti-inflammatory drugs (NSAIDs), inhaled irritants (eg, cigarette smoke, household cleaning fumes, chlorine in a swimming pool), particulate exposure (eg, ambient air pollutants, ice rink pollution), and exposure to cold and exercise.[1–5] Airflow limitation is often reversible, but as asthma symptoms continue, patients may develop "airway remodeling" that leads to chronic irreversible airway obstruction.[6,7] Severe attacks of asthma can also cause irreversible airflow obstruction that can lead to death.[4,8]

The National Heart, Lung, and Blood Institute of the National Institutes of Health launched the National Asthma Education and Prevention Program (NAEPP) in March 1989 to address the increasing prevalence of asthma in the United States and its economic costs to the society; the program was updated in 1997 (as NAEPPII).[1] An updated expert panel report from the NAEPP is expected to be released in 2006. The Global Initiative for Asthma (GINA) was also developed to provide worldwide guidelines for asthma awareness and management.[2] These guidelines are extremely comprehensive and have been regularly updated to reflect advances in the diagnosis and management of asthma. Nevertheless, the guidelines do not describe the role of certified athletic trainers or other allied health care professionals in recognizing and managing asthma in an athletic population.

PURPOSE

The purpose of this position statement is to provide athletic trainers and other allied health care professionals who care for athletes with information to:

1. Identify the characteristics and diagnostic criteria of asth-

ma, especially exercise-induced asthma (EIA) or exercise-induced bronchospasm (EIB).

2. Provide guidelines for referral so that patients with asthma and those in whom asthma is suspected can receive a thorough evaluation.

3. Describe management plans to prevent attacks and to control asthma exacerbations when they occur.

4. Educate certified athletic trainers and athletes about pharmacologic and nonpharmacologic therapies and techniques to help control asthma.

RECOMMENDATIONS

Based on current research and literature, the National Athletic Trainers' Association provides the following guidelines for the identification, examination, management, and prophylaxis of asthma, including EIA, and the education of athletes, parents, coaches, and health care personnel about asthma. Not all individuals who suffer from asthma present in the same manner, nor do they all respond to the same management or treatment plan. Therefore, these recommendations are intended to provide the certified athletic trainer and other health care professionals with an overall guide for a better understanding of the asthmatic condition.

Asthma Identification and Diagnosis

1. All athletes must receive preparticipation screening evaluations sufficient to identify the possible presence of asthma.[9–12] In most situations, this evaluation includes only obtaining a thorough history from the athlete. However, in special circumstances, additional screening evaluations (eg, spirometry testing or the challenge testing described below) should also be performed because the history alone is not reliable.[10]

2. Athletic trainers should be aware of the major signs and symptoms suggesting asthma, as well as the following associated conditions[5,13,14]:
   a. Chest tightness (or chest pain in children)
   b. Coughing (especially at night)
   c. Prolonged shortness of breath (dyspnea)
   d. Difficulty sleeping
   e. Wheezing (especially after exercise)
   f. Inability to catch one's breath
   g. Physical activities affected by breathing difficulty
   h. Use of accessory muscles to breathe
   i. Breathing difficulty upon awakening in the morning
   j. Breathing difficulty when exposed to certain allergens or irritants
   k. Exercise-induced symptoms, such as coughing or wheezing
   l. An athlete who is well conditioned but does not seem to be able to perform at a level comparable with other athletes who do not have asthma
   m. Family history of asthma
   n. Personal history of atopy, including atopic dermatitis/eczema or hay fever (allergic rhinitis)
   Note: Although there is a correlation between the presence of symptoms and EIA, the diagnosis should not be based on history alone.[5] Rather, these symptoms should serve to suggest that an athlete may have asthma.

3. The following types of screening questions can be asked to seek evidence of asthma[13]:

a. Does the patient have breathing attacks consisting of coughing, wheezing, chest tightness, or shortness of breath (dyspnea)?

b. Does the patient have coughing, wheezing, chest tightness, or shortness of breath (dyspnea) at night?

c. Does the patient have coughing, wheezing, or chest tightness after exercise?

d. Does the patient have coughing, wheezing, chest tightness, or shortness of breath (dyspnea) after exposure to allergens or pollutants?

e. Which pharmacologic treatments for asthma or allergic rhinitis, if any, were given in the past, and were they successful?

4. Patients with atypical symptoms, symptoms despite proper therapy, or other complications that can exacerbate asthma (such as sinusitis, nasal polyps, severe rhinitis, gastroesophageal reflux disease, or vocal cord dysfunction) should be referred to a physician with expertise in sports medicine (eg, allergist; ear, nose, and throat physician; cardiologist; or pulmonologist with training in providing care for athletes).[15] Testing might include a stress electrocardiogram, upper airway laryngoscopy or rhinoscopy, echocardiogram, or upper endoscopy.

Pulmonary Function Testing

5. Athletes with a history of asthma or of taking a medication used to treat asthma and those suspected of having asthma should consult a physician for proper medical evaluation and to obtain a classification of asthma severity (Table 1). This evaluation should include pulmonary function testing.[16–18]

6. An exercise challenge test is recommended for athletes who have symptoms suggestive of EIA to confirm the diagnosis.[19]

7. If the diagnosis of asthma remains unclear after the above tests have been performed, then additional testing should be performed to assist in making a diagnosis.[15,20,21] Physicians should be encouraged, when possible, to test the athlete using a sport-specific and environment-specific exercise-challenge protocol, in which the athlete participates in his or her venue to replicate the activity or activities and the environment that may serve to trigger airway hyperresponsiveness.[20,21] In some cases, athletes should also be tested for metabolic gas exchange during strenuous exercise to determine fitness (eg, to assess anaerobic threshold and $\dot{V}O_2$max), especially to rule out the diagnosis of asthma or to rule in another diagnosis (eg, pulmonary fibrosis) for a patient with an unclear diagnosis.[16]

Asthma Management

8. Athletic trainers should incorporate into the existing emergency action plan an asthma action plan for managing and urgently referring all patients who may experience significant or life-threatening attacks of breathing difficulties (Figure 1).[1,2] Immediate access to emergency facilities during practices and game situations should be available. For example, athletic trainers should be familiar with appropriate community resources and must have a fully functional telephone (mobile or cellular) available, preprogrammed with emergency medical care access numbers. A telephone might be the single most important de-

Table 1. National Asthma Education and Prevention Program II: Classification of Asthma Severity*[1]

| | Clinical Features Before Treatment† | | |
	Symptoms‡	Nighttime Symptoms	Lung Function
Step 4 Severe persistent	• Continual symptoms • Limited physical activity • Frequent exacerbations	Frequent	• FEV_1 or PEF ≤60% predicted • PEF variability >30%
Step 3 Moderate persistent	• Daily symptoms • Daily use of inhaled short-acting beta$_2$-agonist • Exacerbations affect activity • Exacerbations ≥2 times/wk; may last days	>1 time/wk	• FEV_1 or PEF >60%–<80% predicted • PEF variability ≥30%
Step 2 Mild persistent	• Symptoms >2 times/wk but <1 time/d • Exacerbations may affect activity	>2 times/mo	• FEV_1 or PEF ≥80% predicted • PEF variability 20–30%
Step 1 Mild intermittent	• Symptoms ≤2 times/wk • Asymptomatic and normal PEF between exacerbations • Exacerbations brief (from a few hours to a few days); intensity may vary	≤2 times/mo	• FEV_1 or PEF ≥80% predicted • PEF variability <20%

*FEV_1 indicates forced expiratory volume in 1 s; PEF, peak expiratory flow.
†The presence of one of the features of severity is sufficient to place a patient in that category. An individual should be assigned to the most severe grade in which any feature occurs. The characteristics noted in this figure are general and may overlap because asthma is highly variable. Furthermore, an individual's classification may change over time.
‡Patients at any level of severity can have mild, moderate, or severe exacerbations. Some patients with intermittent asthma experience severe and life-threatening exacerbations separated by long periods of normal lung function and no symptoms.

vice to have on the practice field for a patient who is experiencing an asthma exacerbation. In addition, athletic trainers should have pulmonary function measuring devices (such as peak expiratory flow meters [PFMs] or portable spirometers) at all athletic venues for athletes for whom such devices have been prescribed and should be familiar with how to use these devices.[22]

9. Patients who are experiencing any degree of respiratory distress (including a significant increase in wheezing or chest tightness, a respiratory rate greater than 25 breaths per minute, inability to speak in full sentences, uncontrolled cough, significantly prolonged expiration phase of breathing, nasal flaring, or paradoxic abdominal movement) should be referred rapidly to an emergency department or to their personal physicians for further evaluation and treatment. Referral to an emergency room or equivalent facility should be sought urgently if the patient is exhibiting signs of impending respiratory failure (eg, weak respiratory efforts, weak breath sounds, unconsciousness, or hypoxic seizures).

10. All patients with asthma should have a rescue inhaler available during games and practices, and the certified athletic trainer should have an extra rescue inhaler for each athlete for administration during emergencies. In case of emergencies, a nebulizer should also be available. With a metered dose inhaler (MDI), athletes should be encouraged to use a spacer to help ensure the best delivery of inhaled therapy to the lungs.[23]

11. Athletic trainers and coaches should consider providing alternative practice sites for athletes with asthma triggered by airborne allergens when practical. Indoor practice facilities that offer good ventilation and air conditioning should be considered for at least part of the practice if this can be accomplished, although in most cases it will not be practical. For example, indoor and outdoor allergens or

irritants, tobacco smoke, and air pollutants might trigger asthma, and attempts should be made to limit exposure to these triggers when possible. Another option is to schedule practices when pollen counts are lowest (eg, in the evening during the ragweed pollen season). Pollen count information can be accessed from the National Allergy Bureau at http://www.aaaai.org/nab.

12. Patients with asthma should have follow-up examinations at regular intervals, as determined by the patient's primary care physician or specialist, to monitor and alter therapy. In general, these evaluations should be scheduled at least every 6 to 12 months, but they may be more frequent if symptoms are not well controlled.

Asthma Pharmacologic Treatment

13. Athletic trainers should understand the various types of pharmacologic strategies used for short- and long-term asthma control and should be able to differentiate controller from rescue or reliever medications (Figure 2).[24–30]

14. Patients with EIA may benefit from the use of short- and long-acting β$_2$-agonists. Rapid-acting agents can be used for prophylaxis during practice and game participation. When the goal is to prevent EIA, a short-acting β$_2$-agonist, such as albuterol, should be inhaled 10 to 15 minutes before exercise. The excessive need (3–4 times per day) for short-acting β$_2$-agonist therapy during practice or an athletic event should cause concern, and a physician should evaluate the patient before return to participation. Long-acting β$_2$-agonists should, in general, only be used for asthma prophylaxis and control and are usually combined with an inhaled corticosteroid. Athletic trainers should understand the use, misuse, and abuse of short-acting β$_2$-agonists.

15. Patients with asthma may also benefit from the use of

Sample (1) Asthma Action Plan

Asthma and Allergy Foundation of America

STUDENT ASTHMA ACTION CARD

National Asthma Education and Prevention Program

EPA

Name:_____ Grade:_____ Age:_____

Homeroom Teacher:_____ Room:_____

Parent/Guardian   Name:_____ Ph: (h):_____

Address:_____ Ph: (w):_____

Parent/Guardian   Name:_____ Ph: (h):_____

Address:_____ Ph: (w):_____

[ID Photo]

Emergency Phone Contact #1 _____
Name   Relationship   Phone

Emergency Phone Contact #2 _____
Name   Relationship   Phone

Physician Treating Student for Asthma:_____ Ph:_____

Other Physician:_____ Ph:_____

EMERGENCY PLAN

Emergency action is necessary when the student has symptoms such as, _____ , _____ , _____ , _____ or has a peak flow reading of _____ .

- **Steps to take during an asthma episode:**
  1. Check peak flow.
  2. Give medications as listed below. Student should respond to treatment in 15-20 minutes.
  3. Contact parent/guardian if _____
  4. Re-check peak flow.
  5. Seek emergency medical care if the student has any of the following:
     - ✓ Coughs constantly
     - ✓ No improvement 15-20 minutes after initial treatment with medication and a relative cannot be reached.
     - ✓ Peak flow of _____
     - ✓ Hard time breathing with:
        - • Chest and neck pulled in with breathing
        - • Stooped body posture
        - • Struggling or gasping
     - ✓ Trouble walking or talking
     - ✓ Stops playing and cannot start activity again
     - ✓ Lips or fingernails are grey or blue

- **Emergency Asthma Medications**

Name	Amount	When to Use
1. _____		
2. _____		
3. _____		
4. _____		

See reverse for more instructions

Figure 1. Sample asthma action plan. Extracted from *Managing Asthma: A Guide for Schools.* National Heart, Lung, and Blood Institute. Available at: http://www.nhlbi.nih.gov/health/prof/lung/asthma/asth_sch.htm. Accessed June 7, 2005.

leukotriene modifiers, inhaled or parenteral corticosteroids, and cromones (such as cromolyn sodium).

16. Pharmacotherapy should be customized for each asthma patient, and a specialist (an allergist or pulmonologist with expertise in sports medicine) should be consulted to maximize therapy when symptoms break through despite apparently optimal therapy.

17. Patients with past allergic reactions or intolerance to aspirin or NSAIDs should be identified and provided with alternative medicines, such as acetaminophen, as needed.

Asthma Nonpharmacologic Treatment

18. Health care providers should identify and consider nonpharmacologic strategies to control asthma, including nose breathing, limiting exposure to allergens or pollutants, and air filtration systems.[31–33] However, these therapies should be expected to provide only limited protection from asthma in most circumstances.

19. Proper warm-up before exercise may lead to a refractory period of as long as 2 hours, which may result in de-

Sample (1) Asthma Action Plan (Continued)

DAILY ASTHMA MANAGEMENT PLAN

- **Identify the things which start an asthma episode (Check each that applies to the student.)**

☐ Exercise ☐ Strong odors or fumes ☐ Other ____________

☐ Respiratory infections ☐ Chalk dust / dust ____________

☐ Change in temperature ☐ Carpets in the room

☐ Animals ☐ Pollens

☐ Food ____________ ☐ Molds

Comments ____________

- **Control of School Environment**

(List any environmental control measures, pre-medications, and/or dietary restrictions that the student needs to prevent an asthma episode.) ____________

- **Peak Flow Monitoring**

Personal Best Peak Flow number: ____________

Monitoring Times: ________ ________ ________ ________

- **Daily Medication Plan**

Name	Amount	When to Use
1.		
2.		
3.		
4.		

COMMENTS / SPECIAL INSTRUCTIONS

____

FOR INHALED MEDICATIONS

☐ I have instructed ____________ in the proper way to use his/her medications. It is my professional opinion that ____________ should be allowed to carry and use that medication by him/herself.

☐ It is my professional opinion that ____________ should not carry his/her inhaled medication by him/herself.

____________ Physician Signature ____________ Date

____________ Parent/Guardian Signature ____________ Date

AAFA • 1233 20th Street, N.W., Suite 402 . Washington, DC 20036 • www.aafa.org • 1-800-7-ASTHMA

02/00

Extracted from "Managing Asthma: A Guide For Schools"

Figure 1. Continued.

creased reliance on medications by some patients with asthma.[34]

20. Patients who have been diagnosed previously as having asthma or suspected of having asthma should follow the recommendations of NAEPPII and GINA for evaluation and everyday management and control.[1,2]

Asthma Education

21. Athletes should be properly educated about asthma, especially EIA, by health care professionals who are knowledgeable about asthma.[35–52] Athletes should be educated about the following:
    a. Recognizing the signs and symptoms of uncontrolled asthma.
    b. Using spirometry recording devices to monitor lung function away from the clinic or athletic training room.
    c. Methods of limiting exposure to primary and secondary smoke and to other recognized or suspicious asthma triggers (eg, pollens, animal allergens, fungi, house dust, and other asthma sensitizers and triggers). Patients with asthma who smoke should be provided with

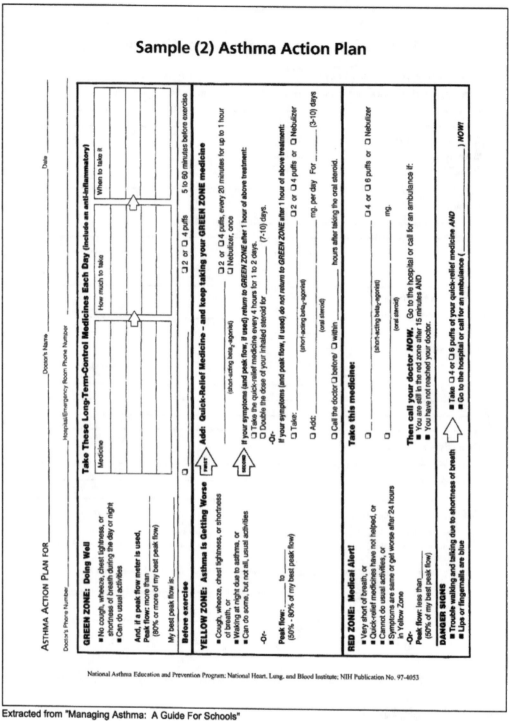

Figure 1. Continued.

information about smoking cessation and encouraged to participate in classes to change socialization patterns.

d. The need for increased asthma rescue medication (eg, short-acting β_2-agonists) as a signal for asthma flare-up. Increased use of short-acting β_2-agonists signals a need for enhanced treatment with asthma controller therapy.

e. The proper techniques for using MDIs, dry powder inhalers, nebulizers, and spacers to control asthma symptoms and to treat exacerbations. Health care professionals should periodically check the patient's medication administration techniques and should examine medication compliance.

f. Asthma and EIA among competitive athletes. These conditions are common, and athletic performance need not be hindered if the patient takes an active role in controlling the disease and follows good practice and control measures.

22. The athletic trainer should also be familiar with vocal cord dysfunction and other upper airway diseases, which can sometimes be confused with asthma.[15,53,54] Vocal cord dysfunction may be associated with dyspnea, chest tight-

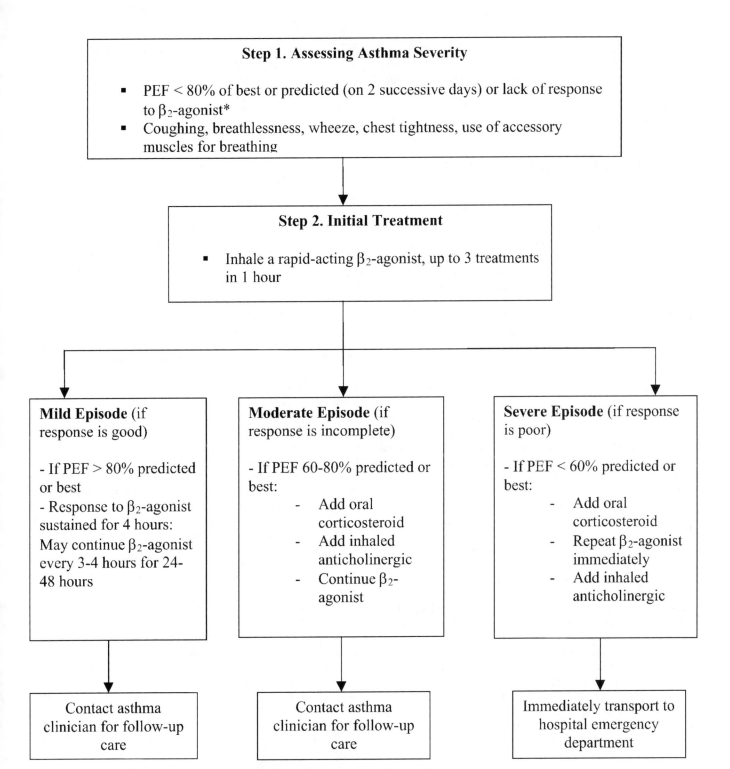

Figure 2. Asthma pharmacologic management.[2] PEF indicates peak expiratory flow.

ness, coughing, wheezing, and inspiratory stridor. In many cases, the condition is triggered with exercise. Visual inspection of the vocal cords by a physician experienced in examining the upper airway during exercise to differentiate vocal cord dysfunction from asthma is recommended.

23. Patients with asthma should be encouraged to engage in exercise as a means to strengthen muscles, improve respiratory health, enhance endurance, and otherwise improve overall well-being.[55]

24. The athletic trainer should differentiate among restricted, banned, and permitted asthma medications. Athletic train-

ers should be familiar with the guidelines of the International Olympic Committee Medical Commission, the United States Anti-Doping Agency, the World Anti-Doping Agency, and the doping committees of the various federations.

25. The athletic trainer should be aware of the various Web sites that provide general information and frequently asked questions on asthma and EIA. These sites include the American Academy of Allergy, Asthma and Immunology (www.aaaai.org); the American Thoracic Society (www.thoracic.org); the Asthma and Allergy Foundation of Amer-

ica (www.aafa.org); the American College of Allergy, Asthma, & Immunology (www.acaai.org); and USA Swimming (http://www.usaswimming.org/USASWeb/_Rainbow/Documents/6c812467-b717-4c16-a32c-a1d9bcc9f444/Asthma-%20Comprehensive%20Guide%2004%20Nov%2029.pdf).

BACKGROUND AND LITERATURE REVIEW

Definition and Pathophysiology of Asthma

Asthma is a common condition that has been recognized for more than 2000 years.[56] Asthma is usually defined operationally as a chronic inflammatory disorder of the airways.[1,2,4,56] In many patients, this chronic inflammation causes an increase in airway hyperresponsiveness, leading to recurrent episodes of wheezing, breathlessness, chest tightness (or chest pain in children), and coughing, particularly at night or in the early morning and after exercise, especially in cold, dry environments. These episodes are associated with widespread but variable airflow obstruction that is often reversible, either spontaneously or with treatment.[1,2,4] This definition implies that asthma has multiple causes, and indeed, it is a complex disorder.

The chronic inflammatory process causes excess mucus production and bronchial smooth muscle constriction,[57-61] which result from a release of inflammatory mediators that include histamine, tryptase, prostaglandin, and leukotrienes from mast cells.[62-66] Airways may also accumulate thick, viscous secretions produced by goblet cells and submucosal glands; moreover, there is leakage of plasma proteins and accumulated cellular debris.[57-61,67] Although airway narrowing affects the tracheobronchial tree, small bronchi (2–5 mm in diameter) are most affected.[68-70] Maximal expiratory flow rate is reduced and residual lung volumes are increased as air is trapped behind the blocked airways.[71] As a result, during an asthma attack, the respiratory rate increases to compensate for the increased obstruction of the airways and the inability of the usually elastic lung to recoil (dynamic hyperinflation). The patient must work harder to breathe as the thorax becomes overinflated. With progression of the attack, the diaphragm and intercostal muscles must compensate and contribute more energy during respiration.[72] In a severe attack, muscle efficiency is eventually lost, and the increased breathing rate leads to respiratory muscle fatigue and physical distress that may result in death. Indeed, as many as 4200 to 5000 people die from asthma each year in the United States.[73]

Environmental Factors

Environmental factors, such as allergens, air pollution, occupational sensitizers, and tobacco smoke, may cause or exacerbate asthma.[74-79] These factors are important triggers that should be considered when evaluating a patient with asthma.[79-83]

Recently, concern about indoor air pollution has been heightened.[79,80,82-84] Indoor ambient air can contain allergens and pollution that can cause or exacerbate asthma and other respiratory ailments when susceptible individuals are exposed to these environments.[85] Many factors should be considered indoors, such as adequacy of ventilation, humidity level, presence of allergens, presence of wall-to-wall carpeting and up-

holstered furniture, and types of building materials.[85-87] Indoor animal allergens (such as from cats, dogs, and other pets) are an important trigger of symptoms in many people.[88] Cockroach allergens are commonly seen indoors (such as in swimming pool locker rooms), and the cockroach allergenic materials can remain for a long period of time, even after extermination.[89-92] Indoor mold and fungal spores, house dust mites, and particulate matter, such as aerosols or smoke from cigarettes, wood, or fossil fuels, also can trigger asthma symptoms.[93-107] Tobacco smoke is a risk factor for the development of asthma, and smoking tobacco appears to increase asthma severity.[108-110]

Other indoor air irritants, such as chlorine, can exacerbate asthma and cause eye and lung irritation.[111,112] School-age children who frequently visit chlorinated pools may have an increased risk of developing asthma, especially if they have other risk factors for asthma.[113] Even individuals who do not usually enter the water but who are exposed to indoor chlorinated pools (eg, lifeguards, coaches) may have respiratory irritation on exposure to chlorine.[114,115]

Many actions can be taken to limit indoor allergen exposure, including prohibiting smoking indoors, using air cleaners equipped with a high-efficiency particulate air cleaner (HEPA) filter, washing walls, vacuuming carpets, and cleaning mattress covers weekly.[116-119] Additional measures include removing carpets and installing linoleum or wood flooring, washing pets (dogs and cats) and their bedding twice a week, keeping pets out of the bedroom or living room at all times to reduce exposure, covering mattresses and pillows, and controlling humidity to help manage dust mites and mold.[81,82,120] Some of these measures, such as the removal of a family pet from the home, can be very difficult, so it is necessary to discuss the effect of these exposures with the asthma patient. Although air filters might help, the house should be cleaned thoroughly before their use and regularly thereafter.[33]

When inhaled, outdoor air pollution, caused by sulfur dioxide, carbon monoxide, nitrogen dioxide, ozone, and particulate matter, can cause pulmonary function decrements, increased reliance on medications, bronchial hyperresponsiveness, and increased asthma symptoms.[121-125] Many pollens (trees, grasses, and weeds) are inhaled into the bronchi and cause allergen-induced asthma.[126,127] Tree pollens predominate in the spring, grass pollens in the late spring or early summer (and fall), and weed pollens in the late summer and fall in the United States, depending on geographic location, but may be present at other times of the year in locations outside of the United States.[128,129] Information about the pollen seasons in the United States can be accessed from the National Allergy Bureau Web site.

Although it is virtually impossible to avoid all outdoor pollution and allergens, some practical precautions can be implemented: move indoors and close all windows, close car windows when traveling, limit exposure when pollen is at its highest levels, monitor local weather stations for allergy reports, and practice indoors if possible when pollen counts are high.

Diagnosis and Classification of Asthma

Asthma can be difficult to diagnose and classify (see Table 1). Some individuals, especially elite athletes, do not display consistent signs or symptoms of asthma.[9,10,130] Asthma symptoms may be present only during certain times (seasons) of the year or only after exercise and may be highly variable, depending upon the athlete, the environment, and the activity.[13]

The first step in determining whether asthma is present is to obtain a detailed medical history. Questions regarding past experiences, symptoms, smoking history, and family history can help to rule out other respiratory disorders such as chronic bronchitis, emphysema, bronchiectasis, allergic rhinitis, upper respiratory infection, congestive heart failure, disorders of the upper airway (eg, vocal cord dysfunction), and nonrespiratory conditions such as anxiety. Most importantly, the athletic trainer should ask general questions as listed in Recommendation 3 to assist in making a proper diagnosis.[13] If a patient appears to have one or more symptoms suggestive of asthma, then lung function testing should be performed (see Table 1).[9] However, it is important to recognize that the history and baseline physical examination will fail to identify many patients with EIA.[9,10,12]

Lung function tests are essential to assess asthma severity and airflow limitation and to determine whether the obstruction is fully reversible with treatment.[16–18,131–133] The most common measures of airway function are the forced expiratory volume in 1 second (FEV_1), the forced vital capacity (FVC), and the peak expiratory flow rate (PEFR). These tests can be performed while the patient is at rest or after a challenge. The FEV_1 measures the volume of air in liters forcefully exhaled out of the airway in 1 second after a full inspiration. The FVC measures the total volume of air in liters forcefully exhaled out of the airway when the breath continues (usually for a period of 6 or more seconds). The FVC procedure is effort dependent and requires the patient to fully understand that he or she needs to inhale a deep breath and then "blast" the air out of the lungs into the measurement device. The FVC testing also requires considerable expertise by the technician and the ability to communicate with the patient. The PEFR measures the maximal flow rate of air (in L/s or L/min) out of the airways and is easier to perform than an FEV_1 or FVC maneuver, although PEFR testing is also effort dependent. A flow volume curve (flow loop) provides a graphic depiction of the breathing effort in which flow rate is plotted against volume (in L/s) of air exhaled and inhaled (in L), as shown in Figure 3. A volume-time curve (called a spirogram) is another way to plot the breath, in which the volume of air exhaled (in L) is plotted against time (in seconds). The FEV_1/FVC ratio is also examined, along with a variety of measures of flow, such as the flow between 25% and 75% of the FVC (called the FEF_{25-75}).

Asthma is an example of an obstructive lung disease in which the airways obstruct the outflow of air. In contrast, pulmonary fibrosis is an example of a restrictive lung disease in which the functional size of the lungs decreases. In obstructive lung diseases, the FEV_1 decreases, whereas the FVC remains relatively normal, so the FEV_1/FVC ratio decreases (until late in the disease or with severe exacerbations, when the FVC may also decrease).[131] In restrictive lung disease, both the FEV_1 and the FVC decrease proportionally (so that the FEV_1/FVC ratio is normal). Nomograms exist to provide guidance as to normal ranges for FEV_1 and FVC based on age, size and race.[134,135] It is important to recognize racial differences in the normal values for these tests. Generally, levels should be at least 80% of the predicted values to be considered "normal." The FEV_1/FVC ratio should also be above 80%. An increase of 12% or more in FEV_1 after an inhaled bronchodilator (eg, a β_2-agonist such as albuterol) suggests reversible airway dis-

ease and may be used as a diagnostic criterion of asthma.[131] A decrease in FEV_1 after a challenge (such as after inhalation of methacholine or running on a treadmill) suggests that the airways are reactive to the stimulus.[19] It is important to determine a patient's personal best FEV_1, FVC, and PEFR, which are identified by plotting these values over time. These values can also demonstrate variability between morning and evening and over time, which may reflect airway hyperreactivity.

Spirometers are used in the clinic or training room to determine these pulmonary function values.[136] Patients may also be given a PFM to measure PEFR away from the clinic or athletic training room (Tables 2 and 3). The PFM is a small, handheld device that measures maximal flow rate during forced exhalation.[137–140] Maximal flow rate usually occurs within the first 120 to 150 milliseconds of a forced exhalation.[140] When used properly, a PFM can be somewhat helpful in following the course of asthma and might even be useful in suggesting the presence of asthma. The PFM can also be used to identify asthma triggers and to monitor medication changes, and it may help to reduce asthma morbidity.[141–147] The device allows the asthmatic patient to measure lung variability over time to assist in determining when to seek medical attention. The PFM should be used at least daily (in the morning after awakening) and preferably also in the late afternoon or evening.[1,2,148] At least 2 or 3 trials should be performed at each specified time and the highest value recorded. The device should be used before taking any medications and at least 4, but preferably 8, hours after inhalation of a bronchodilator, if possible. The device should be used for at least a 2- to 3-week monitoring period. Some devices record the PEFR electronically, which can assist the patient in keeping the data secure and available. Over time, the patient's personal best value will be determined. Subsequently, if the PEFR value is less than 80% of the personal best or if daily variability is greater than 20% of the morning value, then the patient should be reevaluated in an attempt to find better control measures. If the PEFR value is less than 50% of the personal best, the individual should seek immediate attention (see Table 2).[1] Spirometry, including the use of PFMs, may be especially useful in patients who do not perceive the severity of their symptoms.[149,150]

The PFM should be used regularly, even if asthma symptoms appear to be well controlled.[132,151–153] Patients who have good PFM technique (see Table 3) adhere to their treatment plan and control their symptoms better than those who have poor technique. The PFM should be available in all athletic training facilities and on the field in medical kits.

Unfortunately, some reports suggest that PFM recordings are not always reliable indicators of airflow obstruction.[154–159] In certain cases, elite or well-trained athletes may possess large lung capacities, which may exceed the measuring capacity of the PFM. In addition, it appears that PFM values are not consistent from one to another PFM from the same manufacturer, across different PFM devices, when men and women use PFMs, with different techniques while using a single PFM, and at high altitudes.[159–164] The most accurate spirometry testing is performed with office-based spirometry testing equipment.[140] However, as noted above, spirometry testing requires training[22,165] and may be impractical for everyday asthma management, especially in primary care settings in which most patients are not being seen for asthma.[140]

If baseline lung function tests are within normal values and

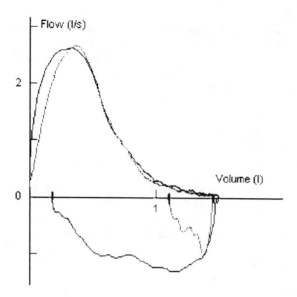

(a)   Flow volume loop plots flow (in liters per second) against volume (in liters).

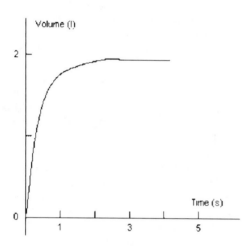

(b)   Volume time curve (spirogram) plots volume (in liters) against time (in seconds).

Figure 3. Flow volume loop and volume time curve.

Table 2. Peak Flow Zones for Asthma Management*

Green zone
- PEF values are between 80% and 100% of personal best
- No asthma management changes are necessary at this time

Yellow zone
- PEF values are between 50% and 80% of personal best
- Caution is warranted; use of medications is required

Red zone
- PEF values are less than 50% of personal best
- Danger: emergency action is needed, including medications or hospital visit

*Adapted with permission from Li JTC.[140] PEF indicates peak expiratory flow.

Table 3. General Instructions for Using a Mechanical Peak Flow Meter*

1. The movable indicator is placed at the beginning of the numbered scale.
2. The patient stands or sits tall and straight.
3. The patient then inhales maximally.
4. The patient places his or her lips tightly around the mouthpiece.
5. The patient is told to "blast" the air out of his or her lungs and into the device. The patient then forcefully exhales as fast and hard as possible.
6. The value is recorded.
7. Steps 1–6 are repeated 2 more times.
8. The highest number is marked as the value for that time period.

*For example, a Mini-Wright peak flow meter (Clement Clarke International Ltd, Essex, UK). Adapted with permission from Li JTC.[140]

Table 4. National Asthma Education and Prevention Program II: Usual Dosages for Long-Term Control Medications*[1]

Medication	Dosage Form	Adult Dose	Child Dose
Inhaled corticosteroids			
Systemic corticosteroids			
Methylprednisolone	2, 4, 8, 16, 32 mg tablets	• 7.5–60 mg daily in a single dose in AM or qod as needed for control	• 0.25–2 mg/kg daily in single dose in AM or qod as needed for control
Prednisolone	5 mg tablets 5 mg/5 cc 15 mg/5 cc	• Short-course "burst" to achieve control; 40–60 mg/d as single or 2 divided doses for 3–10 d	• Short-course "burst": 1–2 mg/kg/d, maximum 60 mg/day for 3–10 days
Prednisone	1, 2.5, 5, 10, 20, 50 mg tablets: 5 mg/cc, 5 mg/5cc		
Long-acting inhaled beta$_2$-agonists (Should not be used for symptom relief or for exacerbations. Use with inhaled corticosteroids.)			
Salmeterol	MDI 21 mcg/puff DPI 50 mcg/blister	2 puffs q12h 1 blister q12h	1–2 puffs q12h 1 blister q12h
Formoterol	DPI 12 mcg/single-use capsule	1 capsule q12 h	1 capsule q12h
Combined medication			
Fluticasone/salmeterol	DPI 100, 250, or 500 mcg/50 mcg	1 inhalation bid; dose depends on severity of asthma	1 inhalation bid; dose depends on severity of asthma
Cromolyn and nedocromil			
Cromolyn	MDI 1 mg/puff Nebulizer 20 mg/ampule	2–4 puffs tid–qid 1 ampule tid–qid	1–2 puffs tid–qid 1 ampule tid–qid
Nedocromil	MDI 1.75 mg/puff	2–4 puffs bid–qid	1–2 puffs bid-qid
Leukotriene modifiers			
Montelukast	4 or 5 mg chewable tablet 10 mg tablet	10 mg qhs	4 mg qhs (2–5 yrs) 5 mg qhs (6–14 yrs) 10 mg qhs (>14 yrs)
Zafirlukast	10 or 20 mg tablet	40 mg daily (20 mg tablet bid)	20 mg daily (7–11 yrs) (10 mg tablet bid)
Zileuton	300 or 600 mg tablet	2,400 mg daily (give tablets qid)	
Methylxanthines (Serum monitoring is important [serum concentration of 5–15 mcg/mL at steady state])			
Theophylline	Liquids, sustained-release tablets, and capsules	Starting dose 10 mg/kg/d up to 300 mg max; usual max 800 mg/d	Starting dose 10 mg/kg/d; usual max: • <1 year of age: 0.2 (age in wk) +5 = mg/kg/d • ≥1 year of age: 16 mg/kg/d

*qod indicates every other day; bid, twice a day; tid, 3 times a day; qid, 4 times a day; qhs, at bedtime; MDI, metered dose inhaler; DPI, dry powder inhaler.

the reversibility test with a β$_2$-agonist is equivocal, then a challenge test (eg, with methacholine) may be performed to test for bronchial hyperresponsiveness.[19] During these tests, progressively increasing concentrations of the aerosolized drug are administered during a multistage procedure.[19] After each stage, spirometry testing is performed to determine whether a 20% reduction in FEV$_1$ from baseline is obtained. If the reduction is less than 20% after all stages have been performed, then the test is considered negative, and the patient is determined not to have bronchial hyperresponsiveness. It is important to note, however, that these tests alone are not diagnostic of asthma. A positive test must be interpreted in the context of other information to make the definitive diagnosis of asthma.

Exercise challenge and other surrogate challenges (such as eucapnic hyperventilation) are described in the EIA section of this statement.[19,21]

Pharmacotherapy for Asthma

It is important to ascertain the correct diagnosis before medications are prescribed and for the health care professional to know the types of medications that are prescribed.[1,2,24–30,166,167] Only a small percentage of asthmatic patients take their medications precisely as prescribed by their physician; the most

common cause of treatment failure is failure to use the prescribed treatment.[167] Regardless, asthma can be managed through various medications to prevent or control symptoms; for an updated medication list, refer to the NAEPPII and GINA guidelines.[1,2] The medications used to treat asthma are classified as either controller or rescue (reliever) medications.

Controller Medications. Controller medications are daily, long-term interventions used prophylactically to manage the symptoms of mild, moderate, and severe asthma and generally should not be used to manage acute asthmatic symptoms.[1,2,25–28] Examples include inhaled corticosteroids, systemic corticosteroids, cromones (sodium cromolyn and nedocromil sodium), long-acting inhaled β$_2$-agonists, theophylline, and leukotriene modifiers (Table 4 provides sample agents).

Inhaled corticosteroids are effective controller medications for treating persistent mild, moderate, and severe asthma.[1,2] They act by decreasing airway inflammation, mucus production, and bronchial hyperresponsiveness.[168–173] Proper use of inhaled corticosteroids can lead to a decrease in the number and severity of asthma exacerbations, improve lung function, lessen bronchial hyperresponsiveness, and reduce the need for symptom relief with short-acting β$_2$-agonists.[174–180] Inhaled corticosteroids should not be used to treat acute asthmatic attacks.[25] Their adverse effects include hoarseness, coughing, and occasionally thrush or oral candidiasis.[177,181] However, rinsing the mouth after inhalation and using a spacer generally help to prevent oral candidiasis.

Systemic corticosteroids are administered orally or parenterally for individuals who have severe persistent asthma that remains poorly responsive to inhaler therapy.[182] Systemic therapy has the same mechanisms of action as inhaled corticosteroids. However, long-term use of systemic agents can cause more significant systemic adverse events than inhaled corticosteroids, including osteoporosis, glucose intolerance, glaucoma, weight gain, skin thinning, bruising, fluid and electrolyte abnormalities, growth suppression, and muscle weakness.[1,2,183] To minimize these adverse events, oral corticosteroids are often taken daily in the morning or every other day, and patients should be monitored closely by a physician.[183] Oral corticosteroids are used much less frequently today than in the past since the advent of high-potency inhaled corticosteroids such as fluticasone and budesonide.[1,2]

The cromones, cromolyn sodium and nedocromil sodium, are inhaled asthma medications used to control mild persistent asthma and are considered less effective anti-inflammatory agents than inhaled corticosteroids.[25,26,184] Although the exact mechanisms of action are poorly understood, they are thought to inhibit IgE-mediated mediator release from mast cells and, thus, to inhibit acute airflow limitations induced by exercise, cold air, and allergens. The cromones are generally used to treat mild persistent asthma and to prevent EIA.[1,2] Cromones should be used as second-line drug therapy alternatives for treating mild persistent asthma, perhaps combined with an inhaled β_2-agonist; however, several doses each day are usually needed to control asthma.[1,2] Only minimal adverse events are seen with these agents, including occasional coughing and an unpleasant taste, particularly with nedocromil sodium.

Long-acting inhaled β_2-agonists (eg, salmeterol and formoterol) have the same mechanisms of action as short-acting β_2-agonists but a 12-hour duration of action, compared with 4 to 6 hours for the short-acting agents.[185–190] A single dose of formoterol or salmeterol before exercise can protect the athlete from asthma symptoms associated with exercise for up to 12 hours.[191–193] Formoterol has a shorter onset of action than salmeterol, approximately 5 minutes as compared with 15 to 30 minutes.[192,194] All β_2-agonists, including formoterol and salmeterol, are restricted asthma medications according to the International Olympic Committee, World Anti-Doping Agency, and United States Anti-Doping Agency; elite athletes taking these medications, their physicians, and their athletic trainers should review the guidelines posted by these agencies.

Patients using long-acting β_2-agonists regularly may display a decrease in the duration of action.[195–197] In one study, formoterol had a shortened duration of action by day 14 of regular daily use.[198] Thus, patients should not expect these drugs to remain effective over the 12-hour dosing interval after regular, daily, extended use. Studies also show that the use of long-acting β_2-agonists does not affect persistent airway inflammation.[199] These agents should only be used in combination with inhaled corticosteroids, which may be more beneficial than ingesting each drug separately.[200–202] Combination therapy (an inhaled, long-acting β_2-agonist and an inhaled corticosteroid) has been shown to decrease the need for short-acting β_2-agonists, decrease nocturnal asthma, improve lung function, decrease asthma exacerbations, and prevent EIA.[200,202–205]

Leukotriene modifiers, taken orally, block leukotriene synthesis or block leukotriene receptors.[206–208] Leukotriene modifiers can be used to control allergen-, aspirin-, and exercise-induced bronchoconstriction; improve lung function; and decrease asthma exacerbations.[209–215] Used primarily as second-line therapy, leukotriene modifiers can reduce the dose of an inhaled corticosteroid required to treat mild persistent asthma and may improve asthma control.[214–217] Adverse events are usually minimal, with reports of headaches and gastrointestinal discomfort. However, zileuton (Zyflo, Abbott Laboratories, Abbott Park, IL) may be associated with liver toxicity; therefore, liver function should be monitored regularly when using this medication.[218] Unlike β_2-agonists, the duration of action of the leukotriene modifiers does not diminish over time.[215] In the past, theophylline has been used alone as a controller agent, but now it is usually used in combination with another agent, such as an inhaled corticosteroid.[219]

Finally, some patients who have allergic asthma may benefit over the long term from the administration of various forms of allergy immunotherapy.[220–222] The decision to initiate such therapy must be made by the patient and physician after a careful evaluation. Even in the most successful cases, additional medical therapy is often required in conjunction with immunotherapy.

Rescue (Reliever) Medications. Rescue medications act rapidly to treat acute bronchoconstriction and associated symptoms of coughing, wheezing, shortness of breath (dyspnea), and chest tightness.[1,2,25–28] Several classes of drugs act in this manner, including rapid-acting inhaled β_2-agonists, inhaled anticholinergics, and short-acting theophylline.

Rapid-acting inhaled β_2-agonists are the most commonly used reliever therapy for chronic asthma. These β_2-agonists act quickly to cause bronchodilation by relaxing airway smooth muscle, decreasing vascular permeability, and modifying mediator release from mast cells.[185] Rapid-acting inhaled β_2-agonists are also the most frequently used agents to prevent EIA and to treat its symptoms.[223] These medications can be used as "rescue therapy" at times of an acute attack. However, because of their relatively short duration of action (2–4 hours), repeat treatments may be necessary for EIA. Some authors[224,225] suggest that repeated use of short-acting β_2-agonists can lead to tolerance and less effectiveness over time. Furthermore, the chronic use of long-acting inhaled β_2-agonists can decrease the effectiveness of the short-acting inhaled β_2-agonists.[189,225]

Inhaled anticholinergic agents (eg, ipratropium) may be used as bronchodilators.[226] These agents block acetylcholine release from cholinergic innervation in airway smooth muscle but have no anti-inflammatory action.

Short-acting theophylline is a bronchodilator that has been used for many years to relieve asthma exacerbations.[29,227] Theophylline's onset of action is delayed when compared with that of β_2-agonists, and so it is not currently used as first-line rescue therapy.[1,2] Theophylline is a controversial drug because its benefits might be outweighed by potential adverse events such as seizures.[228] Adverse events can be serious and severe if dosing is not closely monitored. Short-acting theophylline should not be administered to patients who are already receiving chronic therapy with sustained-release theophylline therapy.

Short-acting oral β_2-agonists, although rarely used, function primarily by relaxing airway smooth muscle within a few minutes after administration and for a period of up to 4 hours; however, they have no anti-inflammatory actions.[24,29] Adverse events include tachycardia, hypertension, and decreased appetite. If used chronically, increasing doses of short-acting oral β_2-agonists might indicate loss of control of asthma.[1,2] All athletes using short-acting oral β_2-agonists should be advised that many sporting organizations restrict or prohibit the use of these agents.

Finally, systemic glucocorticosteriods are administered orally or parenterally for individuals who have acute asthma exacerbations. The mechanisms of action are similar to those for corticosteroids used to treat chronic severe asthma.[1,2]

Asthma Medication Delivery Techniques

Many of the newer asthma medications are delivered to the lungs by inhalation devices.[23] The most common types of inhalers are MDIs and dry powder inhaler devices. The MDIs release a specific amount of a drug from a pressurized canister to propel medication into the lungs when the patient takes a breath. When using MDIs, patients must exhale first, then place the inhaler at or slightly in front of the lips, and slowly inhale at the same time that they are activating the inhaler to release the drug. Patients hold their breath for a few seconds (approximately 10) before exhaling. Patients who have difficulty coordinating MDI activation with breathing generally benefit from the use of a spacer.[229–231] A spacer is attached to the MDI device to reduce side effects of inhaled corticosteroids in the mouth and for patients who have difficulty coordinating the activation of an MDI and breathing. Dry powder inhalers are often easier to use than MDIs, and they do not permit use of a spacer.

Aspirin, Nonsteroidal Anti-Inflammatory Drugs, and Asthma

Aspirin-sensitive athletes may manifest nasal congestion; itchy, watery, or swollen eyes; coughing; difficulty breathing; wheezing; urticaria; and possible shock when they ingest aspirin or other NSAIDs.[232–236] This is not a true allergy because it is not caused by IgE, but it is treated in the same manner as an allergic reaction. Athletic trainers should also be aware of triad syndrome: athletes with asthma, nasal polyps, and aspirin sensitivity may have a severe asthma attack when they take an NSAID.[237]

Although only a small percentage of the population has aspirin-sensitive asthma,[238–240] this condition is particularly concerning in an athletic population because many athletes who have asthma use anti-inflammatory drugs to treat injuries. Therefore, athletic trainers must understand that some patients who have asthma could suffer fatal consequences if they take aspirin or NSAIDs.

Aspirin-sensitive athletes should also avoid COX-2 inhibitors, but acetaminophen in moderate doses can usually be taken without difficulty.[241] Salsalate, choline magnesium trisalicylate, and dextropropoxyphene may be used as substitute medication in patients with aspirin sensitivity if tolerated.[240,242] Athletic trainers should be familiar with the many prescription and over-the-counter products that contain aspirin and other NSAIDs, including ibuprofen (eg, Motrin, McNeil-PPC, Fort Washington, PA; Advil, Wyeth, Madison, NJ) and naproxen (eg, Aleve, Bayer, Morristown, NJ). Health care professionals should supply as much information to the patient as possible, including a list of products to avoid (Table 5).

Table 5. Sample Nonsteroidal Anti-Inflammatory Drugs

Generic Name	Brand Name(s)	Manufacturer
Diclofenac, miso-prostol	Arthrotec	GD Searle LLC, Chicago, IL
Celecoxib	Celebrex	GD Searle LLC
Diclofenac	Voltaren	Novartis Pharmaceuticals Corp, East Hanover, NJ
Diclofenac	Cataflam	Novartis Pharmaceuticals Corp
Diflunisal	Dolobid	Merck & Co, Inc, West Point, PA
Etodolac	Lodine	Wyeth-Ayerst International Inc, Madison, NJ
Flurbiprofen	Ansaid	Pharmacia & Upjohn Co, Kalamazoo, MI
Ibuprofen	Motrin	McNeil-PPC, Fort Washington, PA
	Advil	Wyeth, Madison, NJ
Indomethacin	Indocin	Merck & Co, Inc
Ketoprofen	Orudis	Rhône-Poulenc Rorer New Zealand Ltd, Auckland, New Zealand
Ketorolac	Toradol	Roche Pharmaceuticals, Nutley, NJ
Nabumetone	Relafen	GlaxoSmithKline, Research Triangle Park, NC
Naproxen	Naprosyn	Roche Pharmaceuticals
	Aleve	Bayer, Morristown, NJ
Oxaprozin	Daypro	GD Searle LLC
Piroxicam	Feldene	Pfizer Inc, New York, NY
Rofecoxib	Vioxx	Merck & Co, Inc
Salsalate	Disalcid	3M Pharmaceuticals, Northridge, CA
Sulindac	Clinoril	Merck & Co, Inc

Nonpharmacologic Treatment for Asthma

Athletes with asthma need to keep their asthma under optimal control to prevent exercise-induced breathing symptoms.[31,32,243,244] Masks and nose breathing help to warm and moisturize inhaled air before it reaches the smaller airways. This may decrease the inflammatory reaction in the airways and thus decrease the frequency and intensity of EIA. These maneuvers are effective for some but not all athletes.[224] Nose breathing is not effective at high ventilation rates. Limiting environmental exposures (eg, to cold air and pollen) may decrease symptoms in susceptible athletes; however, this may not be practical in some sports.

Theoretically, exercise training might decrease symptoms by conditioning the body to exercise, but research has not supported this theory.[245,246] Nevertheless, an asthmatic individual should participate in exercise programs tailored to his or her capacity to perform.[55]

A refractory period can occur after exercise, when the airway response to exercise is inhibited for up to 2 to 3 hours. Some athletes have taken advantage of this phenomenon to help control EIA.[31,32,34,247–251] However, there are no specific guidelines to follow, and each athlete must experiment to determine the best individual protocol.

Because hyperosmolarity plays a role in mediating EIA, limiting sodium in the diet has received some attention. Restricting dietary salt may cause a relative decrease in airway obstruction.[252,253] Both sodium and chloride appear to play roles, but this remains an area of active investigation, and no specific guidelines are available.[254] A diet supplemented with n-3 polyunsaturated fatty acid in fish oil has shown favorable results in elite athletes with EIA.[255]

Exercise-Induced Asthma or Bronchospasm

Most asthmatic individuals have a flare of their asthma after exercise.[256,257] Some individuals only have asthma signs and symptoms associated with exercise.[13] By definition, a temporary narrowing of the airways (bronchospasm) induced by strenuous exercise in which the patient has no symptoms is known as EIB.[13] When symptoms are present, EIB is described as EIA.[13] This section reviews the incidence of EIA and EIB in the athletic population and considers special diagnostic or therapeutic measures that should be taken in an athletic population.

Exercise-induced asthma is commonly seen in athletes in all levels of athletic competition.[5,9,10,31,243,244,258–269] In most patients who have chronic asthma (at least 80%), exercise is a trigger for bronchoconstriction.[13,243] Exercise-induced asthma can also occur in patients who do not otherwise have asthma, such as in about 40% of patients who suffer from allergic rhinitis in season.[243,270,271] The incidence of EIA in the general population has been estimated to be between 12% and 15%.[13,271] Rates as high as 23% have been reported in school-age children, and the incidence in athletes may also be this high.[258,262,263,265] Exercise-induced asthma may be more common in urban environments than in rural areas.[261] Other factors, such as high ozone levels, might also account for increased EIA rates.[272]

Exercise-induced asthma can be a significant disability for the athlete, especially in endurance sports.[262,263,273] For example, EIA is relatively common in cross-country skiers, and some studies suggest that the cold air athletes breathe while cross-country skiing may provoke inflammation.[274,275] Similarly, athletes who participate in swimming and long-distance running have a high incidence of asthma.[262] Among Olympic athletes, asthma appears to be more common in those who participate in winter sports than in those who participate in summer sports.[262,263] At least 1 in 5 United States athletes who participated in the 1998 Winter Olympics had the condition, compared with 1 in 6 at the 1996 Summer Olympic Games.[262,263] Wilber et al[265] found a 23% overall incidence of EIA among athletes in the 7 winter sports tested. In addition, more females than males participating in the Winter Games reported an asthma condition or medication use.[262,263,265] Of the winter sports athletes tested, females had an incidence of 26%, compared with 18% in males.[265]

Although EIA impairs performance, it can be overcome. Amy Van Dyken, an athlete who suffered from relatively severe asthma, won 4 gold medals in swimming in the 1996 Olympic Games.[273] Other well-known elite athletes have also been able to excel when their asthma was under good control.[273]

Pathophysiology of Exercise-Induced Asthma

Two major theories exist to explain EIA: the cooling/warming hypothesis and the drying hypothesis.[31,256,257,260,276–287] As ventilation increases, airways progressively cool, which results in bronchoconstriction. This theory is supported by the higher incidence of EIA in athletes participating in cold environments.[263] In addition to cooling, the increased ventilation can lead to airway dehydration as inhaled air is humidified. The main effect of inhaling cold air is actually attributable to the fact that cold air carries less moisture. As with chronic asthma, inflammatory cells and mediators may increase in the lung in response to exercise in patients with EIA.[248,279,288–290]

Environmental allergens may enhance the likelihood of bronchoconstriction, and irritants such as sulfur dioxide, nitrogen dioxide, ozone, and chlorine have been implicated as causing patients to have exercise-induced symptoms.[31,243,291]

Exercise-Induced Asthma Diagnosis

Two requirements are needed to diagnose EIA: symptoms and obstructed airways, both associated with exercise.[13,269]

First, the patient has any of a constellation of symptoms associated with exercise, including shortness of breath (dyspnea), coughing, chest tightness (or chest pain in children), wheezing, and decreased exercise tolerance.[13,262,263] Symptoms generally occur 5 to 8 minutes after sufficiently intense exercise starts. The EIA may be associated with specific sports as well as specific environments.[262–267] Where allergens are present, outdoor activities and cold air exposure may be more likely to foster the appearance of EIA, which would not occur in other environments.

Second, the patient should have objective evidence of airway obstruction associated with exercise.[224] Generally, a drop from baseline of at least 10% to 15% in FEV_1 after a challenge test supports the diagnosis of EIA.[19,292] Pulmonary function should be monitored 5, 10, 15, and 30 minutes after the challenge.[19] The exercise needs to last for 6 to 8 minutes at an intensity level high enough to raise the athlete's heart rate to at least 80% of maximum[19] and ventilation to approximately 40% to 60% of maximum.[19] Exercise challenges can be performed in a laboratory (using a treadmill, a cycle ergometer, a rowing machine, or a free running asthma screening test [FRAST]).[293] Alternatively, an exercise challenge test in the laboratory can attempt to mimic the conditions and intensity of the sport.[20,21] Indeed, 78% of cross-country skiers reported a false-negative test during standard laboratory exercise challenges, suggesting that the standard tests are not as sensitive as sport-specific exercise challenge tests for endurance athletes.[20,21] Cold, dry air and near-maximal exercise intensity (greater than 90% peak heart rate) are required to provoke a positive result, especially in the cold-weather athlete. Time of day can be important: in a group of asthmatics, a greater drop in pulmonary function (FEV_1) to exercise challenge was measured in the evening than in the morning.[294]

Additional challenge tests include eucapnic voluntary hyperventilation or inhalation of hypertonic saline.[21,269,295] The former test requires the athlete to hyperventilate dry air containing 5% carbon dioxide, 21% oxygen, and the balance of nitrogen at 30 times FEV_1 for 6 minutes.[21]

It is important to evaluate athletes with atypical EIA symptoms because upper airway conditions such as vocal cord dysfunction or abnormal movement of the arytenoids region may be the cause.[15,53] The signs and symptoms of vocal cord dysfunction can be similar to asthma and can be confused with EIA.[54,296,297] This laryngeal disorder involves the unintentional paradoxic adduction of the vocal cords with breathing and can be triggered by exercise.[296,297] The patient is often female and may also have gastroesophageal reflux disease or a psychiatric illness. Vocal cord dysfunction often occurs with asthma, making control of EIA difficult. Diagnosis of vocal cord dysfunction involves the direct visualization of the paradoxic vocal cord motion, but the condition is often suspected when voice changes and inspiratory stridor occur during an attack, as well as when the inspiratory (bottom) portion of the flow volume loop is truncated.

Table 6. National Asthma Education and Prevention Program II: Treatment of Exercise-Induced Asthma*[1]

One goal of management is to enable patients to participate in any activity they choose without experiencing asthma symptoms. EIB should not limit either participation or success in vigorous activities.

Recommended treatments include:
- Beta$_2$-agonists will prevent EIB in more than 80 percent of patients.
  - Short-acting inhaled beta$_2$-agonists used shortly before exercise (or as close to exercise as possible) may be helpful for 2 to 3 hours.
  - Salmeterol has been shown to prevent EIB for 10 to 12 hours (Kemp et al 1994[301]).
- Cromolyn and nedocromil, taken shortly before exercise, are also acceptable for preventing EIB.
- A lengthy warmup period before exercise may benefit patients who can tolerate continuous exercise with minimal symptoms. The warmup may preclude a need for repeated medications.
- Long-term–control therapy, if appropriate.
  - There is evidence that appropriate long-term control of asthma with anti-inflammatory medication will reduce airway responsiveness, and this is associated with a reduction in the frequency and severity of EIB (Vathenen et al, 1991[302]).

Teachers and coaches need to be notified that a child has EIB, should be able to participate in activities, and may need inhaled medication before activity. Individuals involved in competitive athletics need to be aware that their medication use should be disclosed and should adhere to standards set by the U.S. Olympic Committee (Nastasi et al, 1995[303]). The U.S. Olympic Committee's Drug Control Hotline is 1-800-233-0393.

EIB indicates exercise-induced bronchospasm.

Table 7. United States Anti-Doping Agency Regulated Asthma Medications

Drug class: β$_2$-agonists:
  Advair* (GlaxoSmithKline, Research Triangle Park, NC)
  albuterol*
  bambuterol
  bitolterol
  Brethaire* (Riker Laboratories, Inc, Northridge, CA)
  Combivent* (Boehringer Ingelheim Pharmaceuticals Inc, Ridgefield (CT)
  fenoterol
  Foradil* (Novartis Pharmaceuticals Corp, East Hanover, NJ)
  formoterol*
  metaproterenol
  orciprenaline
  pirbuterol
  Proventil* (Schering-Plough Corp, Kenilworth, NJ)
  reproterol
  salbutamol*
  salmeterol*
  Serevent* (GlaxoSmithKline)
  terbutaline*
  Ventolin* (GlaxoSmithKline)
  Xopenex* (Sepracor, Marlborough, MA)

Available at: http://www.usantidoping.org. Accessed June 6, 2005.
*Allowed by inhaler or nebulizer only to prevent or treat asthma or exercise-induced asthma. Abbreviated Therapeutic Use Exemption (TUE) must be on file with United States Anti-Doping Agency or international federations, as appropriate. A salbutamol (albuterol) level greater than 1000 ng/mL is prohibited even with abbreviated TUE.

Exercise-Induced Asthma Treatment

Most of the drugs described for the treatment of chronic asthma are used to prevent EIA attacks.[1,2,269,298–300] Table 6 contains recommendations from the NAEPPII for the treatment of EIA.[1] The key feature is that a β$_2$-agonist can be used both to prevent attacks and to treat them when they occur. Once an asthmatic individual meets the requirements for stage 1 through 4 asthma, the NAEPPII treatment guidelines should be followed.

Asthma Education

Throughout this position statement, information has been presented to inform and educate the athletic trainer and allied health personnel about asthma and asthma management. Of particular importance is a properly prepared asthma management plan. Educating athletes about asthma and having a written management plan will help control their disease.[1,2,304] Several groups[35–44,48–51] have shown that an effectively written management plan can reduce medication errors, asthma exacerbations, and hospital visits. Without a written asthma action plan, many patients have a difficult time controlling their asthma symptoms.[45–47,305] It is also imperative that an accessible line of communication between the patient and health care professional be identified.

An effective management plan should include a written document that addresses the following: (1) goals of the patient, (2) proper use and frequency of PEFR monitoring, (3) guidelines for altering medications based upon readings from PFMs or asthma symptoms, (4) contact numbers for all health care professionals, including emergency numbers, and (5) environmental factors to avoid or monitor. The health care professionals developing the asthma management plan should dis-

cuss all goals or expectations with the athlete. This education empowers the athlete and promotes better compliance.

Athletic trainers working with elite or Olympic athletes must be familiar with International Olympic Committee, World Anti-Doping Agency, and United States Anti-Doping Agency medication guidelines (Table 7). Certain asthma medications may be banned, restricted, or permitted, depending on the organization and the medication. A banned medication is one the athlete cannot take. In some cases, a prohibited substance is prohibited at all times or only prohibited in competition, meaning the athlete must allow sufficient time for the substance to clear the system before competition. Restricted medications must have prior physician approval and completion of forms (such as the Therapeutic Use Exemption, or TUE) before the athlete can compete. For example, the United States Anti-Doping Agency lists salbutamol/albuterol, salmeterol, terbutaline, and formoterol as restricted β$_2$-agonists that require a TUE before competition.

Additional information about the diagnosis and management of asthma can be obtained at the National Asthma Education and Prevention Program Web site (http://www.nhlbi.nih.gov/health/prof/lung/index.htm or http://www.nhlbi.nih.gov/about/naepp/) and the GINA Web site (www.ginasthma.com).

CONCLUSIONS

Asthma can affect individuals regardless of age, sex, or socioeconomic status. This National Athletic Trainers' Association asthma position statement is designed to present guidelines for the recognition, prophylaxis, and management of asthma. The information should lead to improvements in the quality of care certified athletic trainers and other health care providers can offer to patients with asthma, particularly athletes and especially those with EIA. In the end, these guidelines should reduce the incidence of asthma complications and improve the quality of life for patients with asthma, especially those in whom exercise is an important trigger.

DISCLAIMER

The NATA publishes its position statements as a service to promote the awareness of certain issues to its members. The information contained in the position statement is neither exhaustive not exclusive to all circumstances or individuals. Variables such as institutional human resource guidelines, state or federal statutes, rules, or regulations, as well as regional environmental conditions, may impact the relevance and implementation of these recommendations. The NATA advises its members and others to carefully and independently consider each of the recommendations (including the applicability of same to any particular circumstance or individual). The position statement should not be relied upon as an independent basis for care but rather as a resource available to NATA members or others. Moreover, no opinion is expressed herein regarding the quality of care that adheres to or differs from NATA's position statements. The NATA reserves the right to rescind or modify its position statements at any time.

ACKNOWLEDGMENTS

We gratefully acknowledge the efforts of Michael C. Koester, MD, ATC; James L. Moeller, MD, FACSM; Kenneth W. Rundell, PhD; Chad Starkey, PhD, ATC; Randall L. Wilber, PhD; and the Pronouncements Committee in the preparation of this document.

REFERENCES

1. National Asthma Education and Prevention Program. *Expert Panel Report II: Guidelines for the Diagnosis and Management of Asthma.* Bethesda, MD: National Institutes of Health; 1997. Publication No. 97-4051:12–18.
2. *Global Strategy for Asthma Management and Prevention.* Bethesda, MD: National Institutes of Health, National Heart, Lung, and Blood Institute; 2002. NIH publication No. 02-3659.
3. Nystad W. Asthma. *Int J Sports Med.* 2000;21(suppl):S-98–S-102.
4. Balatbat JH. Asthma: an overview from prevalence to plan. *J Contin Educ Top Issues.* 2002;2:80–92.
5. Rundell KW, Im J, Mayers LB, Wilber RL, Szmedra L, Schmitz HR. Self-reported symptoms and exercise-induced asthma in the elite athlete. *Med Sci Sports Exerc.* 2001;33:208–213.
6. Tiddens H, Silverman M, Bush A. The role of inflammation in airway disease: remodeling. *Am J Respir Crit Care Med.* 2000;162(2, pt 2):S-7–S-10.
7. Bousquet J, Jeffery PK, Busse WW, Johnson M, Vignola AM. Asthma: from bronchoconstriction to airways inflammation and remodeling. *Am J Respir Crit Care Med.* 2000;161:1720–1745.
8. Wenzel S. Severe asthma in adults. *Am J Respir Crit Care Med.* 2005; 172:149–160.
9. Rupp NT, Guill NF, Brudno DS. Unrecognized exercise-induced bronchospasm in adolescent athletes. *Am J Dis Child.* 1992;146:941–944.
10. Rupp NT, Brudno DS, Guill MF. The value of screening for risk of exercise-induced asthma in high school athletes. *Ann Allergy.* 1993;70: 339–342.
11. Hammerman SI, Becker JM, Rogers J, Quedenfeld TC, D'Alonzo GE Jr. Asthma screening of high school athletes: identifying the undiagnosed and poorly controlled. *Ann Allergy Asthma Immunol.* 2002;88:380–384.
12. Hallstrand TS, Curtis JR, Koepsell TD, et al. Effectiveness of screening examinations to detect unrecognized exercise-induced bronchoconstriction. *J Pediatr.* 2002;141:343–348.
13. Weiler JM. Exercise-induced asthma: a practical guide to definitions, diagnosis, prevalence, and treatment. *Allergy Asthma Proc.* 1996;17: 315–325.
14. Lacroix VJ. Exercise-induced asthma. *Physician Sportsmed.* 1999; 27(12):75–91.
15. Abu-Hasan M, Tannous B, Weinberger M. Exercise-induced dyspnea in children and adolescents: if not asthma then what? *Ann Allergy Asthma Immunol.* 2005;94:366–371.
16. West JB. *Respiratory Physiology: The Essentials.* Philadelphia, PA: Lippincott Williams & Wilkins; 2000.
17. Kanner RE, Morris AH, eds. *Clinical Pulmonary Function Testing: A Manual of Uniform Laboratory Procedures.* Salt Lake City, UT: Intermountain Thoracic Society; 1975.
18. Petty TL. Simple office spirometry. *Clin Chest Med.* 2001;22:845–859.
19. Crapo RO, Casaburi R, Coates AL, et al. Guidelines for methacholine and exercise challenge testing—1999. *Am J Respir Crit Care Med.* 2000; 161:309–329.
20. Rundell KW, Wilber RL, Szmedra L, Jenkinson DM, Mayers LB, Im J. Exercise-induced asthma screening of elite athletes: field versus laboratory exercise challenge. *Med Sci Sports Exerc.* 2000;32:309–316.
21. Rundell KW, Anderson SD, Spiering BA, Judelson DA. Field exercise vs laboratory eucapnic voluntary hyperventilation to identify airway hyperresponsiveness in elite cold weather athletes. *Chest.* 2004;125:909–915.
22. Peak flow meters and spirometers in general practice. *Drug Ther Bull.* 1997;35:52–55.
23. Meadows-Oliver M, Banasiak NC. Asthma medication delivery devices. *J Pediatr Health Care.* 2005;19:121–123.
24. Im J. Asthma. *RxConsultant.* 2003;12:1–8.
25. Baker VO, Friedman J, Schmitt R. Asthma management, part II: pharmacologic management. *J Sch Nurs.* 2002;18:257–269.
26. Self TH, Kelly HW. Asthma. In: Young LY, Koda-Kimble MA, eds. *Applied Therapeutics: The Clinical Use of Drugs.* 6th ed. Vancouver, WA: Applied Therapeutics, Inc; 1995:19-1–19-31.
27. Drugs for asthma. *Med Lett Drugs Ther.* 1999;41:5–10.
28. Szilagyi PG, Kemper KJ. Management of chronic childhood asthma in the primary care office. *Pediatr Ann.* 1999;28:43–52.
29. Sherman J, Hendeles L. Practical pharmacology for pediatric asthma. *Pediatr Ann.* 2000;29:768–773.
30. Houglum JE. Asthma medications: basic pharmacology and use in the athlete. *J Athl Train.* 2000;35:179–187.
31. Hough DO, Dec KL. Exercise-induced asthma and anaphylaxis. *Sports Med.* 1994;18:162–172.
32. Gong H Jr. Breathing easy: exercise despite asthma. *Physician Sportsmed.* 1992;20(3):158–167.
33. McDonald E, Cook D, Newman T, Griffith L, Cox G, Guyatt G. Effect of air filtration systems on asthma: a systematic review of randomized trials. *Chest.* 2002;122:535–1542.
34. Reiff DB, Choudry NB, Pride NB, Ind PW. The effect of prolonged submaximal warm-up exercise on exercise-induced asthma. *Am Rev Respir Dis.* 1989;139:479–484.
35. Turner MO, Taylor D, Bennett R, Fitzgerald JM. A randomized trial comparing peak expiratory flow and symptom self-management plans for patients with asthma attending a primary care clinic. *Am J Respir Crit Care Med.* 1998;157:540–546.
36. Kolbe J, Vamos M, James F, Elkind G, Garrett J. Assessment of practical knowledge of self-management of acute asthma. *Chest.* 1996;109:86–90.
37. Lieu TA, Quesenberry CP Jr., Capra AM, Sorel ME, Martin KE, Mendoza GR. Outpatient management practices associated with reduced risk of pediatric asthma hospitalization and emergency department visits. *Pediatrics.* 1997;100(3, pt 1):334–341.
38. Gibson PG, Wlodarczyk J, Hensley MJ, Murree-Allen K, Olson LG, Saltos N. Using quality-control analysis of peak expiratory flow recordings to guide therapy for asthma. *Ann Intern Med.* 1995;123:488–492.
39. Boggs PB, Hayati F, Washburne WF, Wheeler DA. Using statistical process control charts for the continual improvement of asthma care. *Jt Comm J Qual Improv.* 1999;25:163–181.
40. Allen RM, Jones MP, Oldenburg B. Randomised trial of an asthma self-management programme for adults. *Thorax.* 1995;50:731–738.

41. Bailey WC, Richards JM Jr, Brooks CM, Soong SJ, Windsor RA, Manzella BA. A randomized trial to improve self-management practices of adults with asthma. *Arch Intern Med.* 1990;150:1664–1668.

42. Hilton S, Sibbald B, Anderson HR, Freeling P. Controlled evaluation of the effects of patient education on asthma morbidity in general practice. *Lancet.* 1986;1:26–29.

43. Yoon R, McKenzie DK, Bauman A, Miles DA. Controlled trial evaluation of an asthma education programme for adults. *Thorax.* 1993;48:1110–1116.

44. Wilson SR, Scamagas P, German DF, et al. A controlled trial of two forms of self-management education for adults with asthma. *Am J Med.* 1993;94:564–576.

45. Beilby JJ, Wakefield MA, Ruffin RE. Reported use of asthma management plans in South Australia. *Med J Aust.* 1997;166:298–301.

46. Dales RE, Kerr PE, Schweitzer I, Reesor K, Gougeon L, Dickinson G. Asthma management preceding an emergency department visit. *Arch Intern Med.* 1992;152:2041–2044.

47. Scarfone RJ, Zorc JJ, Capraro GA. Patient self-management of acute asthma: adherence to national guidelines a decade later. *Pediatrics.* 2001;108:1332–1338.

48. Adams RJ, Boath K, Homan S, Campbell DA, Ruffin RE. A randomized trial of peak-flow and symptom-based action plans in adults with moderate-to-severe asthma. *Respirology.* 2001;6:297–304.

49. Myers TR. Improving patient outcomes with tools for asthma self-monitoring: a review of the literature. *Dis Manag Health Outcomes.* 2002;10:631–642.

50. Clark NM, Partridge MR. Strengthening asthma education to enhance disease control. *Chest.* 2002;121:1661–1669.

51. Lawrence G. Asthma self-management programs can reduce the need for hospital-based asthma care. *Respir Care.* 1995;40:39–43.

52. Partridge MR. Delivering optimal care to the person with asthma: what are the key components and what do we mean by patient education? *Eur Respir J.* 1995;8:298–305.

53. Bittleman DB, Smith RJH, Weiler JM. Abnormal movment of the arytenoid region during exercise presenting as exercise-induced asthma in an adolescent athlete. *Chest.* 1994;106:615–616.

54. McFadden ER Jr, Zawadski DK. Vocal cord dysfunction masquerading as exercise-induced asthma: a physiologic cause for "choking" during athletic activities. *Am J Respir Crit Care Med.* 1996;153:942–947.

55. Clark CJ, Cochrane LM. Physical activity and asthma. *Curr Opin Pulm Med.* 1999;5:68–75.

56. Guthrie CM, Tingen MS. Asthma: a case study, review of pathophysiology, and management strategies. *J Am Acad Nurse Pract.* 2002;14:457–461.

57. Wiggs BR, Bosken C, Paré PD, James A, Hogg JC. A model of airway narrowing in asthma and in chronic obstructive pulmonary disease. *Am Rev Respir Dis.* 1992;145:1251–1258.

58. Aikawa T, Shimura S, Sasaki H, Ebina M, Takishima T. Marked goblet cell hyperplasia with mucus accumulation in the airways of patients who died of severe acute asthma attack. *Chest.* 1992;101:916–921.

59. Shimura S, Andoh Y, Haraguchi M, Shirato K. Continuity of airway goblet cells and intraluminal mucus in the airways of patients with bronchial asthma. *Eur Respir J.* 1996;9:1395–1401.

60. Huber HL, Koessler KL. The pathology of bronchial asthma. *Arch Intern Med.* 1922;30:689–760.

61. Dunnill MS. The pathology of asthma, with special reference to changes in the bronchial mucosa. *J Clin Pathol.* 1960;13:27–33.

62. Wenzel SE, Westcott JY, Smith HR, Larsen GL. Spectrum of prostanoid release after bronchoalveolar allergen challenge in atopic asthmatics and in control groups: an alteration in the ratio of bronchoconstrictive to bronchoprotective mediators. *Am Rev Respir Dis.* 1989;139:450–457.

63. Persson CG. Role of plasma exudation in asthmatic airways. *Lancet.* 1986;2:1126–1129.

64. Djukanović R, Wilson JW, Britten KM, et al. Quantitation of mast cells and eosinophils in the bronchial mucosa of symptomatic atopic asthmatics and healthy control subjects using immunohistochemistry. *Am Rev Respir Dis.* 1990;142:863–871.

65. Koshino T, Arai Y, Miyamoto Y, et al. Mast cell and basophil number in the airway correlate with the bronchial responsiveness of asthmatics. *Int Arch Allergy Immunol.* 1995;107:378–379.

66. O'Byrne PM. Airway inflammation and asthma. *Aliment Pharmacol Ther.* 1996;10(suppl 2):18–24.

67. Hays SR, Fahy JV. The role of mucus in fatal asthma. *Am J Med.* 2003;115:68–69.

68. Kessler GF, Austin JH, Graf PD, Gamsu G, Gold WM. Airway constriction in experimental asthma in dogs: tantalum bronchographic studies. *J Appl Physiol.* 1973;35:703–708.

69. Carroll N, Elliot J, Morton A, James A. The structure of large and small airways in nonfatal and fatal asthma. *Am Rev Respir Dis.* 1993;147:405–410.

70. Awadh N, Müller NL, Park CS, Abboud RT, FitzGerald JM. Airway wall thickness in patients with near fatal asthma and control groups: assessment with high resolution computed tomographic scanning. *Thorax.* 1998;53:248–253.

71. McFadden ER Jr. Development, structure, and physiology in the normal lung and in asthma. In: Middleton E, Ellis EF, Adkinson NF Jr, Yuninger JW, Reed CH, Busse WW, eds. *Allergy Principles and Practice.* St. Louis, MO: Mosby; 1998:508–519.

72. McFadden ER Jr, Kiser R, DeGroot WJ. Acute bronchial asthma: relations between clinical and physiologic manifestations. *N Engl J Med.* 1973;288:221–225.

73. National Center for Health Statistics. *NCHS Data on Asthma.* Available at: http://www.cdc.gov/nchs/data/factsheets/asthma.pdf. Accessed June 6, 2005.

74. D'Amato G, Liccardi G, Cazzola M. Environment and development of respiratory allergy, I: outdoors. *Monaldi Arch Chest Dis.* 1994;49:406–411.

75. D'Amato G, Liccardi G, D'Amato M. Environment and development of respiratory allergy, II: indoors. *Monaldi Arch Chest Dis.* 1994;49:412–420.

76. Steerenberg PA, Van Amsterdam JGC, Vandebriel BJ, Vos JG, Van Bree L, Van Loveren H. Environmental and lifestyle factors may act in concert to increase the prevalence of respiratory allergy including asthma. *Clin Exp Allergy.* 1999;29:1303–1308.

77. Sunyer J, Antò JM, Kogevinas M, et al. Risk factors for asthma in young adults: Spanish Group of the European Community Respiratory Health Survey. *Eur Respir J.* 1997;10:2490–2494.

78. Grant EN, Wagner R, Weiss KB. Observations on emerging patterns of asthma in our society. *J Allergy Clin Immunol.* 1999;104(2, pt 2):S-1–S-9.

79. Koenig JQ. Air pollution and asthma. *J Allergy Clin Immunol.* 1999;104(4, pt 1):717–722.

80. Custovic A, Simpson A, Woodcock A. Importance of indoor allergens in the induction of allergy and elicitation of allergic disease. *Allergy.* 1998;53(48 suppl):115–20.

81. Jones AP. Asthma and the home environment. *J Asthma.* 2000;37:103–124.

82. Platts-Mills TAE. Allergen avoidance. *J Allergy Clin Immunol.* 2004;113:388–391.

83. Platts-Mills TAE, Ward GW Jr, Sporik R, Gelber LE, Chapman MD, Heymann PW. Epidemiology of the relationship between exposure to indoor allergens and asthma. *Int Arch Allergy Appl Immunol.* 1991;94:339–345.

84. Gruchalla RS, Pongracic J, Plaut M, et al. Inner City Asthma Study: relationships among sensitivity, allergen exposure, and asthma morbidity. *J Allergy Clin Immunol.* 2005;115:478–485.

85. Platts-Mills TAE, Vervloet D, Thomas WR, Aalberse RC, Chapman MD. Indoor allergens and asthma: report of the Third International Workshop. *J Allergy Clin Immunol.* 1997;100:S-1–S-24.

86. Hirsch T, Hering M, Bürkner K, et al. House-dust-mite allergen concentrations (Der f 1) and mold spores in apartment bedrooms before and after installation of insulated windows and central heating systems. *Allergy.* 2000;55:79–83.

87. Schoenwetter WF. Building a healthy house. *Ann Allergy Asthma Immunol.* 1997;79:1–4.

88. Woodfolk JA, Luczynska CH, de Blay F, Chapman MD, Platts-Mills TAE. Cat allergy. *Ann Allergy.* 1992;69:273–275.

89. Sarpong SB, Karrison T. Season of birth and cockroach allergen sensitization in children with asthma. *J Allergy Clin Immunol*. 1998;101(4, pt 1):566–568.

90. Kuster PA. Reducing risk of house dust mite and cockroach allergen exposure in inner-city children with asthma. *Pediatr Nurs*. 1996;22:297–303.

91. Kang BC, Wu CW, Johnson J. Characteristics and diagnosis of cockroach-sensitive bronchial asthma. *Ann Allergy*. 1992;68:237–244.

92. Liccardi G, Cazzola M, D'Amato M, D'Amato G. Pets and cockroaches: two increasing causes of respiratory allergy in indoor environments. Characteristics of airways sensitization and prevention strategies. *Respir Med*. 2000;94:1109–1118.

93. Platt SD, Martin CJ, Hunt SM, Lewis CW. Damp housing, mould growth, and symptomatic health state. *BMJ*. 1989;298:1673–1678.

94. Potter PC, Juritz J, Little F, McCaldin M, Dowdle EB. Clustering of fungal allergen-specific IgE antibody responses in allergic subjects. *Ann Allergy*. 1991;66:149–153.

95. Henderson FW, Henry MM, Ivins SS, et al. Correlates of recurrent wheezing in school-age children: The Physicians of Raleigh Pediatric Associates. *Am J Respir Crit Care Med*. 1995;151:1786–1793.

96. Gergen PJ, Turkeltaub PC. The association of individual allergen reactivity with respiratory disease in a national sample: data from the second National Health and Nutrition Examination Survey, 1976–80 (NHANES II). *J Allergy Clin Immunol*. 1992;90(4, pt 1):579–588.

97. Duffy DL, Mitchell CA, Martin NG. Genetic and environmental risk factors for asthma: a cotwin-control study. *Am J Respir Crit Care Med*. 1998;157(3, pt 1):840–845.

98. Omenaas E, Bakke P, Eide GE, Elsayed S, Gulsvik A. Serum house-dust-mite antibodies and reduced FEV$_1$ in adults of a Norwegian community. *Am J Respir Crit Care Med*. 1995;152(4, pt 1):1158–1163.

99. Omenaas E, Bakke P, Eide GE, Elsayed S, Gulsvik A. Serum house dust mite antibodies: predictor of increased bronchial responsiveness in adults of a community. *Eur Respir J*. 1996;9:919–925.

100. Turner KJ, Stewart GA, Woolcock AJ, Green W, Alpers MP. Relationship between mite densities and the prevalence of asthma: comparative studies in two populations in the Eastern Highlands of Papua New Guinea. *Clin Allergy*. 1988;18:331–340.

101. Vervloet D, Charpin D, Haddi E, et al. Medication requirements and house dust mite exposure in mite-sensitive asthmatics. *Allergy*. 1991;46:554–558.

102. Tariq SM, Matthews SM, Hakim EA, Stevens M, Arshad SH, Hide DW. The prevalence of and risk factors for atopy in early childhood: a whole population birth cohort study. *J Allergy Clin Immunol*. 1998;101:587–593.

103. Call RS, Smith TF, Morris E, Chapman MD, Platts-Mills TAE. Risk factors for asthma in inner city children. *J Pediatr*. 1992;121:862–866.

104. Platts-Mills TAE, Woodfolk JA, Chapman MD, Heymann PW. Changing concepts of allergic disease: the attempt to keep up with real changes in lifestyles. *J Allergy Clin Immunol*. 1996;98(6, pt 3):S-297–S-306.

105. Forastiére F, Corbo GM, Michelozzi P, et al. Effects of environment and passive smoking on the respiratory health in children. *Int J Epidemiol*. 1992;21:66–73.

106. Gortmaker SL, Walker DK, Jacobs FH, Ruch-Ross H. Parental smoking and the risk of childhood asthma. *Am J Public Health*. 1982;72:574–579.

107. Koenig JQ, Larson TV, Hanley QS, et al. Pulmonary function changes in children associated with fine particulate matter. *Environ Res*. 1993;63:26–38.

108. Murray B, Morrison BJ. The effect of cigarette smoke from the mother on bronchial responsiveness and severity of symptoms in children with asthma. *J Allergy Clin Immunol*. 1986;77:575–581.

109. Halken S, Host A, Nilsson L, Taudorf E. Passive smoking as a risk factor for development of obstructive respiratory disease and allergic sensitization. *Allergy*. 1995;50:97–105.

110. Siroux V, Pin I, Oryszczyn MP, Le Moual N, Kauffmann F. Relationships of active smoking to asthma and asthma severity in the EGEA study: Epidemiological Study on the Genetics and Environment of Asthma. *Eur Respir J*. 2000;15:470–477.

111. Bar-Or O, Inbar O. Swimming and asthma: benefits and deleterious effects. *Sports Med*. 1992;14:397–405.

112. Massin N, Bohadana AB, Wild P, Hery M, Toamain JP, Hubert G. Respiratory symptoms and bronchial responsiveness in lifeguards exposed to nitrogen trichloride in indoor swimming pools. *Occup Environ Med*. 1998;55:258–263.

113. Bernard A, Carbonnelle S, Michel O, et al. Lung hyperpermeability and asthma prevalence in schoolchildren: unexpected associations with the attendance at indoor chlorinated swimming pools. *Occup Environ Med*. 2003;60:385–394.

114. Thickett KM, McCoach JS, Gerber JM, Sadhra S, Burge PS. Occupational asthma caused by chloramines in indoor swimming-pool air. *Eur Respir J*. 2002:19:827–832.

115. Nemery B, Hoet PHM, Nowak D. Indoor swimming pools, water chlorination and respiratory health. *Eur Respir J*. 2002;19:790–793.

116. Zwemer RJ, Karibo J. Use of laminar control device as adjunct to standard environmental control measures in symptomatic asthmatic children. *Ann Allergy*. 1973;31:284–290.

117. Villaveces JW, Rosengren H, Evans J. Use of a laminar air flow portable filter in asthmatic children. *Ann Allergy*. 1977;38:400–404.

118. Kooistra JB, Pasch R, Reed CE. The effects of air cleaners on hay fever symptoms in air-conditioned homes. *J Allergy Clin Immunol*. 1978;61:315–319.

119. Wood RA, Mudd KE, Egglestone PA. The distribution of cat and dust mite allergens on wall surfaces. *J Allergy Clin Immunol*. 1992;89(1, pt 1):126–130.

120. Shirai T, Matsui T, Suzuki K, Chida K. Effect of pet removal on pet allergic asthma. *Chest*. 2005;127:1565–1571.

121. Folinsbee LJ. Does nitrogen dioxide exposure increase airways responsiveness? *Toxicol Ind Health*. 1992;8:273–283.

122. Pope CA III, Dockery DW, Spengler JD, Raizenne ME. Respiratory health and PM$_{10}$ pollution: a daily time series analysis. *Am Rev Respir Dis*. 1991;144(3, pt 1):668–674.

123. Delfino RJ, Coate BD, Zeiger RS, Seltzer JM, Street DH, Koutrakis P. Daily asthma severity in relation to personal ozone exposure and outdoor fungal spores. *Am J Respir Crit Care Med*. 1996;154(3, pt 1):633–641.

124. Delfino RJ, Zeiger RS, Seltzer JM, Street DH. Symptoms in pediatric asthmatics and air pollution: differences in effects by symptoms severity, anti-inflammatory medication use and particulate averaging time. *Environ Health Perspect*. 1998;106:751–761.

125. Koenig JQ, Pierson WE, Horike M, Frank R. Effects of SO$_2$ plus NaCl aerosol combined with moderate exercise on pulmonary function in asthmatic adolescents. *Environ Res*. 1981;25:340–348.

126. Suphioglu C, Singh MB, Taylor P, et al. Mechanism of grass-pollen-induced asthma. *Lancet*. 1992;339:569–572.

127. Helenius I, Haahtela T. Allergy and asthma in elite summer sport athletes. *J Allergy Clin Immunol*. 2000;106:444–452.

128. Solomon WR. Airborne pollen prevalence in the United States. In: Grammer LC, Greenberger PA, eds. *Patterson's Allergic Diseases*. Philadelphia, PA: Lippincott Williams & Wilkins; 2002:131–144.

129. D'Amato G, Spieksma FT, Liccardi G, et al. Pollen-related allergy in Europe. *Allergy*. 1998;53:567–578.

130. Rundell KW, Spiering BA, Evans TM, Baumann JM. Baseline lung function, exercise-induced bronchoconstriction, and asthma-like symptoms in elite women ice hockey players. *Med Sci Sports Exerc*. 2004;36:405–410.

131. Lung function testing: selection of reference values and interpretative strategies. American Thoracic Society. *Am Rev Respir Dis*. 1991;144:1202–1218.

132. Ferguson GT, Enright PL, Buist AS, Higgins MW. Office spirometry for lung health assessment in adults: a consensus statement from the National Lung Health Education Program. *Respir Care*. 2000;45:513–530.

133. Guidelines for the measurement of respiratory function: recommendations of the British Thoracic Society and the Association of Respiratory Technicians and Physiologists. *Respir Med*. 1994;88:165–194.

134. Crapo RO, Morris AH, Gardner RM. Reference spirometric values using techniques and equipment that meet ATS recommendations. *Am Rev Respir Dis*. 1981;123:659–664.

135. Polgar G, Promadhat V. *Pulmonary Function Testing in Children*. Philadelphia, PA: WB Saunders; 1971.

136. Standardization of spirometry: 1994 update. American Thoracic Society. *Am Respir Crit Care Med*. 1995;152:1107–1136.

137. Koyama H, Nishimura K, Ikeda A, Tsukino M, Izumi T. Comparison of four types of portable peak flow meters (Mini-Wright, Assess, Pulmograph and Wright Pocket meters). *Respir Med*. 1998;92:505–511.

138. Kelly CA, Gibson GJ. Relation between FEV_1 and peak expiratory flow in patients with chronic airflow obstruction. *Thorax*. 1988;43:335–336.

139. Ladebauche P. Peak flow meters: child's play. *Office Nurse*. 1996:22–28.

140. Li JTC. Do peak flow meters lead to better asthma control? *J Respir Dis*. 1995;16:381–398.

141. Ignacio-Garcia JM, Gonzales-Santos P. Asthma self-management education program by home monitoring of peak expiratory flow. *Am J Respir Crit Care Med*. 1995;151:353–359.

142. Measuring peak flow at home. *Drug Ther Bull*. 1991;29:87–88.

143. Lahdensuo A, Haahtela T, Herrala J, et al. Randomised comparison of cost effectiveness of guided self management and traditional treatment of asthma in Finland. *BMJ*. 1998;316:1138–1139.

144. Lahdensuo A, Haahtela T, Herrala J, et al. Randomised comparison of guided self management and traditional treatment of asthma over one year. *BMJ*. 1996;312:748–752.

145. Wagner MH, Jacobs J. Improving asthma management with peak flow meters. *Contemp Pediatr*. 1997;14:111–119.

146. Bheekie A, Syce JA, Weinberg EG. Peak expiratory flow rate and symptom self monitoring of asthma initiated from community pharmacies. *J Clin Pharm Ther*. 2001;26:287–296.

147. Cowie RL, Revitt SG, Underwood MF, Field SK. The effect of a peak flow-based action plan in the prevention of exacerbations of asthma. *Chest*. 1997;112:1534–1538.

148. Rachelefsky G, Fitzgerald S, Page D, Santamaria B. An update on the diagnosis and management of pediatric asthma: based on the National Heart, Lung, and Blood Institute expert panel report. *Nurse Pract*. 1993; 18:51–62.

149. Killian KJ, Watson R, Otis J, St Amand TA, O'Bryne PM. Symptom perception during acute bronchoconstriction. *Am J Respir Crit Care Med*. 2000;162(2, pt 1):490–496.

150. Kendrick AH, Higgs CMB, Whitfield MJ, Laszlo G. Accuracy of perception of severity of asthma: patients treated in general practice. *BMJ*. 1993;307:422–424.

151. Klements EM. Monitoring peak flow rates as a health-promoting behavior in managing and improving asthma. *Clin Excell Nurse Pract*. 2001; 5:147–151.

152. Malo JL, L'Archevêque J, Trudeau C, d'Aquino C, Cartier A. Should we monitor peak expiratory flow rates or record symptoms with a simple diary in the management of asthma? *J Allergy Clin Immunol*. 1993;91: 702–709.

153. Verschelden P, Cartier A, L'Archevêque J, Trudeau C, Malo JL. Compliance with and accuracy of daily self-assessment of peak expiratory flows (PEF) in asthmatic subjects over a three month period. *Eur Respir J*. 1996;9:880–885.

154. Sawyer G, Miles J, Lewis S, Fitzharris P, Pearce N, Beasley R. Classification of asthma severity: should the international guidelines be changed? *Clin Exp Allergy*. 1998;28:1565–1570.

155. Eid N, Yandell B, Howell L, Eddy M, Sheikh S. Can peak expiratory flow predict airflow obstruction in children with asthma? *Pediatrics*. 2000;105:354–358.

156. Brand PL, Duiverman EJ, Waalkens HJ, van Essen-Zandvliet EE, Kerrebijn KF. Peak flow variation in childhood asthma: correlation with symptoms, airways obstruction, and hyperresponsiveness during long term treatment with inhaled corticosteroids: Dutch CNSLD Study. *Thorax*. 1999;54:103–107.

157. Folgering H, vd Brink W, v Heeswijk O, v Herwaarden C. Eleven peak flow meters: a clinical evaluation. *Eur Respir J*. 1998;11:188–193.

158. Jain P, Kavuru MS. Peak expiratory flow vs spirometry in a patient with asthma. *Respir Care*. 2000;45:969–970.

159. Nolan S, Tolley E, Leeper K, Strayhorn Smith V, Self T. Peak expiratory flow associated with change in positioning of the instrument: comparison of five peak flow meters. *J Asthma*. 1999;36:291–294.

160. Connolly CK, Murthy NK, Tighe E, Alcock S, Harding T. Mini and Wright peak flow meters. *Thorax*. 1991;46:289P.

161. Dickinson SA, Hitchins DJ, Miller MR. Accuracy of measurement of peak flow using different peak flow meters. *Thorax*. 1991;46:289P.

162. Jain P, Kavuru MS. Peak expiratory flow vs spirometry in a patient with asthma. *Respir Care*. 2000;45:969–970.

163. Gardner RM, Crapo RO, Jackson BR, Jensen RL. Evaluation of accuracy and reproducibility of peak flow meters at 1,400 m. *Chest*. 1992; 101:948–952.

164. Chafin CC, Tolley E, George C, et al. Are there gender differences in the use of peak flow meters? *J Asthma*. 2001;38:541–543.

165. den Otter JJ, Knitel M, Akkermans RPM, Van Schayck CP, Folgering HTM, van Weel C. Spirometry in general practice: the performance of practice assistants scored by lung function technicians. *Br J Gen Pract*. 1997;47:41–42.

166. Flood-Page P, Barnes NC. What are the alternatives to increasing inhaled corticosteroids for the long term control of asthma? *BioDrugs*. 2001;15: 185–198.

167. Spector SL, Kinsman R, Mawhinney H, et al. Compliance of patients with asthma with an experimental aerosolized medication: implications for controlled clinical trials. *J Allergy Clin Immunol*. 1986;77(1, pt 1): 65–70.

168. Jeffery PK, Godfrey RW, Ädelroth E, Nelson F, Rogers A, Johansson SA. Effects of treatment on airway inflammation and thickening of basement membrane reticular collagen in asthma: a quantitative light and electron microscopic study. *Am Rev Respir Dis*. 1992;145(4, pt 1):890–899.

169. Djukanović R, Wilson JW, Britten KM, et al. Effect of an inhaled corticosteroid on airway inflammation and symptoms in asthma. *Am Rev Respir Dis*. 1992;145:669–674.

170. Laitinen LA, Laitinen A, Haahtela T. A comparative study of the effects of an inhaled corticosteroid, budesonide, and a β_2-agonist, terbutaline, on airway inflammation in newly diagnosed asthma: a randomized, double-blind, parallel-group controlled trial. *J Allergy Clin Immunol*. 1992; 90:32–42.

171. van Essen-Zandvliet EE, Hughes MD, Waalkens HJ, Duiverman EJ, Pocock SJ, Kerrebijn KF. Effects of 22 months of treatment with inhaled corticosteroids and/or beta2-agonists on lung function, airway responsiveness, and symptoms in children with asthma: the Dutch Chronic Non-Specific Lung Disease Study Group. *Am Rev Respir Dis*. 1992;146: 547–554.

172. Munck A, Mendel DB, Smith LI, Orti E. Glucocorticoid receptors and actions. *Am Rev Respir Dis*. 1990;141(2, pt 2):S-2–S-10.

173. Schleimer RP. Effects of glucocorticosteroids on inflammatory cells relevant to their therapeutic applications in asthma. *Am Rev Respir Dis*. 1990;141(2, pt 2):S-59–S-69.

174. Shelhamer JH, Levine SJ, Wu T, Jacoby DB, Kaliner MA, Rennard SL. NIH conference: airway inflammation. *Ann Intern Med*. 1995;123:288–304.

175. Haahtela T, Järvinen M, Kava T, et al. Comparison of a β_2-agonist, terbutaline, with an inhaled corticosteroid, budesonide, in newly detected asthma. *N Engl J Med*. 1991;325:388–392.

176. Barnes PJ, Pedersen S, Busse WW. Efficacy and safety of inhaled corticosteroids. New developments. *Am J Respir Crit Care Med*. 1998; 157(3, pt 2):S-1–S-53.

177. Barnes PJ, Pedersen S. Efficacy and safety of inhaled corticosteroids in asthma: report of a workshop held in Eze, France, October 1992. *Am Rev Respir Dis*. 1993;148(4, pt 2):S-1–S-26.

178. Long-term effects of budesonide or nedocromil in children with asthma: The Childhood Asthma Management Program Research Group. *N Engl J Med*. 2000;343:1054–1063.

179. Greenberger PA, Tatum AJ, D'Epiro P. Asthma: acute and long-term concerns. *Patient Care*. 1999;15:154–174.

180. Bleecker ER, Welch MJ, Weinstein SF, et al. Low-dose inhaled fluticasone propionate versus oral zafirlukast in the treatment of persistent asthma. *J Allergy Clin Immunol*. 2000;105:1123–1129.

181. Williamson IJ, Matusiewicz SP, Brown PH, Greening AP, Crompton GK.

Frequency of voice problems and cough in patients using pressurized aerosol inhaled steroid preparations. *Eur Respir J.* 1995;8:590–592.

182. Mash B, Bheekie A, Jones PW. Inhaled versus oral steroids for adults with chronic asthma (Cochrane Review). In: *The Cochrane Library.* Issue 4. Chichester, UK: John Wiley and Sons, Ltd: 2003.

183. Dunlap NE, Fulmer JD. Corticosteroid therapy in asthma. *Clin Chest Med.* 1984;5:669–683.

184. Serafin WE. Drugs used in the treatment of asthma. In: Hardman JG, Limbird LE, Molinoff PB, Ruddon RW, Gilman AG, eds. *The Pharmacological Basis of Therapeutics.* 9th ed. New York, NY: McGraw-Hill; 1996:659–682.

185. Nelson HS. β-adrenergic bronchodilators. *N Engl J Med.* 1995;333:499–506.

186. Boulet LP. Long versus short-acting beta 2-agonists: implications for drug therapy. *Drugs.* 1994;47:207–222.

187. Pearlman DS, Chervinsky P, LaForce C, et al. A comparison of salmeterol with albuterol in the treatment of mild-to-moderate asthma. *N Engl J Med.* 1992;327:1420–1425.

188. Kesten S, Chapman KR, Broder I, et al. A three-month comparison of twice daily inhaled formoterol versus four times daily inhaled albuterol in the management of stable asthma. *Am Rev Respir Dis.* 1991;144:622–625.

189. Anderson SD, Brannan JD. Long-acting β_2-adrenoceptor agonists and exercise-induced asthma: lessons to guide us in the future. *Paediatr Drugs.* 2004;6:161–175.

190. Wenzel SE, Lumry W, Manning M, et al. Efficacy, safety, and effects on quality of life of salmeterol versus albuterol in patients with mild to moderate persistent asthma. *Ann Allergy Asthma Immunol.* 1998;80:463–470.

191. Selroos O. Formoterol used as needed: clinical effectiveness. *Respir Med.* 2001;95:17–20.

192. Richter K, Jamicki S, Jorres RA, Magnussen H. Acute protection against exercise-induced bronchoconstriction by formoterol, salmeterol, and terbutaline. *Eur Respir J.* 2002;19(suppl B):865–871.

193. Bronsky EA, Yegen Ü, Yeh CM, Larsen LV, Della Cioppa G. Formoterol provides long-lasting protection against exercise-induced bronchospasm. *Ann Allergy Asthma Immunol.* 2002;89:417–412.

194. Ferrari M, Segattini C, Zanon R, et al. Comparison of the protective effect of formoterol and of salmerterol against exercise-induced bronchospasm when given immediately before a cycloergometric test. *Respiration.* 2002;69:509–512.

195. Hancox RJ, Subbarao P, Kamada D, Watson RM, Hargreave FE, Inman MD. Beta2-agonist tolerance and exercise-induced bronchospasm. *Am J Respir Crit Care Med.* 2002;165:1068–1070.

196. Ramage L, Lipworth BJ, Ingram CG, Cree IA, Dhillon DP. Reduced protection against exercise induced bronchoconstriction after chronic dosing with salmeterol. *Respir Med.* 1994;88:363–368.

197. Nelson JA, Strauss L, Skowronski M, Ciufo R, Novak R, McFadden ER Jr. Effect of long-term salmeterol treatment on exercise-induced asthma. *N Engl J Med.* 1998;339:141–146.

198. Garcia R, Guerra P, Feo F, et al. Tachyphylaxis following regular use of formoterol in exercise-induced bronchospasm. *J Investig Allergol Clin Immunol.* 2001;11:176–182.

199. Gardiner PV, Ward C, Booth H, Allison A, Hendrick DJ, Walters EH. Effect of eight weeks of treatment with salmeterol on bronchoalveolar lavage inflammatory indices in asthmatics. *Am J Respir Crit Care Med.* 1994;150:1006–1011.

200. Lemanske RF, Sorkness CA, Mauger EA, et al. Inhaled corticosteroid reduction and elimination in patients with persistent asthma receiving salmeterol: a randomized controlled trial. *JAMA.* 2001;285:2594–2603.

201. Lazarus SC, Boushey HA, Fahy JV, et al. Long-acting β_2-agonist monotherapy vs continued therapy with inhaled corticosteroids in patients with persistent asthma: a randomized controlled trial. *JAMA.* 2001;285:2583–2593.

202. Weiler JM, Nathan RA, Rupp NT, Kalberg CJ, Emmett A, Dorinsky PM. Effect of fluticasone/salmeterol administered via a single device on exercise-induced bronchospasm in patients with persistent asthma. *Ann Allergy Asthma Immunol.* 2005;94:65–72.

203. Shrewsbury S, Pyke S, Britton M. Meta-analysis of increased dose of inhaled steroid or addition of salmeterol in symptomatic asthma (MI-ASMA). *BMJ.* 2000;320:1368–1373.

204. Pauwels RA, Löfdahl CG, Postma DS, et al. Effect of inhaled formoterol and budesonide on exacerbations of asthma: Formoterol and Corticosteroids Establishing Therapy (FACET) International Study Group. *N Engl J Med.* 1997;337:1405–1411.

205. Holimon TD, Chafin CC, Self TH. Nocturnal asthma uncontrolled by inhaled corticosteroids: theophylline or long-acting beta2 agonists? *Drugs.* 2001;61:391–418.

206. Montelukast for persistent asthma. *Med Lett Drugs Ther.* 1998;40:71–73.

207. Stempel DA. Leukotriene modifiers in the treatment of asthma. *Respir Care.* 1998;43:481–489.

208. O'Byrne PM, Israel E, Drazen JM. Antileukotreines in the treatment of asthma. *Ann Intern Med.* 1997;127:472–480.

209. Lipworth BJ. Leukotriene-receptor antagonists. *Lancet.* 1999;353:57–62.

210. Drazen JM, Israel E, O'Byrne PM. Treatment of asthma with drugs modifying the leukotriene pathway. *N Engl J Med.* 1999;340:197–206.

211. Drazen JM. Asthma therapy with agents preventing leukotriene synthesis or action. *Proc Assoc Am Physicians.* 1999;111:547–559.

212. Dahlén B, Margolskee DJ, Zetterström O, Dahlén S. Effect of the leukotriene receptor antagonist MK-0679 on baseline pulmonary function in aspirin sensitive asthmatic subjects. *Thorax.* 1993;48:1205–1210.

213. Barnes NC, Miller CJ. Effect of leukotriene receptor antagonist therapy on the risk of asthma exacerbations in patients with mild to moderate asthma: an integrated analysis of zafirlukast trials. *Thorax.* 2000;55:478–483.

214. Christian Virchow J, Prasse A, Naya I, Summerton L, Harris A. Zafirlukast improves asthma control in patients receiving high-dose inhaled corticosteroids. *Am J Respir Crit Care Med.* 2000;162:578–585.

215. Leff JA, Busse WW, Pearlman D, et al. Montelukast, a leukotriene-receptor antagonist, for the treatment of mild asthma and exercise-induced bronchoconstriction. *N Engl J Med.* 1998;339:147–152.

216. Laviolette M, Malmstrom K, Lu S, et al. Montelukast added to inhaled beclomethasone in treatment of asthma: Montelukast/Beclomethasone Additivity Group. *Am J Respir Crit Care Med.* 1999;160:1862–1868.

217. Löfdahl CG, Reiss TF, Leff JA, et al. Randomised, placebo controlled trial of effect of a leukotriene receptor antagonist, montelukast, on tapering inhaled corticosteroids in asthmatic patients. *BMJ.* 1999;319:87–90.

218. Joshi EM, Heasley BH, Chordia MD, Macdonald TL. In vitro metabolism of 2-acetylbenzothiophene: relevance to zileuton hepatotoxicity. *Chem Res Toxicol.* 2004;17:137–143.

219. Ukena D, Harnest U, Sakalauskas R, et al. Comparison of addition of theophylline to inhaled steroid with doubling of the dose of inhaled steroid in asthma. *Eur Respir J.* 1997;10:2754–2760.

220. Norman PS. Immunotherapy: 1999–2004. *J Allergy Clin Immunol.* 2004;113:1013–1023.

221. Stokes J, Casale TB. Rationale for new treatments aimed at IgE immunomodulation. *Ann Allergy Asthma Immunol.* 2004;93:212–217.

222. Creticos PS, Chen YH, Schroeder JT. New approaches in immunotherapy: allergen vaccination with immunostimulatory DNA. *Immunol Allergy Clin North Am.* 2004;24:569–581.

223. Godfrey S, Bar-Yishay E. Exercise-induced asthma revisited. *Respir Med.* 1993;87:331–344.

224. Holzer K, Brukner P, Douglass J. Evidence-based management of exercise-induced asthma. *Curr Sports Med Rep.* 2002;1:86–92.

225. Sears MR, Lotvall J. Past, present and future–beta2-adrenoceptor agonists in asthma management. *Respir Med.* 2005;99:152–170.

226. Knöpfli BH, Bar-Or O, Araúgo CG. Effect of ipratropium bromide on EIB in children depends on vagal activity. *Med Sci Sports Exerc.* 2005;37:354–359.

227. Weinberger M, Hendeles L. Theophylline in asthma. *N Engl J Med.* 1996;334:1380–1388.

228. Sessler CN. Theophylline toxicity: clinical features of 116 consecutive cases. *Am J Med.* 1990;88:567–576.

229. Dozor AJ. Spacer crusader. *Lancet.* 2005;365:572.

230. Newman SP. Spacer devices for metered dose inhalers. *Clin Pharmacokinet.* 2004;43:349–60.

231. Newman KB, Milne S, Hamilton C, Hall K. A comparison of albuterol administered by metered-dose inhaler and spacer with albuterol by nebulizer in adults presenting to an urban emergency department with acute asthma. *Chest*. 2002;121:1036–1041.

232. Stevenson DD. Aspirin and NSAID sensitivity. *Immunol Allergy Clin North Am*. 2004;24:491–505.

233. Namazy JA, Simon RA. Sensitivity to nonsteroidal anti-inflammatory drugs. *Ann Allergy Asthma Immunol*. 2002;89:542–550.

234. Jawien J. A new insight into aspirin-induced asthma. *Eur J Clin Invest*. 2002;32:134–138.

235. de Almeida MA, Gaspar AP, Carvalho FS, Nogueira JM, Pinto JE. Adverse reactions to acetaminophen, ASA, and NSAIDs in children: what alternatives? *Allergy Asthma Proc*. 1997;18:313–318.

236. Vaszar LT, Stevenson DD. Aspirin-induced asthma. *Clin Rev Allergy Immunol*. 2001;21:71–87.

237. Rivas B. The management of ASA syndrome. *J Invest Allergol Clin Immunol*. 1997;7:392–396.

238. Hedman J, Kaprio J, Poussa T, Nieminen MM. Prevalence of asthma, aspirin intolerance, nasal polyposis and chronic obstructive pulmonary disease in a population-based study. *Int J Epidemiol*. 1999;28:717–722.

239. Levy S, Volans G. The use of analgesics in patients with asthma. *Drug Safe*. 2001;24:829–841.

240. Szczeklik A, Stevenson DD. Aspirin-induced asthma: advances in pathogenesis and management. *J Allergy Clin Immunol*. 1999;104:5–13.

241. Settipane RA, Stevenson DD. Cross sensitivity with acetaminophen in aspirin-sensitive subjects with asthma. *J Allergy Clin Immunol*. 1989; 84:26–33.

242. Szczeklik A, Stevenson DD. Aspirin-induced asthma: advances in pathogenesis, diagnosis, and management. *J Allergy Clin Immunol*. 2003; 111:913–921.

243. Mellion MB, Kobayashi RH. Exercise-induced asthma. *Am Fam Physician*. 1992;45:2671–2677.

244. Rupp NT. Diagnosis and management of exercise-induced asthma. *Physician Sportsmed*. 1996;24(1):77–87.

245. Baker WH, Weiler JM. The role of exercise training and conditioning in patients with asthma. In: Weiler JM, ed. *Allergic and Respiratory Disease in Sports Medicine*. New York, NY: Marcel Dekker; 1997:179–206.

246. Cochrane LM, Clark CJ. Benefits and problems of a physical training programme for asthmatic patients. *Thorax*. 1990;45:345–351.

247. Ben Dov I, Bar-Yishay E, Godfrey S. Refractory period after exercise-induced asthma unexplained by respiratory heat loss. *Am Rev Respir Dis*. 1982;125:530–534.

248. Belcher NG, O'Hickey S, Arm JP, Lee TH. Pathogenetic mechanisms of exercise-induced asthma and the refractory period. *N Engl Reg Allergy Proc*. 1988;9:199–201.

249. McKenzie DC, McLuckie SL, Stirling DR. The protective effects of continuous and interval exercise in athletes with exercise-induced asthma. *Med Sci Sports Exerc*. 1994;26:951–956.

250. Morton AR, Fitch KD, Davis T. The effect of "warm-up" on exercise-induced asthma. *Ann Allergy*. 1979;42:257–260.

251. Schnall RP, Landau LI. Protective effects of repeated short sprints in exercise-induced asthma. *Thorax*. 1980;35:828–832.

252. Mickleborough TD, Gotshall RW, Cordain L, Lindley M. Dietary salt alters pulmonary function during exercise in exercise-induced asthmatics. *J Sports Sci*. 2001;19:865–873.

253. Gotshall RW, Mickleborough TD, Cordain L. Dietary salt restriction improves pulmonary function in exercise-induced asthma. *Med Sci Sports Exerc*. 2000;32:1815–1819.

254. Mickleborough TD, Gotshall RW, Kluka EW, Miller CW, Cordian L. Dietary chloride as a possible determinant of the severity of exercise-induced asthma. *Eur J Appl Physiol*. 2001;85:450–456.

255. Mickleborough TD, Murray RL, Ionescu AA, Lindley MR. Fish oil supplementation reduces severity of exercise-induced bronchoconstriction in elite athletes. *Am J Respir Crit Care Med*. 2003;168:1181–1189.

256. Weiler JM, ed. *Allergic and Respiratory Disease in Sports Medicine*. New York, NY: Marcel Dekker; 1997.

257. McFadden ER Jr, ed. *Exercise-Induced Asthma*. New York, NY: Marcel Dekker; 1999.

258. Homnick DN, Marks JH. Exercise and sports in the adolescent with chronic pulmonary disease. *Adolesc Med*. 1998;9:467–481.

259. Milgrom H, Taussig LM. Keeping children with exercise-induced asthma active. *Pediatrics*. 1999;104:38–42.

260. Langdeau JB, Boulet LP. Prevalence and mechanisms of development of asthma and airway hyperresponsiveness in athletes. *Sports Med*. 2001;31:601–616.

261. Sudhir P, Prasad CE. Prevalence of exercise-induced bronchospasm in schoolchildren: an urban-rural comparison. *J Trop Pediatr*. 2003;49: 104–108.

262. Weiler JM, Layton T, Hunt M. Asthma in United States Olympic athletes who participated in the 1996 Summer Games. *J Allergy Clin Immunol*. 1998;102:722–726.

263. Weiler JM, Ryan EJ III. Asthma in United States Olympic athletes who participated in the 1998 Olympic Winter Games. *J Allergy Clin Immunol*. 2000;106:267–271.

264. Storms WW. Review of exercise-induced asthma. *Med Sci Sports Exerc*. 2003;35:1464–1470.

265. Wilber RL, Rundell KW, Szmedra L, Jenkinson DM, Im J, Drake SD. Incidence of exercise-induced bronchospasm in Olympic winter sport athletes. *Med Sci Sports Exerc*. 2000;32:732–737.

266. Rundell KW, Jenkinson DM. Exercise-induced bronchospasm in the elite athlete. *Sports Med*. 2002;32:583–600.

267. Feinstein RA, LaRussa J, Wang-Dohlman A, Bartolucci AA. Screening adolescent athletes for exercise-induced asthma. *Clin J Sport Med*. 1996; 6:119–123.

268. Tan RA, Spector SL. Exercise-induced asthma. *Sports Med*. 1998;25:1–6.

269. Spector SL. Update on exercise-induced asthma. *Ann Allergy*. 1993;71: 571–577.

270. Bierman EW, Kawabori I, Pierson WE. Incidence of exercise-induced asthma in children. *Pediatrics*. 1975;56(5, pt 2 suppl.):847–850.

271. Kovan JR, Mackowiak TJ. Exercise-induced asthma. *Athl Ther Today*. 2001;6(5):22–25, 34–35,64.

272. McConnell R, Berhane K, Gilliland F, et al. Asthma in exercising children exposed to ozone: a cohort study. *Lancet*. 2002;359:386–391.

273. Peter MM, Silvers WS, Thompson FL, Weiler JM. Case studies of asthma in elite and world-class athletes: the roles of the athletic trainer and physician. In: Weiler JM, ed. *Allergic and Respiratory Disease in Sports Medicine*. New York, NY: Marcel Dekker; 1997:353–375.

274. Karjalainen EM, Laitinen A, Sue-Chu M, Altraja A, Bjermer L, Laitinen LA. Evidence of airway inflammation and remodeling in ski athletes with and without bronchial hyperresponsiveness to methacholine. *Am J Respir Crit Care Med*. 2000;161:2086–91.

275. Larsson K, Ohlsén P, Larsson L, Malmberg P, Rydström P-O, Ulriksen H. High prevalence of asthma in cross country skiers. *BMJ*. 1993;307: 1326–1329.

276. Anderson SD, Daviskas E. Pathophysiology of exercise-induced asthma: the role of respiratory water loss. In: Weiler JM, ed. *Allergic and Respiratory Disease in Sports Medicine*. New York, NY: Marcel Dekker; 1997:87–114.

277. Anderson SD, Holzer K. Exercise-induced asthma: is it the right diagnosis in elite athletes? *J Allergy Clin Immunol*. 2000;106:419–428.

278. McFadden ER Jr, Nelson JA, Skowronski ME, Lenner KA. Thermally induced asthma and airway drying. *Am J Respir Crit Care Med*. 1999; 160:221–226.

279. Makker HK, Holgate ST. Pathophysiology: role of mediators in exercise-induced asthma. In: Weiler JM, ed. *Allergic and Respiratory Disease in Sports Medicine*. New York, NY: Marcel Dekker; 1997:115–136.

280. Anderson SD, Daviskas E. The mechanism of exercise-induced asthma is... *J Allergy Clin Immunol*. 2000;106:453–459.

281. Deal EC Jr., McFadden ER Jr, Ingram RH Jr, Strauss RH, Jaeger JJ. Role of respiratory heat exchange in production of exercise-induced asthma. *J Appl Physiol*. 1979;46:467–475.

282. Chen WY, Horton DJ. Heat and water loss from the airways and exercise-induced asthma. *Respiration*. 1977;34:305–313.

283. Gilbert IA, McFadden ER Jr. Airway cooling and rewarming: the second reaction sequence in exercise-induced asthma. *J Clin Invest*. 1992;90: 699–704.

284. Anderson SD, Kippelen P. Exercise-induced bronchoconstriction: pathogenesis. *Curr Allergy Asthma Rep.* 2005;5:116–122.

285. McFadden ER Jr, Lenner KA, Strohl KP. Postexertional airway rewarming and thermally induced asthma: new insights into pathophysiology and possible pathogenesis. *J Clin Invest.* 1986;78:18–25.

286. Smith CM, Anderson SD, Walsh S, McElrea MS. An investigation of the effects of heat and water exchange in the recovery period after exercise in children with asthma. *Am Rev Respir Dis.* 1989;140:598–605.

287. McFadden ER Jr, Gilbert IA. Exercise-induced asthma. *N Engl J Med.* 1994;330:1362–1367.

288. Beck KC. Control of airway function during and after exercise in asthmatics. *Med Sci Sports Exerc.* 1999;31:S-4–S-11.

289. Makker HK, Holgate ST. Mechanisms of exercise-induced asthma. *Eur J Clin Invest.* 1994;24:571–585.

290. Furuichi S, Hashimoto S, Gon Y, Matsumoto K, Horie T. p38 mitogen-activated protein kinase and C-Jun-NH2 terminal kinase regulate interleukin-8 and RANTES production in hyperosmolarity stimulated human bronchial epithelial cells. *Respirology.* 2002;7:193–200.

291. Rundell KW. Pulmonary function decay in women ice hockey players: is there a relationship to ice rink air quality? *Inhal Toxicol.* 2004;16:117–123.

292. Zainudin NM, Aziz BA, Haifa AL, Deng CT, Omar AH. Exercise-induced bronchoconstriction among Malay schoolchildren. *Respirology.* 2001;6:151–155.

293. Jones A, Bowen M. Screening for childhood asthma using an exercise test. *Br J Gen Pract.* 1994;44:127–131.

294. Vianne EO, Boaventura LC, Terra-Filho J, Nakama GY, Martinez JAB, Martinez RJ. Morning-to-evening variation in exercise-induced bronchospasm. *J Allergy Clin Immunol.* 2002;110:236–240.

295. Anderson SD. Exercise-induced asthma and the use of hypertonic saline aerosol as a bronchial challenge. *Respirology.* 1996;3:175–181.

296. Tilles SA. Vocal cord dysfunction in children and adolescents. *Curr Allergy Asthma Rep.* 2003;3:467–472.

297. Rundell KW, Spiering BA. Inspiratory stridor in elite athletes. *Chest.* 2003;123:468–474.

298. Wilkerson LA. Exercise-induced asthma. *J Am Osteopath Assoc.* 1998; 98:211–215.

299. Smith BW, LaBotz M. Pharmacologic treatment of exercise-induced asthma. *Clin Sports Med.* 1998;17:343–363.

300. Fowler C. Preventing and managing exercise-induced asthma. *Nurse Pract.* 2001;26:25–33.

301. Kemp JP, Dockhorn RJ, Busse WW, Bleecker ER, Van As A. Prolonged effect of inhaled salmeterol against exercise-induced bronchospasm. *Am J Respir Crit Care Med.* 1994;150(6 Pt 1):1612–1615.

302. Vathenen AS, Knox AJ, Wisniewski A, Tattersfield AE. Time course of change in bronchial reactivity with an inhaled corticosteroid in asthma. *Am Rev Respir Dis.* 1991;143:1317–1321.

303. Nastasi KJ, Heinly TL, Blaiss MS, Exercise-induced asthma and the athlete. *J Asthma.* 1995;32:249–257.

304. Finch L. Asthma education is key. *J Respir Care Pract.* 2000:85–116.

305. Dawson KP, Van Asperen P, Higgins C, Sharpe C, Davis A. An evaluation of the action plans of children with asthma. *J Paediatr Child Health.* 1995;31:21–23.

Asthma Management Review Questions:

1. What is asthma and what are the major signs and symptoms that suggest asthma? What factors make asthma difficult to diagnose and classify?

2. Research has identified many environmental factors that can cause or exacerbate asthma. For each of the athletic settings where your athletes participate, consider the environmental factors that may cause or exacerbate an athlete's asthma and then detail steps you can take to minimize the influence of these factors.

3. Describe the components of a comprehensive asthma screening program and explain how each of these components can aid athletic trainers in identifying athletes with asthma or exercise-induced asthma (EIA).

4. Explain the pharmacologic and nonpharmacologic treatment strategies for managing asthma. In addition to understanding recommended pharmacologic and nonpharmacologic treatment strategies, what other responsibilities might an athletic trainer have in managing an athlete who has been diagnosed with asthma?

5. Detail an athletic trainer's roles and responsibilities when it comes to educating athletes about asthma.

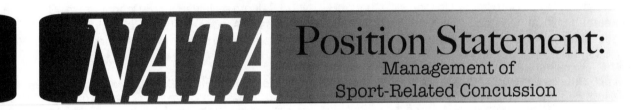

NATA Position Statement:
Management of
Sport-Related Concussion

In This Section: The popularity of contact sports is increasing, and athletic trainers need to be more educated than ever about concussions and other head injuries associated with contact sports. This position statement provides recommendations for management of sport-related concussion and other traumatic brain injuries.

National Athletic Trainers' Association Position Statement: Management of Sport-Related Concussion

Kevin M. Guskiewicz*; Scott L. Bruce†; Robert C. Cantu‡; Michael S. Ferrara§; James P. Kelly‖; Michael McCrea¶; Margot Putukian#; Tamara C. Valovich McLeod**

*University of North Carolina at Chapel Hill, Chapel Hill, NC; †California University of Pennsylvania, California, PA; ‡Emerson Hospital, Concord, MA; §University of Georgia, Athens, GA; ‖University of Colorado, Denver, CO; ¶Waukesha Memorial Hospital, Waukesha, WI; #Princeton University, Princeton, NJ; **Arizona School of Health Sciences, Mesa, AZ

Kevin M. Guskiewicz, PhD, ATC, FACSM; Scott L. Bruce, MS, ATC; Robert C. Cantu, MD, FACSM; Michael S. Ferrara, PhD, ATC; James P. Kelly, MD; Michael McCrea, PhD; Margot Putukian, MD, FACSM; and Tamara C. Valovich McLeod, PhD, ATC, CSCS, contributed to conception and design, acquisition and analysis and interpretation of the data; and drafting, critical revision, and final approval of the article.

Address correspondence to National Athletic Trainers' Association, Communications Department, 2952 Stemmons Freeway, Dallas, TX 75247.

Sport in today's society is more popular than probably ever imagined. Large numbers of athletes participate in a variety of youth, high school, collegiate, professional, and recreational sports. As sport becomes more of a fixture in the lives of Americans, a burden of responsibility falls on the shoulders of the various organizations, coaches, parents, clinicians, officials, and researchers to provide an environment that minimizes the risk of injury in all sports. For example, the research-based recommendations made for football between 1976 and 1980 resulted in a significant reduction in the incidence of fatalities and nonfatal catastrophic injuries. In 1968, 36 brain and cervical spine fatalities occurred in high school and collegiate football. The number had dropped to zero in 1990 and has averaged about 5 per year since then.[1] This decrease was attributed to a variety of factors, including (1) rule changes, which have outlawed spearing and butt blocking, (2) player education about the rule changes and the consequences of not following the rules, (3) implementation of equipment standards, (4) availability of alternative assessment techniques, (5) a marked reduction in physical contact time during practice sessions, (6) a heightened awareness among clinicians of the dangers involved in returning an athlete to competition too early, and (7) the athlete's awareness of the risks associated with concussion.

Research in the area of sport-related concussion has provided the athletic training and medical professions with valuable new knowledge in recent years. Certified athletic trainers, who on average care for 7 concussive injuries per year,[2] have been forced to rethink how they manage sport-related concussion. Recurrent concussions to several high-profile athletes, some of whom were forced into retirement as a result, have increased awareness among sports medicine personnel and the general public. Bridging the gap between research and clinical practice is the key to reducing the incidence and severity of sport-related concussion and improving return-to-play decisions. This position statement should provide valuable information and recommendations for certified athletic trainers (ATCs), physicians, and other medical professionals caring for athletes at the youth, high school, collegiate, and elite levels. The following recommendations are derived from the most recent scientific and clinic-based literature on sport-related concussion. The justification for these recommendations is presented in the summary statement following the recommendations. The summary statement is organized into the following sections: "Defining and Recognizing Concussion," "Evaluating and Making the Return-to-Play Decision," "Concussion Assessment Tools," "When to Refer an Athlete to a Physician After Concussion," "When to Disqualify an Athlete," "Special Considerations for the Young Athlete," "Home Care," and "Equipment Issues."

RECOMMENDATIONS

Defining and Recognizing Concussion

1. The ATC should develop a high sensitivity for the various mechanisms and presentations of traumatic brain injury (TBI), including mild, moderate, and severe cerebral concussion, as well as the more severe, but less common, head injuries that can cause damage to the brain stem and other vital centers of the brain.

2. The colloquial term "ding" should not be used to describe a sport-related concussion. This stunned confusional state is a concussion most often reflected by the athlete's initial confusion, which may disappear within minutes, leaving

no outwardly observable signs and symptoms. Use of the term "ding" generally carries a connotation that diminishes the seriousness of the injury. If an athlete shows concussion-like signs and reports symptoms after a contact to the head, the athlete has, *at the very least,* sustained a mild concussion and should be treated for a concussion.

3. To detect deteriorating signs and symptoms that may indicate a more serious head injury, the ATC should be able to recognize both the obvious signs (eg, fluctuating levels of consciousness, balance problems, and memory and concentration difficulties) and the more common, self-reported symptoms (eg, headache, ringing in the ears, and nausea).

4. The ATC should play an active role in educating athletes, coaches, and parents about the signs and symptoms associated with concussion, as well as the potential risks of playing while still symptomatic.

5. The ATC should document all pertinent information surrounding the concussive injury, including but not limited to (1) mechanism of injury; (2) initial signs and symptoms; (3) state of consciousness; (4) findings on serial testing of symptoms and neuropsychological function and postural-stability tests (noting any deficits compared with baseline); (5) instructions given to the athlete and/or parent; (6) recommendations provided by the physician; (7) date and time of the athlete's return to participation; and (8) relevant information on the player's history of prior concussion and associated recovery pattern(s).[3]

Evaluating and Making the Return-to-Play Decision

6. Working together, ATCs and team physicians should agree on a philosophy for managing sport-related concussion before the start of the athletic season. Currently 3 approaches are commonly used: (1) grading the concussion at the time of the injury, (2) deferring final grading until all symptoms have resolved, or (3) not using a grading scale but rather focusing attention on the athlete's recovery via symptoms, neurocognitive testing, and postural-stability testing. After deciding on an approach, the ATC-physician team should be consistent in its use regardless of the athlete, sport, or circumstances surrounding the injury.

7. For athletes playing sports with a high risk of concussion, baseline cognitive and postural-stability testing should be considered. In addition to the concussion injury assessment, the evaluation should also include an assessment of the cervical spine and cranial nerves to identify any cervical spine or vascular intracerebral injuries.

8. The ATC should record the time of the initial injury and document serial assessments of the injured athlete, noting the presence or absence of signs and symptoms of injury. The ATC should monitor vital signs and level of consciousness every 5 minutes after a concussion until the athlete's condition improves. The athlete should also be monitored over the next few days after the injury for the presence of delayed signs and symptoms and to assess recovery.

9. Concussion severity should be determined by paying close attention to the severity and persistence of *all* signs and symptoms, including the presence of amnesia (retrograde and anterograde) and loss of consciousness (LOC), as well as headache, concentration problems, dizziness, blurred

vision, and so on. It is recommended that ATCs and physicians consistently use a symptom checklist similar to the one provided in Appendix A.

10. In addition to a thorough clinical evaluation, formal cognitive and postural-stability testing is recommended to assist in objectively determining injury severity and readiness to return to play (RTP). No one test should be used solely to determine recovery or RTP, as concussion presents in many different ways.

11. Once symptom free, the athlete should be reassessed to establish that cognition and postural stability have returned to normal for that player, preferably by comparison with preinjury baseline test results. The RTP decision should be made after an incremental increase in activity with an initial cardiovascular challenge, followed by sport-specific activities that do not place the athlete at risk for concussion. The athlete can be released to full participation as long as no recurrent signs or symptoms are present.

Concussion Assessment Tools

12. Baseline testing on concussion assessment measures is recommended to establish the individual athlete's "normal" preinjury performance and to provide the most reliable benchmark against which to measure postinjury recovery. Baseline testing also controls for extraneous variables (eg, attention deficit disorder, learning disabilities, age, and education) and for the effects of earlier concussion while also evaluating the possible cumulative effects of recurrent concussions.

13. The use of objective concussion assessment tools will help ATCs more accurately identify deficits caused by injury and postinjury recovery and protect players from the potential risks associated with prematurely returning to competition and sustaining a repeat concussion. The concussion assessment battery should include a combination of tests for cognition, postural stability, and self-reported symptoms known to be affected by concussion.

14. A combination of brief screening tools appropriate for use on the sideline (eg, Standardized Assessment of Concussion [SAC], Balance Error Scoring System [BESS], symptom checklist) and more extensive measures (eg, neuropsychological testing, computerized balance testing) to more precisely evaluate recovery later after injury is recommended.

15. Before instituting a concussion neuropsychological testing battery, the ATC should understand the test's user requirements, copyright restrictions, and standardized instructions for administration and scoring. All evaluators should be appropriately trained in the standardized instructions for test administration and scoring before embarking on testing or adopting an instrument for clinical use. Ideally, the sports medicine team should include a neuropsychologist, but in reality, many ATCs may not have access to a neuropsychologist for interpretation and consultation, nor the financial resources to support a neuropsychological testing program. In this case, it is recommended that the ATC use screening instruments (eg, SAC, BESS, symptom checklist) that have been developed specifically for use by sports medicine clinicians without extensive

training in psychometric or standardized testing and that do not require a special license to administer or interpret.

16. Athletic trainers should adopt for clinical use only those neuropsychological and postural stability measures with population-specific normative data, test-retest reliability, clinical validity, and sufficient sensitivity and specificity established in the peer-reviewed literature. These standards provide the basis for how well the test can distinguish between those with and without cerebral dysfunction in order to reduce the possibility of false-positive and false-negative errors, which could lead to clinical decision-making errors.

17. As is the case with all clinical instruments, results from assessment measures to evaluate concussion should be integrated with all aspects of the injury evaluation (eg, physical examination, neurologic evaluation, neuroimaging, and player's history) for the most effective approach to injury management and RTP decision making. Decisions about an athlete's RTP should never be based solely on the use of any one test.

When to Refer an Athlete to a Physician After Concussion

18. The ATC or team physician should monitor an athlete with a concussion at 5-minute intervals from the time of the injury until the athlete's condition completely clears or the athlete is referred for further care. Coaches should be informed that in situations when a concussion is suspected but an ATC or physician is not available, their primary role is to ensure that the athlete is immediately seen by an ATC or physician.

19. An athlete with a concussion should be referred to a physician on the day of injury if he or she lost consciousness, experienced amnesia lasting longer than 15 minutes, or meets any of the criteria outlined in Appendix B.

20. A team approach to the assessment of concussion should be taken and include a variety of medical specialists. In addition to family practice or general medicine physician referrals, the ATC should secure other specialist referral sources within the community. For example, neurologists are trained to assist in the management of patients experiencing persistent signs and symptoms, including sleep disturbances. Similarly, a neuropsychologist should be identified as part of the sports medicine team for assisting athletes who require more extensive neuropsychological testing and for interpreting the results of neuropsychological tests.

21. A team approach should be used in making RTP decisions after concussion. This approach should involve input from the ATC, physician, athlete, and any referral sources. The assessment of all information, including the physical examination, imaging studies, objective tests, and exertional tests, should be considered prior to making an RTP decision.

When to Disqualify an Athlete

22. Athletes who are symptomatic at rest and after exertion for at least 20 minutes should be disqualified from returning to participation on the day of the injury. Exertional exercises should include sideline jogging followed by sprinting, sit-ups, push-ups, and any sport-specific, non-contact activities (or positions or stances) the athlete might need to perform on returning to participation. Athletes who return on the same day because symptoms resolved quickly (<20 minutes) should be monitored closely after they return to play. They should be repeatedly reevaluated on the sideline after the practice or game and again at 24 and 48 hours postinjury to identify any delayed onset of symptoms.

23. Athletes who experience LOC or amnesia should be disqualified from participating on the day of the injury.

24. The decision to disqualify from further participation on the day of a concussion should be based on a comprehensive physical examination; assessment of self-reported postconcussion signs and symptoms; functional impairments, and the athlete's past history of concussions. If assessment tools such as the SAC, BESS, neuropsychological test battery, and symptom checklist are not used, a 7-day symptom-free waiting period before returning to participation is recommended. Some circumstances, however, will warrant even more conservative treatment (see recommendation 25).

25. Athletic trainers should be more conservative with athletes who have a history of concussion. Athletes with a history of concussion are at increased risk for sustaining subsequent injuries as well as for slowed recovery of self-reported postconcussion signs and symptoms, cognitive dysfunction, and postural instability after subsequent injuries. In athletes with a history of 3 or more concussions and experiencing slowed recovery, temporary or permanent disqualification from contact sports may be indicated.

Special Considerations for the Young Athlete

26. Athletic trainers working with younger (pediatric) athletes should be aware that recovery may take longer than in older athletes. Additionally, these younger athletes are maturing at a relatively fast rate and will likely require more frequent updates of baseline measures compared with older athletes.

27. Many young athletes experience sport-related concussion. Athletic trainers should play an active role in helping to educate young athletes, their parents, and coaches about the dangers of repeated concussions. Continued research into the epidemiology of sport-related concussion in young athletes and prospective investigations to determine the acute and long-term effects of recurrent concussions in younger athletes are warranted.

28. Because damage to the maturing brain of a young athlete can be catastrophic (ie, almost all reported cases of second-impact syndrome are in young athletes), athletes under age 18 years should be managed more conservatively, using stricter RTP guidelines than those used to manage concussion in the more mature athlete.

Home Care

29. An athlete with a concussion should be instructed to avoid taking medications except acetaminophen after the injury. Acetaminophen and other medications should be given

only at the recommendation of a physician. Additionally, the athlete should be instructed to avoid ingesting alcohol, illicit drugs, or other substances that might interfere with cognitive function and neurologic recovery.

30. Any athlete with a concussion should be instructed to rest, but complete bed rest is not recommended. The athlete should resume normal activities of daily living as tolerated while avoiding activities that potentially increase symptoms. Once he or she is symptom free, the athlete may resume a graded program of physical and mental exertion, without contact or risk of concussion, up to the point at which postconcussion signs and symptoms recur. If symptoms appear, the exertion level should be scaled back to allow maximal activity without triggering symptoms.

31. An athlete with a concussion should be instructed to eat a well-balanced diet that is nutritious in both quality and quantity.

32. An athlete should be awakened during the night to check on deteriorating signs and symptoms only if he or she experienced LOC, had prolonged periods of amnesia, or was still experiencing significant symptoms at bedtime. The purpose of the wake-ups is to check for deteriorating signs and symptoms, such as decreased levels of consciousness or increasing headache, which could indicate a more serious head injury or a late-onset complication, such as an intracranial bleed.

33. Oral and written instructions for home care should be given to the athlete and to a responsible adult (eg, parent or roommate) who will observe and supervise the athlete during the acute phase of the concussion while at home or in the dormitory. The ATC and physician should agree on a standard concussion home-instruction form similar to the one presented in Appendix C, and it should be used consistently for all concussions.

Equipment Issues

34. The ATC should enforce the standard use of helmets for protecting against catastrophic head injuries and reducing the severity of cerebral concussions. In sports that require helmet protection (football, lacrosse, ice hockey, baseball/softball, etc), the ATC should ensure that all equipment meets either the National Operating Committee on Standards for Athletic Equipment (NOCSAE) or American Society for Testing and Materials (ASTM) standards.

35. The ATC should enforce the standard use of mouth guards for protection against dental injuries; however, there is no scientific evidence supporting their use for reducing concussive injury.

36. At this time, the ATC should neither endorse nor discourage the use of soccer headgear for protecting against concussion or the consequences of cumulative, subconcussive impacts to the head. Currently no scientific evidence supports the use of headgear in soccer for reducing concussive injury to the head.

DEFINING AND RECOGNIZING CONCUSSION

Perhaps the most challenging aspect of managing sport-related concussion is recognizing the injury, especially in athletes with no obvious signs that a concussion has actually occurred. The immediate management of the head-injured athlete depends on the nature and severity of the injury. Several terms are used to describe this injury, the most global being TBI, which can be classified into 2 types: focal and diffuse. Focal or posttraumatic intracranial mass lesions include subdural hematomas, epidural hematomas, cerebral contusions, and intracerebral hemorrhages and hematomas. These are considered uncommon in sport but are serious injuries; the ATC must be able to detect signs of clinical deterioration or worsening symptoms during serial assessments. Signs and symptoms of these focal vascular emergencies can include LOC, cranial nerve deficits, mental status deterioration, and worsening symptoms. Concern for a significant focal injury should also be raised if these signs or symptoms occur after an initial lucid period in which the athlete seemed normal.

Diffuse brain injuries can result in widespread or global disruption of neurologic function and are not usually associated with macroscopically visible brain lesions except in the most severe cases. Most diffuse injuries involve an acceleration-deceleration motion, either within a linear plane or in a rotational direction or both. In these cases, lesions are caused by the brain being shaken within the skull.[4,5] The brain is suspended within the skull in cerebrospinal fluid (CSF) and has several dural attachments to bony ridges that make up the inner contours of the skull. With a linear acceleration-deceleration mechanism (side to side or front to back), the brain experiences a sudden momentum change that can result in tissue damage. The key elements of injury mechanism are the velocity of the head before impact, the time over which the force is applied, and the magnitude of the force.[4,5] Rotational acceleration-deceleration injuries are believed to be the primary injury mechanism for the most severe diffuse brain injuries. Structural diffuse brain injury (diffuse axonal injury [DAI]) is the most severe type of diffuse injury because axonal disruption occurs, typically resulting in disturbance of cognitive functions, such as concentration and memory. In its most severe form, DAI can disrupt the brain-stem centers responsible for breathing, heart rate, and wakefulness.[4,5]

Cerebral concussion, which is the focus of this position statement, can best be classified as a mild diffuse injury and is often referred to as mild TBI (MTBI). The injury involves an acceleration-deceleration mechanism in which a blow to the head or the head striking an object results in 1 or more of the following conditions: headache, nausea, vomiting, dizziness, balance problems, feeling "slowed down," fatigue, trouble sleeping, drowsiness, sensitivity to light or noise, LOC, blurred vision, difficulty remembering, or difficulty concentrating.[6] In 1966, the Congress of Neurological Surgeons proposed the following consensus definition of concussion, subsequently endorsed by a variety of medical associations: "Concussion is a clinical syndrome characterized by immediate and transient impairment of neural functions, such as alteration of consciousness, disturbance of vision, equilibrium, etc, due to mechanical forces."[7] Although the definition received widespread consensus in 1966, more contemporary opinion (as concluded at the First International Conference on Concussion in Sport, Vienna, 2001[8]) was that this definition fails to include many of the predominant clinical features of concussion, such as headache and nausea. It is often reported that there is no universal agreement on the standard definition or nature of concussion; however, agreement does exist on several features that incorporate clinical, pathologic, and biomechanical injury constructs associated with head injury:

1. Concussion may be caused by a direct blow to the head or elsewhere on the body from an "impulsive" force transmitted to the head.
2. Concussion may cause an immediate and short-lived impairment of neurologic function.
3. Concussion may cause neuropathologic changes; however, the acute clinical symptoms largely reflect a functional disturbance rather than a structural injury.
4. Concussion may cause a gradient of clinical syndromes that may or may not involve LOC. Resolution of the clinical and cognitive symptoms typically follows a sequential course.
5. Concussion is most often associated with normal results on conventional neuroimaging studies.[8]

Occasionally, players sustain a blow to the head resulting in a stunned confusional state that resolves within minutes. The colloquial term "ding" is often used to describe this initial state. However, the use of this term is not recommended because this stunned confusional state is still considered a concussion resulting in symptoms, although only very short in duration, that should not be dismissed in a cavalier fashion. It is essential that this injury be reevaluated frequently to determine if a more serious injury has occurred, because often the evolving signs and symptoms of a concussion are not evident until several minutes to hours later.

Although it is important for the ATC to recognize and eventually classify the concussive injury, it is equally important for the athlete to understand the signs and symptoms of a concussion as well as the potential negative consequences (eg, second-impact syndrome and predisposition to future concussions) of not reporting a concussive injury. Once the athlete has a better understanding of the injury, he or she can provide a more accurate report of the concussion history.

Mechanisms of Injury

A forceful blow to the resting, movable head usually produces maximum brain injury beneath the point of cranial impact (coup injury). A moving head hitting an unyielding object usually produces maximum brain injury opposite the site of cranial impact (contrecoup injury) as the brain shifts within the cranium. When the head is accelerated before impact, the brain lags toward the trailing surface, thus squeezing away the CSF and creating maximal shearing forces at this site. This brain lag actually thickens the layer of CSF under the point of impact, which explains the lack of coup injury in the moving head. Alternatively, when the head is stationary before impact, neither brain lag nor disproportionate distribution of CSF occurs, accounting for the absence of contrecoup injury and the presence of coup injury.[4,5]

No scientific evidence suggests that one type of injury (coup or contrecoup) is more serious than the other or that symptoms present any differently. Many sport-related concussions are the result of a combined coup-contrecoup mechanism, involving damage to the brain on both the side of initial impact and the opposite side of the brain due to brain lag. Regardless of whether the athlete has sustained a coup, contrecoup, or combined coup-contrecoup injury, the ATC should manage the injury the same.

Three types of stresses can be generated by an applied force to injure the brain: compressive, tensile, and shearing. Compression involves a crushing force in which the tissue cannot absorb any additional force or load. Tension involves pulling or stretching of tissue, whereas shearing involves a force that moves across the parallel organization of the tissue. Brief, uniform compressive stresses are fairly well tolerated by neural tissue, but tension and shearing stresses are very poorly tolerated.[4,9]

Neuroimaging of Cerebral Concussion

Traditionally, computed tomography (CT) and magnetic resonance imaging (MRI) have been considered useful in identifying certain types of brain lesions; however, they have been of little value in assessing less severe head injuries, such as cerebral concussion, and contributing to the RTP decision. A CT scan is often indicated emergently if a focal injury such as an acute subdural or epidural bleed is suspected; this study easily demonstrates acute blood collection and skull fracture, but an MRI is superior at demonstrating an isodense subacute or chronic subdural hematoma that may be weeks old.[10,11] Newer structural MRI modalities, including gradient echo, perfusion, and diffusion-weighted imaging, are more sensitive for structural abnormalities (eg, vascular shearing) compared with other diagnostic imaging techniques.[10] Functional imaging technologies (eg, positron emission tomography [PET], single-photon emission computerized tomography [SPECT], and functional MRI [fMRI]) are also yielding promising early results and may help define concussion recovery.[12] Presently, no neuroanatomic or physiologic measurements can be used to determine the severity of a concussion or when complete recovery has occurred in an individual athlete after a concussion.

EVALUATING AND MAKING THE RETURN-TO-PLAY DECISION

Clinical Evaluation

Results from a thorough clinical examination conducted by both the ATC and the physician cannot be overlooked and should be considered very important pieces of the concussion puzzle. These evaluations should include a thorough *history* (including number and severity of previous head injuries), *observation* (including pupil responses), *palpation,* and *special tests* (including simple tests of memory, concentration, and coordination and a cranial nerve assessment). In many situations, a physician will not be present at the time of the concussion, and the ATC will be forced to act on behalf of the sports medicine team. More formal neuropsychological testing and postural-stability testing should be viewed as adjuncts to the initial clinical and repeat evaluations (see "Concussion Assessment Tools"). The ATC-physician team must also consider referral options to specialists such as neurologists, neurosurgeons, neuropsychologists, and neuro-otologists, depending on the injury severity and situation. Referrals for imaging tests such as CT, MRI, or electronystagmography are also options that sometimes can aid in the diagnosis and/or management of sport-related concussion but are typically used only in cases involving LOC, severe amnesia, abnormal physical or neurologic findings, or increasing or intensified symptoms.

Determining Injury Severity

The definition of concussion is often expanded to include mild, moderate, and severe injuries. Several early grading scales and RTP guidelines early were proposed for classifying and managing cerebral concussions.[6,13–20] None of the scales have been universally accepted or followed with much consistency by the sports medicine community. In addition, most of these classification systems denote the most severe injuries as associated with LOC, which we now know is not always predictive of recovery after a brain injury.[21,22] It is important for the ATC and other health care providers to recognize the importance of identifying retrograde amnesia and anterograde amnesia, LOC, and other signs and symptoms present and to manage each episode independently.

The ATC must recognize that no 2 concussions are identical and that the resulting symptoms can be very different, depending on the force of the blow to the head, the degree of metabolic dysfunction, the tissue damage and duration of time needed to recover, the number of previous concussions, and the time between injuries. All these factors must be considered when managing an athlete suffering from cerebral concussion.[3] The 2 most recognizable signs of a concussion are LOC and amnesia; yet, as previously mentioned, neither is required for an injury to be classified as a concussion. A 2000 study of 1003 concussions sustained by high school and collegiate football players revealed that LOC and amnesia presented infrequently, 9% and 27% of all cases, respectively, whereas other signs and symptoms, such as headache, dizziness, confusion, disorientation, and blurred vision, were much more common.[23] After the initial concussion evaluation, the ATC should determine whether the athlete requires more advanced medical intervention on an emergent basis or whether the team physician should be contacted for an RTP decision (Appendix B). It may be helpful if the injury is graded throughout the process, but this grading is likely to be more important for treating subsequent injuries than the current injury.

Most grading systems rely heavily on LOC and amnesia as indicators of injury severity. Recent research, however, suggests that these 2 factors, either alone or in combination, are not good predictors of injury severity. A number of authors have documented no association between brief (<1 minute) LOC and abnormalities on neuropsychological testing at 48 hours, raising concern for brief LOC as a predictor of recovery after concussion.[8,22,24–27] Studies involving high school and collegiate athletes with concussion revealed no association between (1) LOC and duration of symptoms or (2) LOC and neuropsychological and balance tests at 3, 24, 48, 72, and 96 hours postinjury.[21,28,29] In other words, athletes experiencing LOC were similar to athletes without LOC on these same injury-severity markers.

With respect to amnesia, the issue is more clouded because findings have been inconsistent. Several studies of nonathletes[30–37] suggest that the duration of posttraumatic amnesia correlates with the severity and outcome of severe TBI but not with mild TBI or concussion.[38–40] More contemporary studies of athletes with concussion are also clouded. Two unrelated, prospective studies of concussion suggest that the presence of amnesia best correlates with abnormal neuropsychological testing at 48 hours and with the duration and number of other postconcussion signs and symptoms.[24,41] However, more recently, investigations of high school and collegiate athletes with concussion revealed no association between (1) amnesia and duration of symptoms or (2) amnesia and neuropsychological and balance tests at 3, 24, 48, 72, and 96 hours postinjury.[21,28,29] Of importance in these studies is the significant association between symptom-severity score (within the initial 3 hours postinjury) and the total duration of symptoms (mea-

Table 1. American Academy of Neurology Concussion Grading Scale[6]

Grade 1 (mild)	Transient confusion; no LOC*; symptoms and mental status abnormalities resolve <15 min
Grade 2 (moderate)	Transient confusion; no LOC; symptoms and mental status abnormalities last >15 min
Grade 3 (severe)	Any LOC

*LOC indicates loss of consciousness.

sured until asymptomatic). Although these findings suggest that initial symptom severity is probably a better indicator than either LOC or amnesia in predicting length of recovery, amnesia was recently found to predict symptom and neurocognitive deficits at 2 days postinjury.[42] More research is needed in this area to help improve clinical decision making.

It has been suggested that LOC and amnesia, especially when prolonged, should not be ignored,[43,44] but evidence for their usefulness in establishing RTP guidelines is scarce. Loss of consciousness, whether it occurs immediately or after an initially lucid interval, is important in that it may signify a more serious vascular brain injury. Other postconcussion signs and symptoms should be specifically addressed for presence and duration when the ATC is evaluating the athlete. Determining whether a cervical spine injury has occurred is also of major importance because it is often associated with head injury and should not be missed. If the athlete complains of neck pain or has cervical spine tenderness, cervical spine immobilization should be considered. If a cervical spine injury is ruled out and the athlete is taken to the sideline, a thorough clinical examination should follow, including a complete neurologic examination and cognitive evaluation. The ATC must note the time of the injury and then maintain a timed assessment form to follow the athlete's symptoms and examinations serially. It is often difficult to pay attention to the time that has passed after an injury. Therefore, it is important for one member of the medical team to track time during the evaluation process and record all pertinent information. After an initial evaluation, the clinician must determine whether the injured athlete requires more advanced medical intervention and eventually grade the injury and make an RTP decision that can occur within minutes, hours, days, or weeks of the injury.

There are currently 3 approaches to grading sport-related concussion. One approach is to grade the concussion at the time of the injury on the basis of the signs and symptoms present at the time of the concussion and within the first 15 minutes after injury. The American Academy of Neurology Concussion Grading Scale (Table 1)[6] has been widely used with this approach. It permits the ATC to grade the injury primarily on the basis of LOC and to provide the athlete, coach, and parent with an estimation of injury severity. A disadvantage to this approach is that many injuries behave differently than expected on initial evaluation, potentially creating more difficulties with the athlete, coach, or parent and making the RTP decision more challenging. Another approach is to grade the concussion on the basis of the presence and overall duration of symptoms. This approach is best addressed using the Cantu Evidence-Based Grading Scale (Table 2),[43] which guides the ATC to grade the injury only after all concussion signs and symptoms have resolved. This scale places less emphasis on LOC as a potential predictor of subsequent impairment and additional weight on overall symptom dura-

Table 2. Cantu Evidence-Based Grading System for Concussion[43]

Grade 1 (mild)	No LOC*, PTA† <30 min, PCSS‡ <24 h
Grade 2 (moderate)	LOC <1 min **or** PTA ≥30 min <24 h **or** PCSS ≥24 h <7 d
Grade 3 (severe)	LOC ≥1 min **or** PTA ≥24 h **or** PCSS ≥7 d

*LOC indicates loss of consciousness.
†PTA indicates posttraumatic amnesia (anterograde/retrograde).
‡PCSS indicates postconcussion signs and symptoms other than amnesia.

tion.[3,43] Finally, a third approach to the grading-scale dilemma is to not use a grading scale but rather focus attention on the athlete's recovery via symptoms, neuropsychological tests, and postural-stability tests. This line of thinking is that the ATC should not place too much emphasis on the grading system or grade but should instead focus on whether the athlete is symptomatic or symptom free. Once the athlete is asymptomatic, a stepwise progression should be implemented that increases demands over several days. This progression will be different for athletes who are withheld for several weeks compared with those athletes withheld for just a few days. This multitiered approach was summarized and supported by consensus at the 2001 Vienna Conference on Concussion in Sport.[8]

Making the Return-to-Play Decision

The question raised most often regarding the concussion grading and RTP systems is one of practicality in the sport setting. Many clinicians believe that the RTP guidelines are too conservative and, therefore, choose to base decisions on clinical judgment of individual cases rather than on a general recommendation. It has been reported that 30% of all high school and collegiate football players sustaining concussions return to competition on the same day of injury; the remaining 70% average 4 days of rest before returning to participation.[23] Many RTP guidelines call for the athlete to be symptom free for at least 7 days before returning to participation after a grade 1 or 2 concussion.[6,13,15,17,43,44] Although many clinicians deviate from these recommendations and are more liberal in making RTP decisions, recent studies by Guskiewicz and McCrea et al[21,29] suggest that perhaps the 7-day waiting period can minimize the risk of recurrent injury. On average, athletes required 7 days to fully recover after concussion. Same-season repeat injuries typically take place within a short window of time, 7 to 10 days after the first concussion,[21] supporting the concept that there may be increased neuronal vulnerability or blood-flow changes during that time, similar to those reported by Giza, Hovda, et al[45–47] in animal models.

Returning an athlete to participation should follow a progression that begins once the athlete is completely symptom free. All signs and symptoms should be evaluated using a graded symptom scale or checklist (described in "Concussion Assessment Tools") when performing follow-up assessments and should be evaluated both at rest and after exertional maneuvers such as biking, jogging, sit-ups, and push-ups. Baseline measurements of neuropsychological and postural stability are strongly recommended for comparing with postinjury measurements. If these exertional tests do not produce symptoms, either acutely or in delayed fashion, the athlete can then participate in sport-specific skills that allow return to practice but should remain out of any activities that put him or her at risk for recurrent head injury. For the basketball player, this may

include shooting baskets or participating in walk-throughs, and for the soccer player, this may include dribbling or shooting drills or other sport-specific activities. These restricted and monitored activities should be continued for the first few days after becoming symptom free. The athlete should be monitored periodically throughout and after these sessions to determine if any symptoms develop or increase in intensity. Before returning to full contact participation, the athlete should be reassessed using neuropsychological and postural-stability tests if available. If all scores have returned to baseline or better, return to full participation can be considered after further clinical evaluation. It is strongly recommended that after recurrent injury, especially within-season repeat injuries, the athlete be withheld for an extended period of time (approximately 7 days) after symptoms have resolved.

CONCUSSION ASSESSMENT TOOLS

Sports medicine clinicians are increasingly using standardized methods to obtain a more objective measurement of postconcussion signs and symptoms, cognitive dysfunction, and postural instability. These methods allow the clinician to quantify the severity of injury and measure the player's progress over the course of postinjury recovery. An emerging model of sport concussion assessment involves the use of brief screening tools to evaluate postconcussion signs and symptoms, cognitive functioning, and postural stability on the sideline immediately after a concussion and neuropsychological testing to track recovery further out from the time of injury. Ultimately, these tests, when interpreted with the physical examination and other aspects of the injury evaluation, assist the ATC and other sports medicine professionals in the RTP decision-making process.

Data from objective measures of cognitive functioning, postural stability, and postconcussion signs and symptoms are most helpful in making a determination about severity of injury and postinjury recovery when preinjury baseline data for an individual athlete are available.[3,8,24,29,41] Baseline testing provides an indicator of what is "normal" for that particular athlete while also establishing the most accurate and reliable benchmark against which postinjury results can be compared. It is important to obtain a baseline symptom assessment in addition to baseline cognitive and other ability testing. Without baseline measures, the athlete's postinjury performance on neuropsychological testing and other concussion assessment measures must be interpreted by comparison with available population normative values, which ideally are based on a large sample of the representative population. Normative data for competitive athletes on conventional (ie, paper-and-pencil) and computerized neuropsychological tests and other concussion assessment measures are now more readily available from large-scale research studies, but baseline data on an individual athlete still provide the greatest clinical accuracy in interpreting postinjury test results. When performing baseline testing, a suitable testing environment eliminates all distractions that could alter the baseline performance and enhances the likelihood that all athletes are providing maximal effort. Most important, all evaluators should be aware of a test's user requirements and be appropriately trained in the standardized instructions for test administration and scoring before embarking on baseline testing or adopting a concussion testing paradigm for clinical use.

Several models exist for implementing baseline testing. Ideally, preseason baseline testing is conducted before athletes are exposed to the risk of concussion during sport participation (eg, before contact drills during football). Some programs choose to conduct baseline testing as part of the preparticipation physical examination process. In this model, stations are established for various testing methods (eg, history collection, symptom assessment, neuropsychological testing, and balance testing), and athletes complete the evaluation sequence after being seen by the attending physician or ATC. This approach has the advantage of testing large groups of athletes in 1 session, while they are already in the mindset of undergoing a preseason physical examination. When preseason examinations are not conducted in a systematic group arrangement, alternative approaches can be considered. In any case, it is helpful to conduct all modules of baseline testing on players in 1 session to limit the complications of scheduling multiple testing times and to keep testing conditions constant for the athletes. One should allow adequate planning time (eg, 3 months) to implement a baseline testing module. Often this equates to conducting baseline testing for fall sports during the spring semester, before school is recessed for the summer. The benefits of interpreting postinjury data for an athlete after a concussion far outweigh the considerable time and human resources dedicated to baseline testing.

Collecting histories on individual athletes is also a vital part of baseline testing, especially in establishing whether the athlete has any history of concussion, neurologic disorder, or other remarkable medical conditions. Specifically with respect to concussion, it is important to establish (1) whether the player has any history of concussions and, if so, how many and (2) injury characteristics of previous concussions (eg, LOC, amnesia, symptoms, recovery time, time lost from participation, and medical treatment). For athletes with a history of multiple concussions, it is also important to clarify any apparent pattern of (1) concussions occurring as a result of lighter impacts, (2) concussions occurring closer together in time, (3) a lengthier recovery time with successive concussions, and (4) a less complete recovery with each injury. Documenting a history of attentional disorders, learning disability, or other cognitive development disorders is also critical, especially in interpreting an individual player's baseline and postinjury performance on neuropsychological testing. If resources do not allow for preseason examinations in all athletes, at least a concerted effort to evaluate those athletes with a previous history of concussion should be made because of the awareness of increased risk for subsequent concussions in this group.

Postconcussion Symptom Assessment

Self-reported symptoms are among the more obvious and recognizable ways to assess the effects of concussion. Typical self-reported symptoms after a concussion include but are not limited to headache; dizziness; nausea; vomiting; feeling "in a fog"; feeling "slowed down"; trouble falling asleep; sleeping more than usual; fatigue; drowsiness; sensitivity to light or noise; unsteadiness or loss of balance; feeling "dinged," dazed, or stunned; seeing stars or flashing lights; ringing in the ears; and double vision.[8,26,48] Self-reported symptoms are referenced by many of the concussion grading scales.[10,43,44,49] The presence of self-reported symptoms serves as a major contraindication for RTP, and, based on current recommendations, the athlete should be fully symptom free for at least 7 days at rest and during exertion before returning to play.[43,44]

A number of concussion symptom checklists[43,50–52] and scales[26,41,48,53] have been used in both research and clinical settings. A symptom checklist that provides a list of concussion-related symptoms allows the athlete to report whether the symptom is present by responding either "yes" (experiencing the symptom) or "no" (not experiencing the symptom). A symptom scale is a summative measure that allows the athlete to describe the extent to which he or she is experiencing the symptom. These instruments commonly incorporate a Likert-type scale that allows the player to rate the severity or frequency of postconcussion symptoms. These scores are then summed to form a composite score that yields a quantitative measure of overall injury severity and a benchmark against which to track postinjury symptom recovery. Initial evidence has been provided for the structural validity of a self-report concussion symptom scale.[48] Obtaining a baseline symptom score is helpful to establish any preexisting symptoms attributable to factors other than the head injury (eg, illness, fatigue, or somatization). Serial administration of the symptom checklist is the recommended method of tracking symptom resolution over time (see Appendix A).

Mental Status Screening

Cognitive screening instruments similar to the physician's mini mental status examination objectify what is often a subjective impression of cognitive abnormalities. Various methods have been suggested for a systematic survey of mental status and cognitive function in the athlete with a concussion. The SAC was developed to provide sports medicine clinicians with a brief, objective tool for assessing the injured athlete's mental status during the acute period after concussion (eg, sport sideline, locker room, and clinic).[54] The SAC includes measures of orientation, immediate memory, concentration, and delayed recall that sum to 30 points.[55] Lower scores on the SAC indicate more severe cognitive impairment. The SAC also includes assessments of strength, sensation, and coordination and a standard neurologic examination but should not replace the clinician's thorough physical examination or referral for more extensive neuropsychological evaluation when indicated. Information about the occurrence and duration of LOC and amnesia is also recorded on the SAC. Alternate forms of the SAC are available to minimize the practice effects during retesting. The SAC takes about 5 minutes to administer and should be used only after the clinician's thorough review of the training manual and instructional video on the administration, scoring, and interpretation of the instrument.

The SAC has demonstrated reliability[29,55,56] and validity[29,56,57] in detecting mental status changes after a concussion. Recent evidence suggests that a decline of 1 point or more from baseline classified injured and uninjured players with a level of 94% sensitivity and 76% specificity.[56] The SAC is also sensitive to detecting more severe neurocognitive changes in injured athletes with LOC or amnesia associated with their concussions.[57] The SAC is most useful in the assessment of acute cognitive dysfunction resulting from concussion, with sensitivity and specificity comparable with extensive neuropsychological testing batteries during the initial 2 to 3 days after concussion.[29,58,59] As with neuropsychological testing, sensitivity and specificity of the SAC in concussion assessment are maximized when individual baseline test data are available.[29,55,56,60]

Postural-Stability Assessment

A number of postural-stability tests have been used to assess the effects of concussion in the clinical and laboratory settings. The Romberg and stork stand were basic tests used to assess balance and coordination. Riemann et al[61–62] developed the Balance Error Scoring System (BESS) based on existing theories of posturography. The BESS uses 3 stance positions and tests on both a firm and a foam surface with the eyes closed (for a total of 6 trials). The administration and scoring procedures are found in several publications.[61–63] The BESS has established good test-retest reliability and good concurrent validity when compared with laboratory forceplate measures[52,62] and significant group differences, with an increased number of errors for days 1, 3, and 5 postinjury when compared with controls.[52] Thus, the BESS can be used as a clinical measure in identifying balance impairment that could indicate a neurologic deficit.

The NeuroCom Smart Balance Master System (NeuroCom International, Clackamas, OR) is a forceplate system that measures vertical ground reaction forces produced by the body's center of gravity moving around a fixed base of support. The Sensory Organization Test (SOT, NeuroCom International) is designed to disrupt various sensory systems, including the visual, somatosensory, and vestibular systems. The SOT consists of 6 conditions with 3 trials per condition, for a total of 18 trials, with each trial lasting 20 seconds. The complete administration has been described previously.[52,64] The SOT has produced significant findings related to the assessment of concussion recovery. In a sample of 36 athletes with concussion, the mean stability (composite score) and vestibular and visual ratios demonstrated deficits for up to 5 days postinjury.[52] The greatest deficits were seen 24 hours postinjury, and the athletes with concussion demonstrated a gradual recovery during the 5-day period to within 6% of baseline scores. These results were confirmed by Peterson et al,[65] who found that these deficits continued for up to 10 days after concussion. These findings reveal a sensory interaction problem from the effects of concussion with measurable changes in overall postural stability.

Neuropsychological Testing

Neuropsychological testing has historically been used to evaluate various cognitive domains known to be preferentially susceptible to the effects of concussion and TBI. In recent years, neuropsychological testing to evaluate the effects of sport-related concussion has gained much attention in the sport concussion literature.[20,21,26,29,48,52,58,59,65–69] The work of Barth et al,[70] who studied more than 2000 collegiate football players from 10 universities, was the first project to institute baseline neuropsychological testing. Similar programs are now commonplace among many collegiate and professional teams, and interest is growing at the high school level. Several recent studies have supported the use of neuropsychological testing as a valuable tool to evaluate the cognitive effects and recovery after sport-related concussion,[24,28,29,41,42,50–52,57,65,66,71–75] but its feasibility for sideline use is not likely realistic. As is the case with other concussion assessment tools, baseline neuropsychological testing is recommended, when possible, to establish a normative level of neurocognitive functioning for individual athletes.[24,28,29,41,50–52,57–59,66,69,73–75] Baseline neuropsychological testing typically takes 20 to 30 minutes per athlete.

Before implementing a neuropsychological testing program, the ATC must consider several issues, including test-specific training requirements and methodologic issues, the practicality of baseline testing, the reliability and validity of individual tests comprising the test battery, and the protocol for interpretation of the postinjury test results. Barr[76] provided an excellent review on the methodologic and professional issues associated with neuropsychological testing in sport concussion assessment. Most states require advanced training and licensure to purchase and use neuropsychological tests for clinical purposes. Neuropsychological tests are also copyright protected to prevent inappropriate distribution or use by unqualified professionals. At present, these requirements necessitate that a licensed psychologist, preferably one Board certified in clinical neuropsychology or with clinical experience in the evaluation of sport-related concussion, oversee and supervise the clinical application of neuropsychological testing for sport concussion assessment. These factors likely restrict how widely neuropsychological testing can be used to assess sport-related concussion, especially at the high school level and in rural areas where neuropsychologists are not readily available for consultation.

Neuropsychologists, ATCs, and sports medicine clinicians are faced with the challenge of designing a model that jointly upholds the testing standards of neuropsychology and meets the clinical needs of the sports medicine community without undue burden. The cost of neuropsychological testing, either conventional or computerized, is also a factor in how widely this method can be implemented, especially at the high school level. Consultation fees for the neuropsychologist can be considerable if work is not done on a pro bono basis, and some computerized testing companies charge a consulting fee for interpreting postinjury test results by telephone.

Although no clear indications exist as to which are the best individual neuropsychological tests to evaluate sport concussion, the use of multiple instruments as a "test battery" offers clinicians greater potential for recognizing any cognitive deficits incurred from the injury. A number of neuropsychological tests and test batteries have been used to assess sport-related concussion. Table 3 provides a brief description of the paper-and-pencil neuropsychological tests commonly used by neuropsychologists in the assessment of sport concussion. Sport concussion batteries should include measures of cognitive abilities most susceptible to change after concussion, including attention and concentration, cognitive processing (speed and efficiency), learning and memory, working memory, executive functioning, and verbal fluency. Tests of attention and concentration[50,52,74,77] and memory functioning[41] have been reported as the most sensitive to the acute effects of concussion. The athlete's age, sex, primary language, and level of education should be considered when selecting a test battery.[68]

Computerized Neuropsychological Tests. Recently, a number of computerized neuropsychological testing programs have been designed for the assessment of athletes after concussion. The Automated Neuropsychological Assessment Metrics (ANAM), CogSport, Concussion Resolution Index, and Immediate Postconcussion Assessment and Cognitive Testing (ImPACT) are all currently available and have shown promise for reliable and valid concussion assessment (Table 4).[24,41,51,53,66,71,72,75,78–84] The primary advantages to computerized testing are the ease of administration, ability to baseline test a large number of athletes in a short period of time, and multiple forms used within the testing paradigm to reduce the

Table 3. Common Neuropsychological Tests Used in Sport Concussion Assessment

Neuropsychological Test	Cognitive Domain
Controlled Oral Word Association Test	Verbal fluency
Hopkins Verbal Learning Test	Verbal learning, immediate and delayed memory
Trail Making: Parts A and B	Visual scanning, attention, information processing speed, psychomotor speed
Wechsler Letter Number Sequencing Test	Verbal working memory
Wechsler Digit Span: Digits Forward and Digits Backward	Attention, concentration
Wechsler Digit Symbol Test	Psychomotor speed, attention, concentration
Symbol Digit Modalities Test	Psychomotor speed, attention, concentration
Paced Auditory Serial Addition Test	Attention, concentration
Stroop Color Word Test	Attention, information processing speed

practice effects. Collie et al[71] summarized the advantage and disadvantages of computerized versus traditional paper-and-pencil testing.

As outlined, in the case of conventional neuropsychological testing, several of the same challenges must be addressed before computerized testing becomes a widely used method of sport concussion assessment. Issues requiring further consideration include demonstrated test reliability; validity, sensitivity, and specificity in the peer-reviewed literature; required user training and qualifications; the necessary role of the licensed psychologist for clinical interpretation of postinjury test results; hardware and software issues inherent to computerized testing; and user costs.[71] Progress is being made on many of these issues, but further clinical research is required

to provide clinicians with the most effective neuropsychological assessment tools and maintain the testing standards of neuropsychology.

Neuropsychological Testing Methods. Neuropsychological testing is not a tool that should be used to diagnose the injury (ie, concussion); however, it can be very useful in measuring recovery once it has been determined that a concussion has occurred. The point(s) at which postinjury neuropsychological testing should occur has been a topic of debate. A variety of testing formats has been used to evaluate short-term recovery from concussion.[24,41,50,73,75,82] Two approaches are most common. The first incorporates neuropsychological testing only after the injured player reports that his or her symptoms are completely gone. This approach is based on the conceptual foundation that an athlete should not participate while symptomatic, regardless of neuropsychological test performance. Unnecessary serial neuropsychological testing, in addition to being burdensome and costly to the athlete and medical staff, also introduces practice effects that may confound the interpretation of performance in subsequent postinjury testing sessions.[85] The second approach incorporates neuropsychological testing at fixed time points (eg, postinjury day 1, day 7, and so on) to track postinjury recovery. This approach is often appropriate for prospective research protocols but is unnecessary in a clinical setting when the player is still symptomatic and will be withheld from competition regardless of the neuropsychological test results. In this model, serial testing can be used until neuropsychological testing returns to normal, preinjury levels and the player is completely symptom free.

Measuring "recovery" on neuropsychological tests and other clinical instruments is often a complex statistical matter, further complicated by practice effects and other psychometric dynamics affected by serial testing, even when preinjury baseline data are available for individual athletes. The use of statistical models that empirically identify meaningful change while controlling for practice effects on serial testing may provide the clinician with the most precise benchmark in deter-

Table 4. Computerized Neuropsychological Tests

Neuropsychological Test	Developer (Contact Information)	Cognitive Domains
Automated Neuropsychological Assessment Metrics (ANAM)	National Rehabilitation Hospital Assistive Technology and Neuroscience Center, Washington, DC[84] (jsb2@mhg.edu)	Simple Reaction Metrics Sternberg Memory Math Processing Continuous Performance Matching to Sample Spatial Processing Code Substitution
CogSport	CogState Ltd, Victoria, Australia (www.cogsport.com)	Simple Reaction Time Complex Reaction Time One-Back Continuous Learning
Concussion Resolution Index	HeadMinder Inc, New York, NY (www.headminder.com)	Reaction Time Cued Reaction Time Visual Recognition 1 Visual Recognition 2 Animal Decoding Symbol Scanning
Immediate Postconcussion Assessment and Cognitive Testing (ImPACT)	University of Pittsburgh Medical Center, Pittsburgh, PA (www.impacttest.com)	Verbal Memory Visual Memory Information Processing Speed Reaction Time Impulse Control

Table 5. Factors Influencing Neuropsychological Test Performance[68]*

Previous concussions
Educational background
Preinjury level of cognitive functioning
Cultural background
Age
Test anxiety
Distractions
Sleep deprivation
Medications, alcohol, or drugs
Psychiatric disorders
Learning disability
Attention deficit/hyperactivity
Certain medical conditions
Primary language other than English
Previous neuropsychological testing

*Reprinted with permission of Grindel SH, Lovell MR, Collins MW. The assessment of sport-related concussion: the evidence behind neuropsychological testing and management. *Clin J Sport Med.* 2001; 11: 134–143.

mining postinjury recovery, above and beyond the simple conclusion that the player is "back to baseline." The complexity of this analysis is the basis for the neuropsychologist overseeing the clinical interpretation of test data to determine injury severity and recovery. Further research is required to clarify the guidelines for determining and tracking recovery on specific measures after concussion. The clinician should also be aware that any concussion assessment tool, either brief screening instruments or more extensive neuropsychological testing, comes with some degree of risk for false negatives (eg, a player performs within what would be considered the normal range on the measure before actually reaching a complete clinical recovery after concussion). Therefore, test results should always be interpreted in the context of all clinical information, including the player's medical history. Also, caution should be exercised in neuropsychological test interpretation when preinjury baseline data do not exist. Numerous factors apart from the direct effects of concussion can influence test performance (Table 5).

WHEN TO REFER AN ATHLETE TO A PHYSICIAN AFTER CONCUSSION

Although most sport-related concussions are considered mild head injuries, the potential exists for complications and life-threatening injuries. Each ATC should be concerned about the potential for the condition of an athlete with a concussion to deteriorate. This downward trend can occur immediately (minutes to hours) or over several days after the injury. As discussed earlier, the spectrum of sport-related head injuries includes more threatening injuries, such as epidural and subdural hematomas and second-impact syndrome. Postconcussion syndrome, however, is a more likely consequence of a sport-related concussion. Not every sport-related concussion warrants immediate physician referral, but ATCs must be able to recognize those injuries that require further attention and provide an appropriate referral for advanced care, which may include neuroimaging. Serial assessments and physician follow-up are important parts of the evaluation of the athlete with a concussion. Referrals should be made to medical personnel with experience managing sport-related concussion. The ATC should monitor vital signs and level of consciousness every 5

minutes after a concussion until the athlete's condition stabilizes and improves. The athlete should also be monitored over the next few hours and days after the injury for delayed signs and symptoms and to assess recovery. Appendix B outlines scenarios that warrant physician referral or, in many cases, transport to the nearest hospital emergency department.

WHEN TO DISQUALIFY AN ATHLETE

Return to participation after severe or repetitive concussive injury should be considered only if the athlete is completely symptom free and has a normal neurologic examination, normal neuropsychological and postural-stability examinations, and, if obtained, normal neuroimaging studies (ie, MRI with gradient echo). It may not be practical or even possible to use all these assessments in all athletes or young children, but a cautious clinical judgment should take into account all evaluation options. Each injured athlete should be considered individually, with consideration for factors including age, level of participation, nature of the sport (high risk versus low risk), and concussion history.

Standardized neuropsychological testing, which typically assesses orientation, immediate and delayed memory recall, and concentration may assist the ATC and physician in determining when to disqualify an athlete from further participation.[60] Balance testing may provide additional information to assist the clinician in the decision-making process of whether to disqualify an individual after a concussion.[52] When to disqualify the athlete is one of the most important decisions facing the ATC and team physician when dealing with an athlete suffering from a concussion. This includes not only when to disqualify for a single practice or event but also when to disqualify for the season or for a career.

Disqualifying for the Game or Practice

The decision to disqualify an individual from further participation on the day of the concussive episode is based on the sideline evaluation, the symptoms the athlete is experiencing, the severity of the apparent symptoms, and the patient's past history.[86] The literature is clear: any episode involving LOC or persistent symptoms related to concussion (headache, dizziness, amnesia, and so on), regardless of how mild and transient, warrants disqualification for the remainder of that day's activities.[8,9,13,19,43,60,87] More recent studies of high school and collegiate athletes underscore the importance of ensuring that the athlete is symptom free before returning to participation on the same day; even when the player is symptom free within 15 to 20 minutes after the concussive episode, he or she may still demonstrate delayed symptoms or depressed neurocognitive levels. Lovell et al[88] found significant memory deficits 36 hours postinjury in athletes who were symptom free within 15 minutes of a mild concussion. Guskiewicz et al[21] found that 33% (10/30) of the players with concussion who returned on the same day of injury experienced delayed onset of symptoms at 3 hours postinjury, as compared with only 12.6% (20/158) of those who did not return to play on the same day of injury. Although more prospective work is needed in this area, these studies raise questions as to whether the RTP criteria for grade 1 (mild) concussions are conservative enough.

Disqualifying for the Season

Guidelines from Cantu[43] and the American Academy of Neurology[6] both recommend termination of the season after the third concussion within the same season. The decision is more difficult if one of the injuries was more severe or was a severe injury resulting from a minimal blow, suggesting that the athlete's brain may be at particular risk for recurrent injury. In addition, because many athletes participate in year-round activities, once they are disqualified for the "season," it may be difficult to determine at what point they can resume contact play. Other issues without clear-cut answers in the literature are when to disqualify an athlete who has not been rendered unconscious and whose symptoms cleared rapidly or one who suffered multiple mild to moderate concussions throughout the career and whether youth athletes should be treated differently for initial and recurrent concussive injuries.

Disqualifying for the Career

When to disqualify an athlete for a career is a more difficult question to answer. The duration of symptoms may be a better criterion as to when to disqualify an athlete for the season or longer. Merril Hoge, Eric Lindros, Chris Miller, Al Toon, and Steve Young provide highly publicized cases of athletes sustaining multiple concussions with recurrent or postconcussion signs and symptoms that lasted for lengthy periods of time.[43]

Once an athlete has suffered a concussion, he or she is at increased risk for subsequent head injuries.[21,43,86] Guskiewicz et al[21,23] found that collegiate athletes had a 3-fold greater risk of suffering a concussion if they had sustained 3 or more previous concussions in a 7-year period and that players with 2 or more previous concussions required a longer time for total symptom resolution after subsequent injuries.[21] Players also had a 3-fold greater risk for subsequent concussions in the same season,[23] whereas recurrent, in-season injuries occurred within 10 days of the initial injury 92% of the time.[21] In a similar study of high school athletes, Collins et al[82] found that athletes with 3 or more prior concussions were at an increased risk of experiencing LOC (8-fold greater risk), anterograde amnesia (5.5-fold greater risk), and confusion (5.1-fold greater risk) after subsequent concussion. Despite the increasing body of literature on this topic, debate still surrounds the question of how many concussions are enough to recommend ending the player's career. Some research suggests that the magic number may be 3 concussions in a career.[21,23,82] Although these findings are important, they should be carefully interpreted because concussions present in varying degrees of severity, and all athletes do not respond in the same way to concussive insults. Most important is that these data provide evidence for exercising caution when managing younger athletes with concussion and athletes with a history of previous concussions.

SPECIAL CONSIDERATIONS FOR THE YOUNG ATHLETE

Many epidemiologic studies on concussion have focused on professional or collegiate athletes. However, this focus seems to now be shifting to the high school level and even to youth sports. Special consideration must be given to the young athlete. The fact that the brain of the young athlete is still developing cannot be ignored, and the effect of concussion on the developing brain is still not entirely understood. Even sub-tle damage may lead to deficits in learning that adversely influence development. Therefore, it has been suggested that pediatric athletes suffering a concussion should be restricted from further participation for the day and that additional consideration should be given as to when to return these individuals to activity.[46]

Recent epidemiologic investigations of head-injury rates in high school athletes have shown that 13.3% of all reported injuries in high school football affect the head and neck, whereas the numbers in other sports range from 1.9% to 9.5% in baseball and wrestling, respectively.[89] Guskiewicz et al[23] prospectively examined concussion incidence in high school and collegiate football players and found that the greatest incidence was at the high school level (5.6%), compared with the National Collegiate Athletic Association Division I (4.4%), Division II (4.5%), and Division III (5.5%).

Authors who have tracked symptoms and neuropsychological function after concussion suggest that age-related differences exist between high school and collegiate athletes with regard to recovery. Lovell et al[41] reported that the duration of on-field mental status changes in high school athletes, such as retrograde amnesia and posttraumatic confusion, was related to the presence of memory impairment at 36 hours, 4 days, and 7 days postinjury as well as slower resolution of self-reported symptoms. These findings further emphasize the need to collect these on-field measures after concussion and to use the information wisely in making RTP decisions, especially when dealing with younger athletes. Field et al[90] found that high school athletes who sustained a concussion demonstrated prolonged memory dysfunction compared with collegiate athletes who sustained a concussion. The high school athletes performed significantly worse on select tests of memory than age-matched control subjects at 7 days postinjury when compared with collegiate athletes and their age-matched control subjects. We hope these important studies and others will eventually lead to more specific guidelines for managing concussions in high school athletes.

Very few investigators have studied sport-related injuries in the youth population, and even fewer focused specifically on sport-related concussion. One group[91] reported that 15% of the children (mean = 8.34 ± 5.31 years) who were admitted to hospitals after MTBI suffered from a sport-related mechanism of injury. Another group[92] found that sport-related head injury accounted for 3% of all sport-related injuries and 24% of all serious head injuries treated in an emergency department. Additionally, sport-related concussion represented a substantial percentage of all head injuries in children under the age of 10 years (18.2%) and 10- to 14-year-old (53.4%) and 15- to 19-year-old (42.9%) populations.[92] Thus, sport-related head injury has a relatively high incidence rate and is a significant public health concern in youth athletes, not just participants at higher competitive levels.

Although no prospective investigations in younger athletes (younger than 15 years old) have been undertaken regarding symptom resolution and cognitive or postural-stability recovery, Valovich McLeod et al[93] recently determined the reliability and validity of brief concussion assessment tools in a group of healthy young athletes (9–14 years old). The SAC is valid within 48 hours of injury and reliable for testing of youths above age 5 years, but younger athletes score slightly below high school and collegiate athletes.[55] This issue is remedied, however, if preseason baseline testing is conducted for all players and a preinjury baseline score established for each athlete against which changes resulting from concussion can be detected and other factors that affect test performance can be controlled. Users of standardized clinical tools should be aware of the effects of age and education on cognitive test performance and make certain to select the appropriate normative group for comparison when testing an injured athlete at a specific competitive level. Uncertainties about the effects of concussion on young children warrant further study.

HOME CARE

Once the athlete has been thoroughly evaluated and determined to have sustained a concussion, a comprehensive medical management plan should be implemented. This plan should include frequent medical evaluations and observations, continued monitoring of postconcussion signs and symptoms, and postinjury cognitive and balance testing. If symptoms persist or worsen or the level of consciousness deteriorates at all after a concussion, neuroimaging should be performed. Although scientific evidence for the evaluation and resolution of the concussion is ample, specific management advice to be given to the athlete on leaving the athletic training room is lacking.[94] Athletic trainers and hospital emergency rooms have created various home instruction forms, but minimal scientific evidence supports these instructions. However, despite these limitations, a concussion instruction form (Appendix C) should be given to the athlete and a responsible adult who will have direct contact with the athlete for the initial 24 hours after the injury. This form helps the companion to know what signs and symptoms to watch for and provides useful recommendations on follow-up care.

Medications

At this time, the clinician has no evidence-based pharmacologic treatment options for an athlete with a concussion.[95] Most pharmacologic studies have been performed in severely head-injured patients. It has been suggested that athletes with concussion avoid medications containing aspirin or nonsteroidal anti-inflammatories, which decrease platelet function and potentially increase intracranial bleeding, mask the severity and duration of symptoms, and possibly lead to a more severe injury. It is also recommended that acetaminophen (Tylenol, McNeil Consumer & Specialty Pharmaceuticals, Fort Washington, PA) be used sparingly in the treatment of headache-like symptoms in the athlete with a concussion. Other substances to avoid during the acute postconcussion period include those that adversely affect central nervous function, in particular alcohol and narcotics.

Wake-Ups and Rest

Once it has been determined that a concussion has been sustained, a decision must be made as to whether the athlete can return home or should be considered for overnight observation or admission to the hospital. For more severe injuries, the athlete should be evaluated by the team physician or emergency room physician if the team physician is not available. If the athlete is allowed to return home or to the dormitory room, the ATC should counsel a friend, teammate, or parent to closely monitor the athlete. Traditionally, part of these instructions included a recommendation to wake up the athlete every 3 to 4 hours during the night to evaluate changes in

symptoms and rule out the possibility of an intracranial bleed, such as a subdural hematoma. This recommendation has raised some debate about unnecessary wake-ups that disrupt the athlete's sleep pattern and may increase symptoms the next day because of the combined effects of the injury and sleep deprivation. It is further suggested that the concussed athlete have a teammate or friend stay during the night and that the athlete not be left alone. No documented evidence suggests what severity of injury requires this treatment. However, a good rule to use is if the athlete experienced LOC, had prolonged periods of amnesia, or is still experiencing significant symptoms, he or she should be awakened during the night. Both oral and written instructions should be given to both the athlete and the caregiver regarding waking.[96] The use of written and oral instructions increases the compliance to 55% for purposeful waking in the middle of the night. In the treatment of concussion, complete bed rest was ineffective in decreasing postconcussion signs and symptoms.[97] The athlete should avoid activities that may increase symptoms (eg, staying up late studying and physical education class) and should resume normal activities of daily living, such as attending class and driving, once symptoms begin to resolve or decrease in severity. As previously discussed, a graded test of exertion should be used to determine the athlete's ability to safely return to full activity.

Diet

Evidence is limited to support the best type of diet for aiding in the recovery process after a concussion. A cascade of neurochemical, ionic, and metabolic changes occur after brain injury.[47] Furthermore, some areas of the brain demonstrate glycolytic increases and go into a state of metabolic depression as a result of decreases in both glucose and oxidative metabolism with a reduction in cerebral blood flow. Severely brain-injured subjects ate larger meals and increased their daily caloric intake when compared with controls.[98] Although limited information is available regarding the recommended diet for the management of concussion, it is well accepted that athletes should be instructed to avoid alcohol, illicit drugs, and central nervous system medications that may interfere with cognitive function. A normal, well-balanced diet should be maintained to provide the needed nutrients to aid in the recovery process from the injury.

EQUIPMENT ISSUES

Helmets and Headgear

Although wearing a helmet will not prevent all head injuries, a properly fitted helmet for certain sports reduces the risk of such injuries. A poorly fitted helmet is limited in the amount of protection it can provide, and the ATC must play a role in enforcing the proper fitting and use of the helmet. Protective sport helmets are designed primarily to prevent catastrophic injuries (ie, skull fractures and intracranial hematomas) and are not designed to prevent concussions. A helmet that protects the head from a skull fracture does not adequately prevent the rotational and shearing forces that lead to many concussions.[99]

The National Collegiate Athletic Association requires helmets be worn for the following sports: baseball, field hockey (goalkeepers only), football, ice hockey, women's lacrosse (goalkeepers only), men's lacrosse, and skiing. Helmets are also recommended for recreational sports such as bicycling, skiing, mountain biking, roller and inline skating, and speed skating. Headgear standards are established and tested by the National Operating Committee on Standards for Athletic Equipment and the American Society for Testing and Materials.[99]

Efforts to establish and verify standards continue to be tested and refined, but rarely are the forces and conditions experienced on the field by the athletes duplicated. In addition to direction, speed, and amount of the forces delivered and received by the athlete, conditions not controlled in the testing process include weather conditions, changes in external temperatures and temperatures inside the helmet, humidity levels, coefficient of friction for the surfaces of the equipment and ground, and density of the equipment and ground. However, equipment that does meet the standards is effective in reducing head injuries.[99]

More recently, the issue of headgear for soccer players has received much attention. Although several soccer organizations and governing bodies have approved the use of protective headbands in soccer, no published, peer-reviewed studies support their use. Recommendations supporting the use and performance of headgear for soccer are limited by a critical gap in biomechanical information about head impacts in the sport of soccer. Without data linking the severity and type of impacts and the clinical sequelae of single and repeated impacts, specifications for soccer headgear cannot be established scientifically. These types of headgear may reduce the "sting" of a head impact, yet they likely do not meet other sports headgear performance standards. This type of headgear may actually increase the incidence of injury. Players wearing headgear may have the false impression that the headgear will protect them during more aggressive play and thereby subject themselves to even more severe impacts that may not be attenuated by the headgear.

Mouth Guards

The wearing of a mouth guard is thought by some to provide additional protection for the athlete against concussion by either reducing the risk of injury or reducing the severity of the injury itself.[100] Mouth guards aid in the separation between the head of the condyle of the mandible and the base of the skull. It is thought that wearing an improperly fitted mouth guard or none at all increases this contact point. This theory, which is based on Newtonian laws of physics, suggests that the increased separation between 2 adjacent structures increases the time to contact, thus decreasing the amount of contact and decreasing the trauma done to the brain.[100] However, no biomechanical studies support the theory that the increased separation results in less force being delivered to the brain.

High school football and National Collegiate Athletic Association football rules mandate the wearing of a mouth guard, but the National Football League rulebook does not require players to wear a mouth guard. The National Collegiate Athletic Association requires mouth guards to be worn by all athletes in football, field hockey, ice hockey, and lacrosse. Researchers[101,102] have found no advantage in wearing a custom-made mouth guard over a boil-and-bite mouth guard to reduce the rise of cerebral concussion in athletes. However, ATCs and coaches should mandate the regular use of mouth guards because a properly fitted mouth guard, with no alterations such as cutting off the back part, is of great value in protecting the teeth and preventing fractures and avulsions that could require many years of expensive dental care.

ACKNOWLEDGMENTS

We gratefully acknowledge the efforts of Kent Scriber, PhD, ATC; Scott Anderson, MS, ATC; Michael Collins, PhD; Vito A. Perriello, Jr, MD, PhD; Karen Johnston, MD, PhD; and the Pronouncements Committee in the preparation of this document.

REFERENCES

1. Mueller FO, Cantu RC. *Nineteenth Annual Report of the National Center for Catastrophic Sports Injury Research: Fall 1982–Spring 2001*. Chapel Hill, NC: National Center for Catastrophic Sports Injury Research; 2002.
2. Ferrara MS, McCrea M, Peterson CL, Guskiewicz KM. A survey of practice patterns in concussion assessment and management. *J Athl Train*. 2001;36:145–149.
3. Guskiewicz KM, Cantu RC. The concussion puzzle: evaluation of sport-related concussion. *Am J Med Sports*. 2004;6:13–21.
4. Gennarelli T. Mechanisms of brain injury. *J Emerg Med*. 1993;11(suppl 1):5–11.
5. Schneider RC. *Head and Neck Injuries in Football: Mechanisms, Treatment and Prevention*. Baltimore, MD: Williams & Wilkins; 1973.
6. Practice parameter: the management of concussion in sports (summary statement). Report of the Quality Standards Subcommittee of the American Academy of Neurology. *Neurology*. 1997;48:581–585.
7. Congress of Neurological Surgeons Committee on Head Injury Nomenclature. Glossary of head injury. *Clin Neurosurg*. 1966;12:386–394.
8. Aubry M, Cantu R, Dvorak J, et al. Summary and agreement statement of the First International Conference on Concussion in Sport, Vienna 2001: recommendations for the improvement of safety and health of athletes who may suffer concussive injuries. *Br J Sports Med*. 2002;36: 6–10.
9. Cantu RC. Athletic head injuries. *Clin Sports Med*. 1997;16:531–542.
10. Bailes JE, Hudson V. Classification of sport-related head trauma: a spectrum of mild to severe injury. *J Athl Train*. 2001;36:236–243.
11. Cantu RC. Intracranial hematoma. In: *Neurologic Athletic Head and Spine Injuries*. Philadelphia, PA: WB Saunders; 2000:124–131.
12. Johnston KM, Ptito A, Chankowsky J, Chen JK. New frontiers in diagnostic imaging in concussive head injury. *Clin J Sport Med*. 2001;11: 166–175.
13. Cantu RC. Guidelines for return to contact sports after a cerebral concussion. *Physician Sportsmed*. 1986;14(10):75–83.
14. Report of the Sports Medicine Committee. Guidelines for the management of concussion in sports. Denver, CO: Colorado Medical Society; 1990 (revised May 1991).
15. Jordan, B. Head injuries in sports. In: Jordan B, Tsairis P, Warren R, eds. *Sports Neurology*. Rockville, MD: Aspen Publishers, Inc; 1989.
16. Nelson W, Jane J, Gieck J. Minor head injuries in sports: a new system of classification and management. *Physician Sportsmed*. 1984;12(3): 103–107.
17. Roberts W. Who plays? Who sits? Managing concussion on the sidelines. *Physician Sportsmed*. 1992;20(6):66–72.
18. Torg JS, Vegso JJ, Sennett B, Das M. The National Football Head and Neck Injury Registry: 14-year report on cervical quadriplegia, 1971 through 1984. *JAMA*. 1985;254:3439–3443.
19. Wilberger JE Jr, Maroon JC. Head injuries in athletes. *Clin Sports Med*. 1989;8:1–9.
20. Wojtys EM, Hovda DA, Landry G, et al. Current concepts: concussion in sports. *Am J Sports Med*. 1999;27:676–687.
21. Guskiewicz KM, McCrea M, Marshall SW, et al. Cumulative effects of recurrent concussion in collegiate football players: the NCAA Concussion Study. *JAMA*. 2003;290:2549–2555.
22. Lovell MR, Iverson GL, Collins MW, McKeag D, Maroon JC. Does loss of consciousness predict neuropsychological decrements after concussion? *Clin J Sport Med*. 1999;9:193–198.
23. Guskiewicz KM, Weaver NL, Padua DA, Garrett WE Jr. Epidemiology

of concussion in collegiate and high school football players. *Am J Sports Med*. 2000;28:643–650.

24. Erlanger D, Saliba E, Barth JT, Almquist J, Webright W, Freeman JR. Monitoring resolution of postconcussion symptoms in athletes: preliminary results of a Web-based neuropsychological test protocol. *J Athl Train*. 2001;36:280–287.

25. Leininger BE, Gramling SE, Ferrell AD, Kreutzer JS, Peck EA III. Neuropsychological deficits in symptomatic minor head injury patients after concussion and mild concussion. *J Neurol Neurosurg Psychiatry*. 1990; 53:293–296.

26. Maroon JC, Lovell MR, Norwig J, Podell K, Powell JW, Hartl R. Cerebral concussion in athletes: evaluation and neuropsychological testing. *Neurosurgery*. 2000;47:659–669.

27. McCrory PR, Ariens T, Berkovic SF. The nature and duration of acute concussive symptoms in Australian football. *Clin J Sport Med*. 2000; 10:235–238.

28. Brown CN, Guskiewicz KM, Bleiberg J, McCrea M, Marshall SW, Matthews A. Comprehensive assessment of concussion in high school and collegiate athletes [abstract]. *J Athl Train*. 2003;38:S-24.

29. McCrea M, Guskiewicz KM, Barr W, et al. Acute effects and recovery time following concussion in collegiate football players: the NCAA Concussion Study. *JAMA*. 2003;290:2556–2563.

30. Levin HS, Benton AL, Grossman RG, eds. *Neurobehavioral Consequences of Closed Head Injury*. New York, NY: Oxford University Press; 1982:221–230.

31. Levin HS, O'Donnell VM, Grossman RG. The Galveston Orientation and Amnesia Test: a practical scale to assess cognition after head injury. *J Nerv Ment Dis*. 1979;167:675–684.

32. Richardson JTE. *Clinical and Neuropsychological Aspects of Closed Head Injury*. London, UK: Taylor and Francis; 1990:1–273.

33. Russell WR. The after effects of head injury. *Edinburgh Med J*. 1934; 41:129–144.

34. Russell WR, Nathan P. Traumatic amnesia. *Brain*. 1946;69:280–300.

35. Russell WR, Smith A. Post-traumatic amnesia in closed head injury. *Arch Neurol*. 1961;5:4–17.

36. Sciarra D. Head injury. In: Merritt HH, Rowland LP, eds. *Merritt's Textbook of Neurology*. 7th ed. Philadelphia, PA: Lea & Febiger; 1984:277–279.

37. Smith A. Duration of impaired consciousness as an index of severity in closed head injury: a review. *Dis Nerv Sys*. 1961;22:69–74.

38. Fisher CM. Concussion amnesia. *Neurology*. 1966;16:826–830.

39. Maddocks DL, Dicker GD, Saling MM. The assessment of orientation following concussion in athletes. *Clin J Sport Med*. 1995;5:32–35.

40. Yarnell PR, Lynch S. The 'ding': amnestic states in football trauma. *Neurology*. 1973;23:196–197.

41. Lovell MR, Collins MW, Iverson GL, et al. Recovery from mild concussion in high school athletes. *J Neurosurg*. 2003;98:296–301.

42. Collins MW, Iverson GL, Lovell MR, McKeag DB, Norwig J, Maroon J. On-field predictors of neuropsychological and symptom deficit following sports-related concussion. *Clin J Sport Med*. 2003;13:222–229.

43. Cantu RC. Posttraumatic retrograde and anterograde amnesia: pathophysiology and implications in grading and safe return to play. *J Athl Train*. 2001;36:244–248.

44. Kelly JP. Loss of consciousness: Pathophysiology and implications in grading and safe return to play. *J Athl Train*. 2001;36:249–252.

45. Giza CC, Hovda DA. Ionic and metabolic consequences of concussion. In: Cantu RC, ed. *Neurologic Athletic Head and Spine Injuries*. Philadelphia, PA: WB Saunders; 2000:80–100.

46. Giza CC, Hovda DA. The neurometabolic cascade of concussion. *J Athl Train*. 2001;36:228–235.

47. Hovda DA, Yoshino A, Kawamata T, Katayama Y, Becker DP. Diffuse prolonged depression of cerebral oxidative metabolism following concussive brain injury in the rat: a cytochrome oxidase histochemistry study. *Brain Res*. 1991;567:1–10.

48. Piland SG, Moti RW, Ferrara MS, Peterson CL. Evidence for the factorial and construct validity of a self-report concussion symptom scale. *J Athl Train*. 2003;38:104–114.

49. Guskiewicz KM. Concussion in sport: the grading-system dilemma. *Athl Ther Today*. 2001;6(1):18–27.

50. Echemendia R, Putukian M, Mackin RS, Julian L, Shoss N. Neuropsychological test performance prior to and following sports-related mild traumatic brain injury. *Clin J Sport Med*. 2001;11:23–31.

51. Erlanger D, Kaushik T, Cantu R, et al. Symptom-based assessment of the severity of a concussion. *J Neurosurg*. 2003;98:477–484.

52. Guskiewicz KM, Ross SE, Marshall SW. Postural stability and neuropsychological deficits after concussion in collegiate athletes. *J Athl Train*. 2001;36:263–273.

53. Collins MW, Field M, Lovell MR, et al. Relationship between postconcussion headache and neuropsychological test performance in high school athletes. *Am J Sports Med*. 2003;31:168–173.

54. McCrea M. Standardized mental status assessment of sports concussion. *Clin J Sport Med*. 2001;11:176–181.

55. McCrea M, Randolph C, Kelly JP. *Standardized Assessment of Concussion (SAC): Manual for Administration, Scoring and Interpretation*. Waukesha, WI: CNS Inc; 1997.

56. Barr WB, McCrea M. Sensitivity and specificity of standardized neurocognitive testing immediately following sports concussion. *J Int Neuropsychol Soc*. 2001;7:693–702.

57. McCrea M, Kelly JP, Randolph C, Cisler R, Berger L. Immediate neurocognitive effects of concussion. *Neurosurgery*. 2002;50:1032–1042.

58. McCrea M, Kelly JP, Kluge J, Ackley B, Randolph C. Standardized assessment of concussion in football players. *Neurology*. 1997;48:586–588.

59. McCrea M, Kelly JP, Randolph C, et al. Standardized Assessment of Concussion (SAC): on-site mental evaluation of the athlete. *J Head Trauma Rehabil*. 1998;13:27–35.

60. McCrea M. Standardized mental status testing on the sideline after sport-related concussion. *J Athl Train*. 2001;36:274–279.

61. Riemann BL, Guskiewicz KM. Effects of mild head injury on postural stability as measured through clinical balance testing. *J Athl Train*. 2000; 35:19–25.

62. Riemann BL, Guskiewicz KM, Shields EW. Relationship between clinical and forceplate measures of postural stability. *J Sport Rehabil*. 1999; 8:71–62.

63. Valovich TC, Perrin DH, Gansneder BM. Repeat administration elicits a practice effect with the Balance Error Scoring System but not with the Standardized Assessment of Concussion in high school athletes. *J Athl Train*. 2003;38:51–56.

64. Guskiewicz KM. Postural stability assessment following concussion: one piece of the puzzle. *Clin J Sport Med*. 2001;11:182–189.

65. Peterson CL, Ferrara MS, Mrazik M, Piland SG. An analysis of domain score and posturography following cerebral concussion. *Clin J Sport Med*. 2003;13:230–237.

66. Bleiberg J, Cernich AN, Cameron K, et al. Duration of cognitive impairment after sports concussion. *Neurosurgery*. 2004;54:1073–1080.

67. Bailes JE, Cantu RC. Head injury in athletes. *Neurosurgery*. 2001;48: 26–45.

68. Grindel SH, Lovell MR, Collins MW. The assessment of sport-related concussion: the evidence behind neuropsychological testing and management. *Clin J Sport Med*. 2001;11:134–143.

69. Pottinger L, Cullum M, Stallings RL. Cognitive recovery following concussion in high school athletes. *Arch Clin Neuropsychol*. 1999;14:39–40.

70. Barth JT, Alves WM, Ryan TV, et al. Mild head injury in sports: neuropsychological sequelae and recovery of function. In: Levin HS, Eisenberg HA, Benton AL, eds. *Mild Head Injury*. New York, NY: Oxford University Press; 1989:257–275.

71. Collie A, Darby D, Maruff P. Computerised cognitive assessment of athletes with sports related head injury. *Br J Sports Med*. 2001;35:297–302.

72. Collie A, Maruff P, Makdissi M, McCrory P, McStephen M, Darby D. CogSport: reliability and correlation with conventional cognitive tests used in postconcussion medical evaluations. *Clin J Sport Med*. 2003;13: 28–32.

73. Collins MW, Grindel SH, Lovell MR, et al. Relationship between concussion and neuropsychological performance in college football players. *JAMA*. 1999;282:964–970.

74. Macciocchi SN, Barth JT, Alves WM, Rimel RW, Jane JA. Neuropsy-

chological functioning and recovery after mild head injury in collegiate athletes. *Neurosurgery*. 1996;39:510–514.

75. Makdissi M, Collie A, Maruff P, et al. Computerised cognitive assessment of concussed Australian rules footballers. *Br J Sports Med*. 2001; 35:354–360.

76. Barr WB. Methodologic issues in neuropsychological testing. *J Athl Train*. 2001;36:297–302.

77. Macciocchi SN, Barth JT, Littlefield LM. Outcome after mild head injury. *Clin Sports Med*. 1998;17:27–36.

78. Bleiberg J, Garmoe WS, Halpern EL, Reeves DL, Nadler JD. Consistency of within-day and across-day performance after mild brain injury. *Neuropsychiatry Neuropsychol Behav Neurol*. 1997;10:247–253.

79. Bleiberg J, Halpern EL, Reeves D, Daniel JC. Future directions for the neuropsychological assessment of sports concussion. *J Head Trauma Rehabil*. 1998;13:36–44.

80. Bleiberg J, Kane RL, Reeves DL, Garmoe WS, Halpern E. Factor analysis of computerized and traditional tests used in mild brain injury research. *Clin Neuropsychol*. 2000;14:287–94.

81. Collie A, Maruff P, Darby DG, McStephen M. The effects of practice on the cognitive test performance of neurologically normal individuals assessed at brief test-retest intervals. *J Int Neuropsychol Soc*. 2003;9: 419–428.

82. Collins MW, Lovell MR, Iverson GL, Cantu RC, Maroon JC, Field M. Cumulative effects of concussion in high school athletes. *Neurosurgery*. 2002;51:1175–1181.

83. Daniel JC, Olesniewicz MH, Reeves DL, et al. Repeated measures of cognitive processing efficiency in adolescent athletes: implications for monitoring recovery from concussion. *Neuropsychiatry Neuropsychol Behav Neurol*. 1999;12:167–169.

84. Reeves D, Thorne R, Winter S, Hegge F. Cognitive Performance Assessment Battery (UTC-PAB). Report 89-1. San Diego, CA: Naval Aerospace Medical Research Laboratory and Walter Reed Army Institute of Research; 1989.

85. McCrea M, Barr WB, Guskiewicz KM, et al. Standard regression-based methods for measuring recovery after sport-related concussion. *J Int Neuropsychol Soc*. In press.

86. Oliaro S, Anderson S, Hooker D. Management of cerebral concussion in sports: the athletic trainer's perspective. *J Athl Train*. 2001;36:257–262.

87. Wilberger JE. Minor head injuries in American football: prevention of long term sequelae. *Sports Med*. 1993;15:338–343.

88. Lovell MR, Collins MW, Iverson GL, Johnston KM, Bradley JP. Grade 1 or "ding" concussions in high school athletes. *Am J Sports Med*. 2004; 32:47–54.

89. Powell JW, Barber-Foss KD. Injury patterns in selected high school sports: a review of the 1995–1997 seasons. *J Athl Train*. 1999;34:277–284.

90. Field M, Collins MW, Lovell MR. Does age play a role in recovery from sports related concussion? A comparison of high school and collegiate athletes. *Am J Pediatr*. 2003;142:546–553.

91. Adams J, Frumiento C, Shatney-Leach L, Vane DW. Mandatory admission after isolated mild closed head injury in children: is it necessary? *J Pediatr Surg*. 2001;36:119–121.

92. Kelly KD, Lissel HL, Rowe BH, Vincenten JA, Voaklander DC. Sport and recreation-related head injuries treated in the emergency department. *Clin J Sport Med*. 2001;11:77–81.

93. Valovich McLeod TC, Perrin DH, Guskiewicz KM, Diamond R, Shultz SJ, Gansneder BM. Serial administration of clinical concussion assessments and learning effects in healthy young athletes. *Clin J Sport Med*. In press.

94. McCrory P. What advice should we give to athletes postconcussion? *Br J Sports Med*. 2002;36:316–318.

95. McCrory P. New treatments for concussion: the next millennium beckons. *Clin J Sport Med*. 2001;11:190–193.

96. de Louw A, Twijnstra A, Leffers P. Lack of uniformity and low compliance concerning wake-up advice following head trauma. *Ned Tijdschr Geneeskd*. 1994;138:2197–2199.

97. de Kruijk JR, Leffers P, Meerhoff S, Rutten J, Twijnstra A. Effectiveness of bed rest after mild traumatic brain injury: a randomised trial of no versus six days of bed rest. *J Neurol Neurosurg Psychiatry*. 2002;73: 167–172.

98. Henson MB, De Castro JM, Stringer AY, Johnson C. Food intake by brain-injury humans who are in the chronic phase of recovery. *Brain Inj*. 1993;7:169–178.

99. Halstead DP. Performance testing updates in head, face, and eye protection. *J Athl Train*. 2001;36:322–327.

100. Winters JE Sr. Commentary: role of properly fitted mouthguards in prevention of sport-related concussion. *J Athl Train*. 2001;36:339–341.

101. Labella CR, Smith BW, Sigurdsson A. Effect of mouthguards on dental injuries and concussions in college basketball. *Med Sci Sports Exerc*. 2002;34:41–44.

102. Wisniewski JF, Guskiewicz KM, Trope M, Sigurdsson A. Incidence of cerebral concussions associated with type of mouthguard used in college football. *Dent Traumatol*. 2004;20:143–149.

Graded Symptom Checklist (GSC)

Symptom	Time of injury	2-3 Hours postinjury	24 Hours postinjury	48 Hours postinjury	72 Hours postinjury
Blurred vision					
Dizziness					
Drowsiness					
Excess sleep					
Easily distracted					
Fatigue					
Feel "in a fog"					
Feel "slowed down"					
Headache					
Inappropriate emotions					
Irritability					
Loss of consciousness					
Loss or orientation					
Memory problems					
Nausea					
Nervousness					
Personality change					
Poor balance/ coordination					
Poor concentration					
Ringing in ears					
Sadness					
Seeing stars					
Sensitivity to light					
Sensitivity to noise					
Sleep disturbance					
Vacant stare/glassy eyed					
Vomiting					

NOTE: The GSC should be used not only for the initial evaluation but for each subsequent follow-up assessment until all signs and symptoms have cleared at rest and during physical exertion. In lieu of simply checking each symptom present, the ATC can ask the athlete to grade or score the severity of the symptom on a scale of 0-6, where 0=not present, 1=mild, 3=moderate, and 6=most severe.

Appendix B. Physician Referral Checklist

Day-of-injury referral

1. Loss of consciousness on the field
2. Amnesia lasting longer than 15 min
3. Deterioration of neurologic function*
4. Decreasing level of consciousness*
5. Decrease or irregularity in respirations*
6. Decrease or irregularity in pulse*
7. Increase in blood pressure
8. Unequal, dilated, or unreactive pupils*
9. Cranial nerve deficits
10. Any signs or symptoms of associated injuries, spine or skull fracture, or bleeding*
11. Mental status changes: lethargy, difficulty maintaining arousal, confusion, or agitation*
12. Seizure activity*
13. Vomiting
14. Motor deficits subsequent to initial on-field assessment
15. Sensory deficits subsequent to initial on-field assessment
16. Balance deficits subsequent to initial on-field assessment
17. Cranial nerve deficits subsequent to initial on-field assessment
18. Postconcussion symptoms that worsen
19. Additional postconcussion symptoms as compared with those on the field
20. Athlete is still symptomatic at the end of the game (especially at high school level)

Delayed referral (after the day of injury)

1. Any of the findings in the day-of-injury referral category
2. Postconcussion symptoms worsen or do not improve over time
3. Increase in the number of postconcussion symptoms reported
4. Postconcussion symptoms begin to interfere with the athlete's daily activities (ie, sleep disturbances or cognitive difficulties)

*Requires that the athlete be transported immediately to the nearest emergency department.

Appendix C. Concussion Home Instructions

I believe that _____ sustained a concussion on _____. To make sure he/she recovers, please follow the following important recommendations:

1. Please **remind** _____ to report to the athletic training room tomorrow at _____ for a follow-up evaluation.

2. Please **review** the items outlined on the enclosed **Physician Referral Checklist.** If any of these problems develop prior to his/her visit, please call _____ at _____ or contact the local emergency medical system or your family physician. Otherwise, you can follow the instructions outlined below.

It is OK to:
- Use acetaminophen (Tylenol) for headaches
- Use ice pack on head and neck as needed for comfort
- Eat a light diet
- Return to school
- Go to sleep
- Rest (no strenuous activity or sports)

There is NO need to:
- Check eyes with flashlight
- Wake up every hour
- Test reflexes
- Stay in bed

Do NOT:
- Drink alcohol
- Eat spicy foods

Specific recommendations:

Recommendations provided to: _____

Recommendations provided by: _____ Date: _____ Time: _____

Please feel free to contact me if you have any questions. I can be reached at: _____

Signature: _____ Date: _____

Concussion Management Review Questions:

1. What is meant by the term 'ding' and why should this term be avoided?

2. What are the signs of a more serious head injury?

3. What are some techniques for assessing a concussion?

4. True or false: Recovery from concussion takes longer in older athletes than younger athletes.

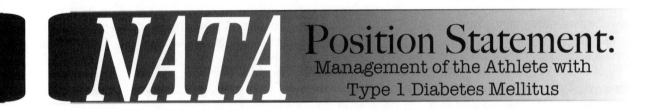

NATA Position Statement:
Management of the Athlete with Type 1 Diabetes Mellitus

In This Section: This position statement is intended to help certified athletic trainers manage type 1 diabetes in athletes. It details the causes of the disease and explains the essential components of a treatment plan for diabetes mellitus.

National Athletic Trainers' Association Position Statement: Management of the Athlete With Type 1 Diabetes Mellitus

Carolyn C. Jimenez, PhD, ATC*; Matthew H. Corcoran, MD, CDE†;
James T. Crawley, MEd, PT, ATC‡; W. Guyton Hornsby, Jr, PhD, CDE‖;
Kimberly S. Peer, EdD, LATC¶; Rick D. Philbin, MBA, MEd, ATC#;
Michael C. Riddell, PhD**

*West Chester University, West Chester, PA; †Lehigh Valley Hospital, Allentown, PA; ‡Dominican College, Orangeburg, NY; ‖West Virginia University, Morgantown, WV; ¶Kent State University, Kent, OH; #Animas Corp, West Chester, PA; **York University, Toronto, ON

Objective: To present recommendations for the certified athletic trainer in the management of type 1 diabetes in the athlete.

Background: In managing diabetes, the most important goal is to keep blood glucose levels at or as close to normal levels as possible without causing hypoglycemia. This goal requires the maintenance of a delicate balance among hypoglycemia, euglycemia, and hyperglycemia, which is often more challenging in the athlete due to the demands of physical activity and competition. However, effectively managing blood glucose, lipid, and blood pressure levels is necessary to en-suring the long-term health and well-being of the athlete with diabetes.

Recommendations: These recommendations are intended to provide the certified athletic trainer participating in the management of an athlete with type 1 diabetes mellitus with the specific knowledge and problem-solving skills needed. Athletic trainers have more contact with the athlete with diabetes than most members of the diabetes management team do and so must be prepared to assist the athlete as required.

Key Words: hypoglycemia, hyperglycemia, insulin replacement therapy

Effective management of glycemic, lipid, and blood pressure control plays an important role in the health outcomes of persons with diabetes mellitus. The primary goal of diabetes management is to consistently maintain blood glucose levels in a normal or near-normal range without provoking undue hypoglycemia.[1–5] Although several exercise guidelines for persons with diabetes have been published (American Diabetes Association's "Physical Activity/Exercise and Type 2 Diabetes,"[6] American College of Sports Medicine's "Exercise and Type 2 Diabetes,"[7] and the joint statement of the American College of Sports Medicine and the American Diabetes Association, "Diabetes Mellitus and Exercise"[8]), none address issues of concern for athletic trainers (eg, blood glucose management strategies during injury or the effect of therapeutic modalities on blood glucose control). The following position statement and recommendations provide relevant information on type 1 diabetes mellitus and specific recommendations for athletic trainers who work with patients with diabetes.

RECOMMENDATIONS

Based on current research and literature, the National Athletic Trainers' Association (NATA) suggests the following guidelines for management of athletes with type 1 diabetes mellitus. These recommendations have been organized into the following categories: diabetes care plan; supplies for athletic training kits; preparticipation physical examination (PPE); recognition, treatment, and prevention of hypoglycemia; recognition, treatment, and prevention of hyperglycemia; insulin administration; travel recommendations; and athletic injury and glycemic control.

Diabetes Care Plan

1. Each athlete with diabetes should have a diabetes care plan for practices and games. The plan should include the following:

   a. Blood glucose monitoring guidelines. Address frequency of monitoring and pre-exercise exclusion values.

   b. Insulin therapy guidelines. Should include the type of insulin used, dosages and adjustment strategies for planned activities types, as well as insulin correction dosages for high blood glucose levels.

   c. List of other medications. Include those used to assist with glycemic control and/or to treat other diabetes-related conditions.

   d. Guidelines for hypoglycemia recognition and treatment. Include prevention, signs, symptoms, and treatment of hypoglycemia, including instructions on the use of glucagon.

   e. Guidelines for hyperglycemia recognition and treatment. Include prevention, signs, symptoms, and treatment of hyperglycemia and ketosis.

f. Emergency contact information. Include parents' and/or other family member's telephone numbers, physician's telephone number, and consent for medical treatment (for minors).

g. Athletes with diabetes should have a medic alert tag with them at all times.

Supplies for Athletic Training Kits

2. Supplies to treat diabetes-related emergencies should be available at all practices and games. The athlete (or athlete's parents/guardians, in the case of minors) provides the following items:

   a. A copy of the diabetes care plan.

   b. Blood glucose monitoring equipment and supplies. The athletic trainer should check the expiration dates of supplies, such as blood glucose testing strips and insulin, on a regular basis. Blood glucose testing strips have a code number located on the outside of the test strip vial. The code number on the blood glucose meter and test strip vial must match.

   c. Supplies to treat hypoglycemia, including sugary foods (eg, glucose tablets, sugar packets) or sugary fluids (eg, orange juice, non-diet soda) and a glucagon injection kit.

   d. Supplies for urine or blood ketone testing.

   e. A "sharps" container to ensure proper disposal of syringes and lancets.

   f. Spare batteries (for blood glucose meter and/or insulin pump) and, if applicable, spare infusion sets and reservoirs for insulin pumps.

Preparticipation Physical Examination

3. Athletes with type 1 diabetes should have a glycosylated hemoglobin (HbA1c) assay every 3 to 4 months to assess overall long-term glycemic control. However, the HbA1c value is not used to make day-to-day decisions concerning participation.

4. An annual examination for retinopathy, nephropathy, and neuropathy is recommended along with an annual foot examination to check sensory function and ankle reflexes. Screening for cardiovascular disease should occur at intervals recommended by the athlete's endocrinologist or cardiologist. Exercise limitations or restrictions for athletes with diabetes-related complications should be determined by the athlete's physician.[9–11]

Recognition, Treatment, and Prevention of Hypoglycemia

5. Strategies to recognize, treat, and prevent hypoglycemia typically include blood glucose monitoring, carbohydrate supplementation, and/or insulin adjustments. Athletes with diabetes should discuss with their physicians specific carbohydrate qualities and quantities as well as the use of an insulin reduction plan for activity (Appendix 1).

6. Athletic trainers should know the signs, symptoms, and treatment guidelines for mild and severe hypoglycemia. Hypoglycemia is defined as mild if the athlete is conscious and able to swallow and follow directions or severe if the athlete is unable to swallow, follow directions, or eat as directed or is unconscious. Treatment of severe hypoglycemia requires a glucagon injection, and athletic trainers should be trained in mixing and administering glucagon. The athlete, athlete's family, or physician can provide appropriate training (Appendix 2).

Recognition, Treatment, and Prevention of Hyperglycemia

7. Athletes with type 1 diabetes and athletic trainers are advised to follow the American Diabetes Association (ADA) guidelines for avoiding exercise during periods of hyperglycemia (Appendix 3).

8. Athletes with type 1 diabetes who experience hyperglycemia during short-term, intense, and stressful periods of exercise should consult with their physicians concerning an increased basal rate or the use of small insulin boluses to counteract this phenomenon.[30]

9. Athletes should drink noncarbohydrate fluids when blood glucose levels exceed the renal glucose threshold (180 mg/dL, or 10 mmol/L), which may lead to increased urination, fluid loss, and dehydration.

Insulin Administration

10. Insulin should be administered into the subcutaneous tissue. The abdomen, upper thigh, and upper arms are common sites for injection. Intramuscular injections of insulin should always be avoided as muscle contractions may accelerate insulin absorption.[12]

11. Depending on the type of insulin used by the athlete, heat and cold should be avoided for 1 to 3 hours after an injection of rapid-acting insulin (eg, lispro, aspart, or glulisine) and up to 4 hours for fast-acting (eg, regular) insulin.[31,32] Heat may increase insulin absorption rates. Thus, athletes with type 1 diabetes should avoid warm whirlpools, saunas, showers, hot tubs, and baths after injection. Local heat-producing modalities such as moist hot packs, diathermy, and thermal ultrasound should not be applied directly over an infusion or injection site. By contrast, cold may decrease insulin absorption rates. Therefore, athletes with type 1 diabetes should avoid using ice and cold sprays directly over the injection or infusion site after insulin administration. Similarly, cold whirlpools should be avoided after insulin injection.

12. Insulin pump users should replace insulin infusion sets every 2 to 3 days to reduce skin and infusion site irritation.

13. Extreme ambient temperature ($<36°F$ or $>86°F$ [$<2.2°C$ or $>30°C$]) can reduce insulin action. Athletes with type 1 diabetes are advised to check blood glucose levels frequently and replace the entire insulin-filled cartridge and infusion set if any signs of unusual hyperglycemia occur in extreme environmental conditions.

Travel Recommendations

14. Athletic trainers should review the advice provided by the Transportation Security Administration (TSA) in conjunction with the ADA for airline passengers with diabetes traveling within the United States.[33] In addition, athletes are advised to carry diabetes supplies with them and have prescriptions available in the event that medication or supplies need to be replaced. Due to extreme temperature

fluctuations that could affect insulin action, insulin should not be stored in the cargo hold of the airplane.

15. When traveling, athletes with type 1 diabetes are advised to carry prepackaged meals and snacks in case food availability is interrupted. If travel occurs over several time zones, insulin therapy may need to be adjusted to coordinate with changes in eating and activity patterns.

Athletic Injury and Glycemic Control

16. Trauma, even in persons without diabetes, often causes a hyperglycemic state. Hyperglycemia is known to impair the wound healing process; thus, for athletes with type 1 diabetes, an individualized blood glucose management protocol should be developed for use during injury recovery, including frequency of blood glucose monitoring.

BACKGROUND

Diabetes mellitus is a chronic endocrine disorder characterized by hyperglycemia. Persons with diabetes are at risk for macrovascular, microvascular, and neuropathic complications. For those without diabetes, normal fasting blood glucose levels are 60 to 100 mg/dL (3.3 to 5.5 mmol/L); normal postprandial levels are less than 140 mg/dL (7.8 mmol/L) 2 hours after a meal. Chronic hyperglycemia leads to long-term damage, dysfunction, and failure of various organs, especially the eyes, kidneys, nerves, and heart.[34] The literature supports the importance of a consistent, near-normal blood glucose level, as well as blood pressure and lipid control, for preventing diabetes-related complications and improving quality of life.[2–5]

Currently, approximately 20.8 million persons are living with diabetes in the United States.[35] It is estimated that approximately 90% have type 2 diabetes and approximately 10% have type 1 diabetes.[35] Type 2 diabetes typically occurs in adults 40 years of age and older; however, the incidence of type 2 diabetes in children is increasing, especially among American Indian, African American, and Hispanic/Latino populations. Type 1 diabetes typically occurs in children and young adults.[35,36]

Type 1 diabetes is the rarer form of the disease, but athletic trainers working in middle schools, secondary schools, colleges, and many professional settings are more likely to encounter athletes with type 1 than type 2 diabetes. This position statement focuses on recommendations for the athlete with type 1 diabetes, although athletic trainers can also play a crucial role in the diabetes-management plan of a person with type 2 diabetes.

Type 1 diabetes is characterized by absolute insulin deficiency. It is considered an autoimmune disorder resulting from a combination of genetic and unknown environmental factors. The signs and symptoms of type 1 diabetes develop rapidly and are related to hyperglycemia. Symptoms include frequent urination, thirst, hunger and polyphagia, weight loss, visual disturbances, fatigue, and ketosis.[37] Usually, athletes are able to resume exercise and sports within weeks of starting insulin treatment as long as a treatment plan is developed and a support team exists. The treatment plan for persons with type 1 diabetes focuses on a self-care plan predicated on exogenous insulin, monitoring of blood glucose, healthy nutrition, and exercise.

DIABETES MANAGEMENT TEAM AND THE DIABETES CARE PLAN

Proper management of blood glucose levels during practices and games allows the athlete with diabetes to compete in a safe and effective manner. Maintaining a near-normal blood glucose level (100 to 180 mg/dL, or 5.5 mmol/L to 10 mmol/L) reduces the risk of dehydration, lethargy, hypoglycemia, and autonomic counterregulatory failure. This goal is best achieved through a team approach. The team-management approach to providing support for patients with diabetes is well established in the allied health literature.[38–46] In school-aged athletes, the team should include the school nurse, coach, and school administrators. In adult athletes, diabetes is best managed by a team that includes several health professionals.[39,41–43,47,48] Creating this team requires a deliberate, well-designed plan, which defines the role of each individual in the supervision and care of the athlete with diabetes. All members of the team should be trained and willing to assist an athlete who is experiencing a diabetes-related emergency.

Critical roles for the athletic trainer include prevention, recognition, and immediate care of hypoglycemia and hyperglycemia (with and without ketoacidosis); exercise nutrition; hydration counseling; and helping the athlete to recognize the intensity of the exercise session in order to adjust glucose and insulin levels accordingly.[41,49–51] The athletic trainer also facilitates communication among the other members of the diabetes management team.

Athletes with type 1 diabetes should have a diabetes care plan for practices and games.[40] The plan should identify blood glucose targets for practices and games, including exclusion thresholds; strategies to prevent exercise-associated hypoglycemia, hyperglycemia, and ketosis; a list of medications used for glycemic control or other diabetes-related conditions; signs, symptoms, and treatment protocols for hypoglycemia, hyperglycemia, and ketosis; and emergency contact information. The athlete must have access to supplies for managing glycemic emergencies at all times. When the athlete requires assistance, the athletic trainer and/or other members of the diabetes management team (eg, coach) must have immediate access to these supplies. The athlete or parent/guardian should provide the necessary supplies and equipment.

PREPARTICIPATION PHYSICAL EXAMINATION FOR ATHLETES WITH TYPE 1 DIABETES

A thorough PPE should begin with the team or primary care physician. This examination should include a sports history, assessment of the level of diabetes self-care skills and knowledge, general physical examination emphasizing screening of diabetes-related complications, and discussion of how sports participation will affect blood glucose and blood pressure control. As part of the PPE, the athlete's endocrinologist or primary care physician should provide an assessment of the current level of glycemic control, information concerning the presence and status of diabetes-related complications, and blood glucose management strategies. Completion of the PPE may require consultation with other specialists (eg, cardiologist, ophthalmologist), especially in the case of diabetes-related complications.[52] Athletic trainers are referred to the *Handbook of Exercise in Diabetes*,[53] published by the American Diabetes Association, for further readings on prescreening of the active individual with type 1 diabetes.

Preparticipation Physical Examination and Glycemic Control

The athlete's level of long-term glycemic control should be listed on the PPE. Long-term glycemic control is assessed by an HbA1c test every 3 to 4 months.[54] Normal HbA1c levels, depending on the laboratory assay, are generally between 4.0% and 6.0%. The ADA recommends a target HbA1c level of 7% or less for adults on intensive insulin therapy and 7.5% or less for teens and adolescents.[55] An HbA1c level of 7% correlates with an average blood glucose level of approximately 150 mg/dL (8.3 mmol/L). Other organizations, such as the American Association of Clinical Endocrinologists, set more stringent recommendations, such as 6.5% (approximately 135 mg/dL [7.5 mmol/L]) or less in adults.[56] In general, a lower HbA1c level correlates with a lower risk of diabetes-related complications at the expense of an increased risk of hypoglycemia.[2] The athletic trainer should understand that although the HbA1c level provides a long-term perspective of glycemic control, it is not used to make day-to-day participation decisions.

Preparticipation Physical Examination and Screening for Diabetes-Related Complications

Athletic trainers should be aware that an athlete with type 1 diabetes may be chronologically young but may have had the disease for many years and, as such, may experience diabetes-related complications. Common diabetes-related complications are retinopathy, nephropathy, neuropathy, and cardiovascular disease.

The ADA recommends an initial dilated and comprehensive ophthalmologic examination 3 to 5 years after the diagnosis of type 1 diabetes and an annual screening thereafter for retinopathy, glaucoma, and cataracts.[11,57] Decisions regarding activity limitations for the athlete are based on the presence and degree of retinopathy and are made by the athlete's physician.

Diabetic nephropathy is characterized by increased urinary protein excretion. An initial examination is recommended 5 years after the diagnosis of type 1 diabetes and annually thereafter.[9,58] The athlete's physician may limit exercise based upon the presence and degree of nephropathy.

Peripheral neuropathy is characterized by bilateral sensory involvement with dull perception of vibration, pain, and temperature, particularly in the lower extremities. This is of particular concern for the athlete performing weight-bearing activities. Athletic trainers should instruct the athlete with diabetes to inspect the feet on a daily basis for any reddened areas, blisters, abrasions, or lacerations. Cutting toenails straight across, not walking barefoot, and avoiding poor-fitting or tight shoes are all recommendations the athletic trainer should provide.[53] Initial screening for peripheral neuropathy is recommended 5 years after diagnosis.[10] Thereafter, an annual examination for peripheral neuropathy (ie, examining sensory function of the feet and checking the ankle reflexes) is recommended.[10] The athlete's physician may limit certain physical activities in the presence of peripheral neuropathy.

Autonomic neuropathy may affect the cardiovascular, gastrointestinal, and neuroendocrine systems. This may predispose the athlete with diabetes to exercise intolerance, orthostatic hypotension, and hypoglycemic unawareness (a failure to effectively recognize the signs and symptoms of low blood sugar). The ADA recommends an initial screening for autonomic neuropathy 5 years after the diagnosis of type 1 diabetes and annually thereafter.[10] Suspected autonomic neuropathy should be evaluated by the athlete's endocrinologist and/or cardiologist for exercise recommendations.[59]

Cardiovascular complications include myocardial infarction, stroke, and peripheral arterial disease. The ADA recommends that persons who have had type 1 diabetes for more than 15 years or have any other risk factor for coronary artery disease, microvascular disease, peripheral vascular disease, or autonomic neuropathy undergo a graded exercise stress test to evaluate cardiovascular function.[59] For those athletes with, or suspected of having, cardiovascular disease, referral to an endocrinologist and/or cardiologist for further assessment and treatment is warranted.

INSULIN REPLACEMENT THERAPY

The objective of insulin replacement therapy is the near-normalization of blood glucose levels while minimizing the risks of hypoglycemia and weight gain. The standard of care is "intensive insulin therapy."[2] Intensive insulin therapy uses basal and bolus insulin doses to regulate blood glucose levels during fasting, feeding, and hyperglycemic periods. Basal insulin is used to maintain glycemic stability during fasting periods and delivers a steady, low dose of insulin 24 hours a day. Bolus insulin is used to control elevations in blood glucose levels that occur after eating or to lower blood glucose levels during hyperglycemia. Bolus insulin doses are determined by several factors, including the prevailing blood glucose level, carbohydrate content of the meal, and anticipated exercise.

Insulin pumps and multiple daily injections (MDI) are the primary methods used to deliver basal and bolus therapy. Insulin pump therapy uses novel technology to deliver rapid-acting or fast-acting insulin to provide both basal and bolus doses (see Appendix 4 for examples of fast-acting and rapid-acting insulins). However, rapid-acting insulins are considered the standard of care in insulin pump therapy because of their physiologic profile. In insulin pump therapy, basal insulin is continuously administered via preset basal infusion rates (ie, 1.2 units of insulin per hour) over a 24-hour period. At meals or to correct hyperglycemia, the athlete uses a bolus-dosing menu on the insulin pump to dispense insulin dosages (ie, 5 units of insulin).

The MDI plans require patients with diabetes to inject both basal and bolus insulins. Typically, basal insulin is injected 1 or 2 times a day. Unlike insulin pump basal infusion rates, basal therapy with MDI consists of injecting a fixed amount of long-acting insulin, such as 6.5 units. Optimal basal insulin use with MDI has a long biological activity (18 to 24 hours) and a relatively peakless profile. Patients with diabetes may use 2 to 4 injections of rapid-acting or fast-acting insulin to provide bolus coverage at mealtimes or to correct hyperglycemia. Bolus dosing with MDI is similar to that with insulin pump therapy in that a fixed amount of insulin (ie, 5 units of insulin) is administered based upon the current blood glucose level, carbohydrate content of the meal, and any anticipated exercise.

The choice to use an insulin pump or MDI is made by the athlete in consultation with the physician. Each method of delivery has distinct advantages and disadvantages. Advantages of insulin pump therapy include the use of a single rapid-acting insulin to achieve a more physiologic insulin profile; the ability to alter the basal rate before or during exercise; the ability to suspend or disconnect the pump; "smart pumps" that use internal calculators to determine an estimated amount of insulin in circulation, which may help to prevent excessive insulin dosing; allowance for flexible meal schedules; and avoiding the regular use of needles for insulin administration. Disadvantages of insulin pump therapy include possible damage during contact sports; risk of hyperglycemia and ketosis if the insulin pump malfunctions or is inadvertently disconnected from the athlete; infusion set displacement, as heavy sweating or water contact may reduce the ability of adhesives to hold the infusion set in place; movement or contact leading to irritation at the infusion site, especially in those using metal needle infusion sets; and extreme ambient temperatures (<36°F [2.22°C] or >86°F [30°C]), which can affect insulin housed within the pump and interfere with insulin action.[65]

The advantages of MDI include a lower cost of operation compared with insulin pumps and the absence of a connection to a device. Disadvantages include the inability to manipulate basal insulin levels during exercise, the need for regular injections, and the lack of flexibility regarding meal timing and unplanned exercise.

Insulin absorption is the rate-limiting step in insulin activity for both the insulin pump and MDI, and many factors may affect the absorption rate.[66] Athletes should use consistent sites for injections to eliminate absorption differences among body regions (ie, abdomen versus triceps). Appendix 5 lists some of the variables that can affect absorption rates.

The athlete and diabetes management team should be aware of insulin-specific pharmacokinetic and pharmacodynamic properties. For example, rapid-acting insulin analogs (lispro, aspart, glulisine) all reach peak circulating levels within 90 minutes of administration. This peak represents the maximal glucose-lowering effect and greatest risk for hypoglycemia. See Appendix 4 for pharmacokinetic properties of commonly used basal and bolus insulins.

HYPOGLYCEMIA

Hypoglycemia is the most severe acute complication of intensive insulin therapy in diabetes, and exercise is its most frequent cause.[1,68] Intensive insulin therapy is associated with a 2-fold to 3-fold increase in severe hypoglycemia (ie, the person with diabetes requires assistance).[2] The risk of severe hypoglycemia is higher in males, adolescents, and those who have already had a severe episode.[2] Although responses are individualized, signs and symptoms of hypoglycemia typically occur when blood glucose levels fall below 70 mg/dL (3.9 mmol/L).

Under most circumstances, hypoglycemia is the result of overinsulinization, both during and after exercise. Several factors contribute to overinsulinization. First, the rate at which subcutaneously injected insulin is absorbed increases with exercise due to increases in body temperature and in subcutaneous and skeletal muscle blood flow.[69] Second, exogenously administered insulin levels do not decrease during exercise in persons with type 1 diabetes. This is in contrast to exercise in persons without diabetes, in whom insulin levels decrease during exercise to prevent hypoglycemia. The inability to decrease plasma insulin levels during exercise in type 1 diabetes causes relative hyperinsulinemia, which impairs hepatic glucose production and initiates hypoglycemia, usually within 20 to 60 minutes after the onset of exercise.[13,14,70] Third, hypoglycemia during exercise can result from impaired release of glucose-counterregulatory hormones (ie, glucagon and catecholamines) caused by either a previous bout of exercise or hypoglycemic episode.[68] As a result, athletes with type 1 diabetes who experience hypoglycemia on the days preceding

competition may be at risk for exercise-associated hypoglycemia.[68] Finally, exercise improves insulin sensitivity in skeletal muscle. Exercise-associated improvements in insulin sensitivity may last for several hours to days after exercise. Thus, some athletes experience a phenomenon known as postexercise late-onset hypoglycemia, which may occur while the athlete is sleeping. Athletes who experience nighttime hypoglycemia require additional blood glucose monitoring in addition to a snack.[15,71]

Managing blood glucose levels during practices and games and preventing hypoglycemia are challenges. Typically, hypoglycemia prevention uses a 3-pronged approach of blood glucose monitoring, carbohydrate supplementation, and insulin adjustments. Appendix 1 lists strategies to prevent hypoglycemia during and after practices and games. The athlete and the diabetes management team should work together to determine which strategies to employ.

Hypoglycemia normally produces noticeable autonomic or neurogenic symptoms. Autonomic symptoms include tachycardia, sweating, palpitations, hunger, nervousness, headache, trembling, and dizziness. These symptoms typically occur at blood glucose levels <70 mg/dL (<3.9 mmol/L) in persons with diabetes and are related to the release of epinephrine and acetylcholine.[26,27] As glucose continues to fall, symptoms of brain neuronal glucose deprivation (neurogenic symptoms) occur and may cause blurred vision, fatigue, difficulty thinking, loss of motor control, aggressive behavior, seizures, convulsions, and loss of consciousness; if hypoglycemia is prolonged and severe, brain damage and even death can result. Symptoms of hypoglycemia can be unique to a person with diabetes.[72] Thus, the athletic training staff should be familiar with athlete-specific symptoms of hypoglycemia and be prepared to act appropriately. Hypoglycemia can cause some athletes to be especially aggressive and unwilling to cooperate with instructions. Treatment guidelines for mild and severe cases of hypoglycemia are presented in Appendix 2.

ACUTE HYPERGLYCEMIA AND KETOSIS

Hyperglycemia with or without ketosis can occur during exercise in athletes with type 1 diabetes. Hyperglycemia during exercise is related to several factors. First, exercise (especially high-intensity exercise at 70% VO_2 max or >85% of maximal heart rate) can cause additional increases in blood glucose concentrations and possible ketoacidosis in athletes with poor glycemic control and those who are underinsulinized. Without adequate insulin levels, blood glucose levels continue to rise due to exaggerated hepatic glucose production and impairments in exercise-induced glucose utilization.[73] Second, even in well-controlled athletes with type 1 diabetes, high-intensity exercise may result in hyperglycemia. High-intensity exercise may lead to significant increases in catecholamines, free fatty acids, and ketone bodies, all of which impair muscle glucose utilization and increase blood glucose levels.[74] This exercise-associated rise in glucose levels is usually transient in the well-controlled diabetic athlete, declining as counterregulatory hormone levels decrease, typically within 30 to 60 minutes.[15] Third, the psychological stress of competition is frequently associated with increases in blood glucose levels before competition. Although data do not exist for those with type 1 diabetes, it is likely that excessive increases in counterregulatory hormones occur before exercise, when anticipatory stress is high.[75] Athletes may find that blood glucose management strategies that work on practice days actually result in hyperglycemia on game days due to psychological stress. Frequent blood glucose monitoring and either small boluses of rapid-acting insulin or a temporary increase in basal rate insulin may be required to recover from these hyperglycemic episodes. Finally, limited data exist regarding competition and training in hot and humid environments by athletes with type 1 diabetes. Athletes may find that training or competing in these environments elevates blood glucose levels, likely because of exaggerated increases in glucose counterregulatory hormones.[76]

Effects vary from one athlete to another, but hyperglycemic signs and symptoms include nausea, dehydration, reduced cognitive performance, slowing of visual reaction time, and feelings of sluggishness and fatigue.[16] The symptoms of hyperglycemia with ketoacidosis may include those listed above as well as rapid breathing (also known as Kussmaul breathing), fruity odor to the breath, unusual fatigue, sleepiness, inattentiveness, loss of appetite, increased thirst, and frequent urination. Athletic trainers should also be aware that some athletes with type 1 diabetes may intentionally train and compete in a hyperglycemic state (>180 mg/dL [10 mmol/L]) to avoid hypoglycemia. Competing in a hyperglycemic state places the athlete at risk for dehydration, reduced athletic performance, and possibly ketosis.[77]

The ADA provides guidelines for exercise during hyperglycemic periods (Appendix 3). Athletes should work with their physicians to determine the need for insulin adjustments for periods of hyperglycemia before, during, and after exercise. In addition, dehydration is possible when blood glucose levels exceed the renal glucose threshold (180 mg/dL [10 mmol/L]) as urinary output increases to excrete excess glucose. During these periods, athletes may need to increase consumption of noncarbohydrate fluids.

TRAVEL FOR THE ATHLETE WITH TYPE 1 DIABETES

The athlete with diabetes must take special precautions to ensure that blood glucose management is not disrupted by travel. If travel is by airplane, the athlete is advised to study and be prepared for all current regulations and advice from the TSA of the United States Department of Homeland Security before departure. The following advice has been provided by the TSA in conjunction with the ADA for airline passengers with diabetes traveling within the 50 United States[78]:

Athletes with diabetes should notify airport security screeners of their medical condition and need to carry on board all diabetes equipment and supplies. The TSA allows the following diabetes materials through the checkpoint:

1. Clearly identified and labeled, with pharmaceutical labels, insulin and insulin-loaded dispensing products, including vials or a box of individual vials, jet injectors, pens, infusers, and preloaded syringes.
2. An unlimited number of unused syringes when accompanied by insulin or other injectable medication.
3. Lancets, blood glucose meters, test strips, alcohol swabs, and meter-testing solutions.
4. Insulin pump and supplies such as cleaning agents, batteries, plastic tubing, and infusion kit catheter and needle.
5. Glucagon emergency kit, clearly identified and labeled.

6. Ketone testing supplies.
7. An unlimited number of used syringes as long as they are transported in a "sharps" disposable container or other similar hard-surface container.[79]

Before travel, the athlete should obtain prescriptions for insulin and other medications along with a letter from the physician, on letterhead, explaining the need for diabetes medications, equipment, and supplies. Travel may result in medications, equipment, and supplies becoming lost, damaged, or destroyed. Thus, it is advisable for the athlete to travel with twice the amount of medications and supplies needed for the trip. The athlete should also carry a health insurance card that has the insurance company name, policy number, and emergency phone numbers.

Travel may affect the accessibility to meals and snacks, as well as when and where food may be eaten. Athletes with diabetes should carry prepackaged meals and/or snacks in the event that meals are delayed. If travel occurs over several time zones, insulin therapy may need to be adjusted to coordinate with changes in eating and activity patterns. The athlete should be instructed to discuss the travel plans with his or her diabetes health care team before departure.

It is advisable that everyone with diabetes wear or carry some form of medical identification, especially when traveling. If the trip includes stops in non–English-speaking countries, the ADA can provide identification cards translated into almost any language.[80] However, it may be helpful to learn phrases for requesting medical attention, such as "I need a doctor," "I need sugar," or "I have diabetes."[81-88]

INJURY AND GLYCEMIC CONTROL

Trauma is associated with dramatic increases in the secretion of stress hormones (adrenocorticotropic hormone, cortisol, growth hormone, catecholamines, and glucagon) and an increase in blood glucose levels. In persons without diabetes, these changes ensure a steady supply of fuel that assists with the recovery process. Patients with type 1 diabetes appear to have an exaggerated hyperglycemic response to trauma, especially with preexisting hyperglycemia and/or hypoinsulinemia. Numerous authors[87,88] have demonstrated that poor blood glucose control is associated with an increased risk of infection, as well as poor wound and fracture healing. These deficits can be corrected by the administration of insulin and proper blood glucose management.[89,90] Athletes with diabetes should strive to maintain near-normal blood glucose levels via proper insulin administration during the injury process.[91]

Athletes with diabetes should strive for tight blood glucose control in order to minimize the deleterious effects of trauma on glycemic control. Although no researchers have directly addressed the issue of blood glucose control and insulin therapy for common athletic injuries (eg, sprains, strains), the guidelines developed by the ADA for blood glucose control in noncritical patients could be applied to injured athletes with diabetes.[91] The guidelines recommend a premeal blood glucose target of 110 mg/dL (6.1 mmol/L) and a postmeal blood glucose level of <180 mg/dL (10 mmol/L) in noncritical patients. The ADA guidelines listed above can serve as a starting point to assist the diabetes care team in developing glycemic goals.

SUMMARY

Although the literature supports the benefits of physical activity for persons with type 1 diabetes, exercise training and competition can cause major disturbances to blood glucose management. Maintaining the delicate balance among hypoglycemia-euglycemia-hyperglycemia is best achieved through a team approach. Special considerations for glycemic control, medication, travel, and recovery from injury are needed for the athlete with type 1 diabetes. The certified athletic trainer, who has more contact with the athlete with diabetes than most members of the diabetes management team, is an integral component of the team. Athletes with diabetes can benefit from a well-organized plan that may allow them to compete on equal ground with their teammates and competitors without diabetes.

DISCLAIMER

The NATA publishes its position statements as a service to promote the awareness of certain issues to its members. The information contained in the position statement is neither exhaustive nor exclusive to all circumstances or individuals. Variables such as institutional human resource guidelines, state or federal statutes, rules, or regulations, as well as regional environmental conditions, may impact the relevance and implementation of these recommendations. The NATA advises its members and others to carefully and independently consider each of the recommendations (including the applicability to any particular circumstance or individual). The position statement should not be relied upon as an independent basis for care but rather as a resource available to NATA members or others. Moreover, no opinion is expressed herein regarding the quality of care that adheres to or differs from NATA's position statements. The NATA reserves the right to rescind or modify its position statements at any time.

ACKNOWLEDGMENTS

We gratefully acknowledge the efforts of Ann Albright, PhD, RD; Rebecca M. Lopez, MS, ATC; Mark A. Merrick, PhD, ATC; Stephen H. Schneider, MD; and the Pronouncements Committee in the preparation of this document.

REFERENCES

1. Wasserman DH, Davis SN, Zinman B. Fuel metabolism during exercise in health and diabetes. In: Ruderman N, Devlin JT, Schneider SH, Kriska A, eds. *Handbook of Exercise in Diabetes*. Alexandria, VA: American Diabetes Association; 2002:63–100.
2. The Diabetes Control and Complications Trial Research Group. The effect of intensive treatment of diabetes on the development and progression of long-term complications in insulin-dependent diabetes mellitus. *N Engl J Med*. 1993;329:977–986.
3. UK Prospective Diabetes Study (UKPDS) Group. Intensive blood-glucose control with sulphonylureas or insulin compared with conventional treatment and risk of complications in patients with type 2 diabetes (UKPDS 33). *Lancet*. 1998;352:837–853.
4. Ludvigsson J, Nordfeldt S. Hypoglycaemia during intensified insulin therapy of children and adolescents. *J Pediatr Endocrinol Metab*. 1998; 11(suppl 1):159–166.
5. The Diabetes Control and Complications Trial Research Group. Hypoglycemia in the Diabetes Control and Complications Trial. *Diabetes*. 1997;46:271–286.
6. Sigal RJ, Kenny GP, Wasserman DH, Castaneda-Sceppa C, White RD. Physical activity/exercise and type 2 diabetes: a consensus statement from the American Diabetes Association. *Diabetes Care*. 2006;29:1433–1438.
7. Albright A, Franz M, Hornsby G, et al. American College of Sports Medicine position stand: exercise and type 2 diabetes. *Med Sci Sports Exerc*. 2000;32:1345–1360.
8. American College of Sports Medicine and American Diabetes Association joint position statement: diabetes mellitus and exercise. *Med Sci Sports Exerc*. 1997;29:i–iv.
9. Molitch ME, DeFronzo RA, Franz MJ, et al. Nephropathy in diabetes. *Diabetes Care*. 2004;27(suppl 1):S79–S83.
10. Boulton AJ, Vinik AI, Arezzo JC, et al. Diabetic neuropathies: a statement by the American Diabetes Association. *Diabetes Care*. 2005;28:956–962.
11. Fong DS, Aiello L, Gardner TW, et al. Retinopathy in diabetes. *Diabetes Care*. 2004;27(suppl 1):S84–S87.
12. Berger M. Adjustments of insulin and oral agent therapy. In: Ruderman N, Devlin JT, Schneider SH, Kriska A, eds. *Handbook of Exercise in Diabetes*. Alexandria, VA: American Diabetes Association; 2002:365–376.
13. Schiffrin A, Parikh S. Accommodating planned exercise in type I diabetic patients on intensive treatment. *Diabetes Care*. 1985;8:337–342.
14. Schiffrin A, Parikh S, Marliss EB, Desrosiers MM. Metabolic response to fasting exercise in adolescent insulin-dependent diabetic subjects treated with continuous subcutaneous insulin infusion and intensive conventional therapy. *Diabetes Care*. 1984;7:255–260.
15. Riddell MC, Perkins BA. Type 1 diabetes and exercise, part I: applications of exercise physiology to patient management during vigorous activity. *Can J Diabetes*. 2006;30:63–71.
16. Zinman B, Ruderman N, Campaigne BN, Devlin JT, Schneider SH. Physical activity/exercise and diabetes. *Diabetes Care*. 2004;27(suppl 1):S58–S62.
17. Wright DA, Sherman WM, Dernbach AR. Carbohydrate feedings before, during, or in combination improve cycling endurance performance. *J Appl Physiol*. 1991;71:1082–1088.
18. Kalergis M, Schiffrin A, Gougeon R, Jones PJ, Yale JF. Impact of bedtime snack composition on prevention of nocturnal hypoglycemia in adults with type 1 diabetes undergoing intensive insulin management using lispro insulin before meals: a randomized, placebo-controlled, crossover trial. *Diabetes Care*. 2003;26(1):9–15.
19. Zinman B. Insulin pump with continuous subcutaneous insulin infusion and exercise in patients with type 1 diabetes. In: Ruderman N, Devlin JT, Schneider SH, Kriska A, eds. *Handbook of Exercise in Diabetes*. Alexandria, VA: American Diabetes Association; 2002:377–381.
20. Zinman B, Tildesley H, Chiasson JL, Tsui E, Strack T. Insulin lispro in CSII: results of a double-blind crossover study. *Diabetes*. 1997;46:440–443.
21. Francescato MP, Geat M, Fusi S, Stupar G, Noacco C, Cattin L. Carbohydrate requirement and insulin concentration during moderate exercise in type 1 diabetic patients. *Metabolism*. 2004;53:1126–1130.
22. Franz MJ. Nutrition, physical activity, and diabetes. In: Ruderman N, Devlin JT, Schneider SH, Kriska A, eds. *Handbook of Exercise in Diabetes*. Alexandria, VA: American Diabetes Association; 2002:321–338.
23. Wasserman DH, Zinman B. Exercise in individuals with IDDM. *Diabetes Care*. 1994;17:924–937.
24. Franz MJ, Bantle JP, Beebe CA, et al. Nutrition principles and recommendations in diabetes. *Diabetes Care*. 2004;27(suppl 1):S36–S46.
25. Brubaker PL. Adventure travel and type 1 diabetes: the complicating effects of high altitude. *Diabetes Care*. 2005;28:2563–2572.
26. Cryer PE, Davis SN, Shamoon H. Hypoglycemia in diabetes. *Diabetes Care*. 2003;26:1902–1912.
27. Bolli GB. How to ameliorate the problem of hypoglycemia in intensive as well as nonintensive treatment of type 1 diabetes. *Diabetes Care*. 1999; 22(suppl 2):B43–B52.
28. American Diabetes Association. Preventing and treating severe hypoglycemia. Available at: http://www.diabetes.org/preventing.jsp. Accessed September 10, 2007.
29. American Diabetes Association. Hypoglycemia. Available at: http://www.diabetes.org/type-1-diabetes/hypoglycemia.jsp. Accessed September 10, 2007.
30. Perkins BA, Riddell MC. Type I diabetes and exercise: using the insulin pump to maximum advantage. *Can J Diabetes*. 2006;30:72–79.
31. Berger M, Cuppers HJ, Hegner H, Jorgens V, Berchtold P. Absorption kinetics and biologic effects of subcutaneously injected insulin preparations. *Diabetes Care*. 1982;5:77–91.
32. Gossain VV. Insulin analogs and intensive insulin therapy in type 1 diabetes. *Int J Diab Dev Ctries*. 2003;23:26–36.
33. U.S. Department of Homeland Security Transportation Security Administration. Hidden disabilities: travelers with disabilities and medical con-

ditions. Available at: http://www.tsa.gov/travelers/airtravel/specialneeds/editorial_1347.shtm. Accessed September 10, 2007.

34. Gavin JR, Alberti KGMM, Davidson MB, et al. Report of the Expert Committee on the Diagnosis and Classification of Diabetes Mellitus. *Diabetes Care.* 1997;20(7):1183–1197.

35. American Diabetes Association. All about diabetes. Available at: http://www.diabetes.org/about-diabetes.jsp. Accessed September 10, 2007.

36. Centers for Disease Control and Prevention. National diabetes fact sheet: general information and national estimates on diabetes in the United States, 2003. Available at: http://www.cdc.gov/diabetes/pubs/factsheet.htm. Accessed September 10, 2007.

37. American Diabetes Association. *Medical Management of Insulin-Dependent (Type I) Diabetes.* 2nd ed. Alexandria, VA: American Diabetes Association; 1994.

38. Siminerio LM, Koerbel G. A diabetes education program for school personnel. *Practical Diabetes Int.* 2000;17:174–177.

39. Khan MA, Longley J. Psychosocial aspects of diabetes: the diabetologists' perspective. *Semin Clin Neuropsychiatry.* 1997;2:94–98.

40. American Diabetes Association. Care of children with diabetes in the school and day care setting. *Diabetes Care.* 1999;22:163–166.

41. Jimenez CC. Diabetes and exercise: the role of the athletic trainer. *J Athl Train.* 1997;32:339–343.

42. Stoller WA. Individualizing insulin management: three practical cases, rules for regimen adjustment. *Postgrad Med.* 2002;111: 51–54,59,60,63–66.

43. Brink SJ. How to apply the experience from the diabetes control and complications trial to children and adolescents? *Ann Med.* 1997;29:425–438.

44. The Diabetes Control and Complications Trial Research Group. Influence of intensive diabetes treatment on body weight and composition of adults with type 1 diabetes in the Diabetes Control and Complications Trial. *Diabetes Care.* 2001;24:1711–1721.

45. Kollipara S, Warren-Boulton E. Diabetes and physical activity in school. *School Nurse News.* 2004;21:12–16.

46. Katz G, Strain GW, Rodriguez M, Roman SH. Influence of an interdisciplinary diabetes specialist team on short-term outcomes of diabetes at a community health center. *Endocr Pract.* 1998;4:27–31.

47. Kanner S, Hamrin V, Grey M. Depression in adolescents with diabetes. *J Child Adolesc Psychiatr Nurs.* 2003;16:15–24.

48. Draznin MB. Type 1 diabetes and sports participation: strategies for training and competing safely. *Physician Sportsmed.* 2000;28(12):49–56.

49. Hopkins D. Exercise-induced and other daytime hypoglycemic events in patients with diabetes: prevention and treatment. *Diabetes Res Clin Pract.* 2004;65(suppl 1):S35–S39.

50. O'Connor DP. *Clinical Pathology for Athletic Trainers: Recognizing Systemic Disease.* Thorofare, NJ: Slack Inc; 2001.

51. Ciccone CD. *Pharmacology in Rehabilitation.* 2nd ed. Philadelphia, PA: FA Davis; 1996.

52. Skinner JS. *Exercise Testing and Exercise Prescription for Special Cases: Theoretical Basis and Clinical Application.* 3rd ed. Philadelphia, PA: Lippincott Williams & Wilkins; 2005.

53. Schneider SH, Shindler D. Application of the American Diabetes Association's guidelines for the evaluation of the diabetic patient before recommending and exercise program. In: Ruderman N, Devlin JT, Schneider SH, Kriska A, eds. *Handbook of Exercise in Diabetes.* Alexandria, VA: American Diabetes Association; 2002:253–268.

54. Nathan DM, Singer DE, Hurxthal K, Goodson JD. The clinical information value of the glycosylated hemoglobin assay. *N Engl J Med.* 1984; 310:341–346.

55. American Diabetes Association. Standards of medical care in diabetes, 2006. *Diabetes Care.* 2006;29(suppl 1):S4–S42.

56. Lebovitz HE, Austin MM, Blonde L, et al. ACE/AACE consensus conference on the implementation of outpatient management of diabetes mellitus: consensus conference recommendations. *Endocr Pract.* 2006; 12(suppl 1):6–12.

57. Aiello LP, Wong J, Cavallerano JD, Bursell S. Retinopathy. In: Ruderman N, Devlin JT, Schneider SH, Kriska A, eds. *Handbook of Exercise in Diabetes.* Alexandra, VA: American Diabetes Association; 2002:401–413.

58. Gross JL, de Azevedo MJ, Silveiro SP, Canani LH, Caramori ML, Zelmanovitz T. Diabetic nephropathy: diagnosis, prevention, and treatment. *Diabetes Care.* 2005;28:164–176.

59. Waxman S, Nest RW. Cardiovascular complications. In: Ruderman N, Devlin JT, Schneider SH, Kriska A, eds. *Handbook of Exercise in Diabetes.* Alexandra, VA: American Diabetes Association; 2002:415–432.

60. Heinemann L. Variability of insulin absorption and insulin action. *Diabetes Technol Ther.* 2002;4:673–682.

61. Koda-Kimble MA, Carlisle BA. Diabetes mellitus. In: Koda-Kimble MA, Young LY, eds. *Applied Therapeutics: The Clinical Use of Drugs.* Philadelphia, PA: Lippincott Williams & Wilkins; 2001:48–51.

62. Roy B, Chou MC, Field JB. Time-action characteristics of regular and NPH insulin in insulin-treated diabetics. *J Clin Endocrinol Metab.* 1980; 50:475–479.

63. Frohnauer MK, Woodworth JR, Anderson JH. Graphical human insulin time-activity profiles using standardized definitions. *Diabetes Technol Ther.* 2001;3:419–429.

64. Kang S, Brange J, Burch A, Volund A, Owens DR. Absorption kinetics and action profiles of subcutaneously administered insulin analogues S (AspB9GluB27, AspB10, AspB28) in healthy subjects. *Diabetes Care.* 1991;14:1057–1065.

65. American Diabetes Association. Insulin administration. *Diabetes Care.* 2004;27(suppl 1):S106–S107.

66. Binder C, Brange J. Insulin chemistry and pharmacokinetics. In: Porte D, Sherwin RS, eds. *Ellenberg and Rifkin's Diabetes Mellitus.* Stamford, CT: Appleton and Lange; 1997:689.

67. ter Braak EW, Woodworth JR, Bianchi R, et al. Injection site effects on the pharmacokinetics and glucodynamics of insulin lispro and regular insulin. *Diabetes Care.* 1996;19:1437–1440.

68. Camacho RC, Galassetti P, Davis SN, Wasserman DH. Glucoregulation during and after exercise in health and insulin-dependent diabetes. *Exerc Sport Sci Rev.* 2005;33:17–23.

69. Zinman B, Murray FT, Vranic M, et al. Glucoregulation during moderate exercise in insulin treated diabetics. *J Clin Endocrinol Metab.* 1977;45: 641–652.

70. Riddell MC, Bar-Or O, Ayub BV, Calvert RE, Heigenhauser GJ. Glucose ingestion matched with total carbohydrate utilization attenuates hypoglycemia during exercise in adolescents with IDDM. *Int J Sport Nutr.* 1999; 9:24–34.

71. MacDonald MJ. Postexercise late-onset hypoglycemia in insulin-dependent diabetic patients. *Diabetes Care.* 1987;10:584–588.

72. McAulay V, Deary IJ, Frier BM. Symptoms of hypoglycaemia in people with diabetes. *Diabet Med.* 2001;18:690–705.

73. Marliss EB, Vranic M. Intense exercise has unique effects on both insulin release and its roles in glucoregulation: implications for diabetes. *Diabetes.* 2002;51(suppl 1):S271–S283.

74. Mitchell TH, Abraham G, Schiffrin A, Leiter LA, Marliss EB. Hyperglycemia after intense exercise in IDDM subjects during continuous subcutaneous insulin infusion. *Diabetes Care.* 1988;11:311–317.

75. Hargreaves M, Angus D, Howlett K, Conus NM, Febbraio M. Effect of heat stress on glucose kinetics during exercise. *J Appl Physiol.* 1996;81: 1594–1597.

76. Cox DJ, Kovatchev BP, Gonder-Frederick LA, et al. Relationships between hyperglycemia and cognitive performance among adults with type 1 and type 2 diabetes. *Diabetes Care.* 2005;28:71–77.

77. Hornsby WG Jr, Chetlin RD. Management of competitive athletes with diabetes. *Diabetes Spectr.* 2005;18:102–107.

78. American Diabetes Association. Traveling with diabetes supplies. Available at: http://www.diabetes.org/advocacy-and-legalresources/discrimination/public_accommodation/travel.jsp. Accessed September 10, 2007.

79. Dewey CM, Riley WJ. Have diabetes, will travel. *Postgrad Med.* 1999; 105: 111–113,117,118,124–216.

80. Bia FJ, Barry M. Special health considerations for travelers. *Med Clin North Am.* 1992;76:1295–1312.

81. White CB, Turner NS, Lee GC, Haidukewych GJ. Open ankle fractures in patients with diabetes mellitus. *Clin Orthop Relat Res.* 2003;414:37–44.

82. Jani MM, Ricci WM, Borrelli J Jr, Barrett SE, Johnson JE. A protocol

for treatment of unstable ankle fractures using transarticular fixation in patients with diabetes mellitus and loss of protective sensibility. *Foot Ankle Int.* 2003;24:838–844.

83. Bibbo C, Lin SS, Beam HA, Behrens FF. Complications of ankle fractures in diabetic patients. *Orthop Clin North Am.* 2001;32:113–133.

84. Young ME. Malnutrition and wound healing. *Heart Lung.* 1988;17:60–67.

85. Hotter AN. Physiologic aspects and clinical implications of wound healing. *Heart Lung.* 1982;11:522–531.

86. Cooper DM. Optimizing wound healing: a practice within nursing's domain. *Nurs Clin North Am.* 1990;25:165–180.

87. Goodson WH III, Hunt TK. Wound healing in experimental diabetes mellitus: importance of early insulin therapy. *Surg Forum.* 1978;29:95–98.

88. Flynn JM, Rodriguez-del Rio F, Piza PA. Closed ankle fractures in the diabetic patient. *Foot Ankle Int.* 2000;21:311–319.

89. Bagdade JD, Walters E. Impaired granulocyte adherence in mildly diabetic patients: effects of tolazamide treatment. *Diabetes.* 1980;29:309–311.

90. Pierre EJ, Barrow RE, Hawkins HK, et al. Effects of insulin on wound healing. *J Trauma.* 1998;44:342–345.

91. Clement S, Braithwaite SS, Magee MF, et al. Management of diabetes and hyperglycemia in hospitals. *Diabetes Care.* 2004;27:553–591.

Carolyn C. Jimenez, PhD, ATC; Matthew H. Corcoran, MD, CDE; James T. Crawley, MEd, PT, ATC; W. Guyton Hornsby, Jr, PhD, CDE; Kimberly S. Peer, EdD, LATC; Rick D. Philbin, MBA, MEd, ATC; and Michael C. Riddell, PhD, contributed to conception and design; acquisition and analysis and interpretation of the data; and drafting, critical revision, and final approval of the article.

Address correspondence to National Athletic Trainers' Association, Communications Department, 2952 Stemmons Freeway, Dallas, TX 75247. Address e-mail to cjimenez@wcupa.edu.

Appendix 1. Strategies to Prevent Hypoglycemia[1,12–25]

Strategy	Comment
Blood glucose monitoring	Athletes should measure blood glucose levels before, during, and after exercise. Athletes who exercise in extreme heat or cold or at high altitude or experience postexercise late-onset hypoglycemia, which may lead to nighttime hypoglycemia, require additional monitoring. 1. Measure blood glucose levels 2 to 3 times before exercise at 30-min intervals to determine directional glucose movement. 2. Measure glucose levels every 30 min during exercise if possible. 3. Athletes who experience postexercise late-onset hypoglycemia should measure glucose levels every 2 h up to 4 h postexercise. Athletes who experience nighttime hypoglycemia should measure blood glucose values before going to sleep, once during the night, and immediately upon waking.
Carbohydrate supplementation (Note: The athlete should discuss specific carbohydrate quantities and types with his or her physician.)	Before exercise Consumption of carbohydrates before exercise depends on the prevailing blood glucose level. In general, when the blood glucose level is <100 mg/dL (5.5 mmol/L), carbohydrates should be consumed.[26,27] During exercise 1. Additional carbohydrate supplementation may be needed for practices or games lasting >60 min when the pre-exercise insulin dosage has not been reduced by at least 50%. 2. Athletes who are exercising at the peak of insulin activity may require additional carbohydrates. Postexercise Athletes should eat a snack and/or meal shortly after exercise.

Insulin adjustments (Note: These are very important for moderate-intensity to high-intensity exercise sessions of ≥30 min.)	Physician determines insulin reduction strategies.
	1. Insulin pump (may use one or more of the following strategies)
	  a. Reduce basal rate by 20% to 50% 1 to 2 h before exercise.
	  b. Reduce bolus dose up to 50% at the meal preceding exercise.
	  c. Suspend or disconnect the insulin pump at the start of exercise. Note: Athletes should not suspend or disconnect from pump longer than 60 min without supplemental insulin.
	2. Multiple daily injection
	Reduce bolus dose up to 50% at the meal preceding exercise.
	3. Nighttime hypoglycemia
	Reduce evening meal bolus insulin by 50%.

Appendix 2. Treatment Guidelines for Mild and Severe Hypoglycemia[28,29]

Mild Hypoglycemia (Athlete is conscious and able to follow directions and swallow.)	Severe Hypoglycemia (Athlete is unconscious or unable to follow directions or swallow.)
1. Administer 10 g to 15 g of fast-acting carbohydrate: eg, 4 to 8 glucose tablets, 2 T honey.	1. Activate emergency medical system.
2. Measure blood glucose level.	2. Prepare glucagon for injection following directions in glucagon kit. The glucagon kit has either (1) a fluid-filled syringe and a vial of glucagon powder, or (2) a syringe, 1 vial of glucagon powder, and 1 vial of fluid.
3. Wait approximately 15 min and remeasure blood glucose.	• Inject the fluid into the vial of glucagon. Note: If the vial of fluid is separate, draw the fluid into the syringe and inject it into the vial of glucagon powder.
4. If blood glucose level remains low, administer another 10 g to 15 g of fast-acting carbohydrate.	• Gently shake the vial until the glucagon powder dissolves and the solution is clear.
5. Recheck blood glucose level in approximately 15 min.	• Draw fluid back into the syringe and then inject glucagon into the arm, thigh, or buttock.*
6. If blood glucose level does not return to the normal range after second dosage of carbohydrate, activate emergency medical system.	• Glucagon administration may cause nausea and/or vomiting when the athlete awakens. Place the athlete on his or her side to prevent aspiration.
7. Once blood glucose level is in the normal range, athlete may wish to consume a snack (eg, sandwich, bagel)	• The athlete should become conscious within 15 min of administration.
	3. Once the athlete is conscious and able to swallow, provide food.

*Athletic trainers should be trained in the mixing and administration of glucagon. The athlete or athlete's family can provide training. In addition, a video demonstrating the preparation and administration of glucagon is available at http://www.diabetes.org/type-2-diabetes/hypoglycemia.jsp.[29]

Appendix 3. American Diabetes Association Guidelines Concerning Hyperglycemia and Exercise[16]

Blood Glucose Level	Comment
Fasting* blood glucose level is ≥250 mg/dL (13.9 mmol/L).	Test urine and/or blood for ketones. If ketones present, exercise is contraindicated. If ketones not present, exercise is not contraindicated.
Blood glucose value is ≥300 mg/dL (16.7 mmol/L) and without ketones.	Exercise with caution, and continue to monitor blood glucose levels.

*Fasting is defined as 4 h or more after eating a meal.

Appendix 4. Pharmacokinetics of Commonly Used Insulin Preparations[60–64]

Product	Action Type	Basal or Bolus Use	Onset	Peak Effect	Duration
Humalog (lispro; Eli Lilly and Co, Indianapolis, IN)	Rapid acting	Bolus in MDI*	5–15 min	45–75 min	3–5 h
Novolog (aspart; Novo Nordisk Inc, Princeton, NJ)		Basal and bolus in insulin pump			
Apidra (glulisine; Sanofi-Aventis, Bridgewater, NJ)					
Humulin (regular; Eli Lilly and Co)	Fast acting	Bolus in MDI	30 min	2–4 h	5–8 h
Novolin (regular; Novo Nordisk Inc)		Basal and bolus in insulin pump			
Humulin N (NPH; Eli Lilly and Co)†	Intermediate acting	Basal insulin in MDI	1–2 h	4–10 h	14+ h
Novolin N (NPH; Novo Nordisk Inc)†					
Lantus (glargine; Sanofi-Aventis)†	Long acting	Basal in MDI	1.5–2 h	Flat	18–24 h
Detemir (levimir; Novo Nordisk Inc) †					

*Indicates multiple daily injections.
†Indicates not used in insulin pump therapy.

Appendix 5. Variables That Affect Insulin Absorption Rate[31,32,60,61,66,67]

Variable	Notes
Exercise of the injected area	Exercise of injected area within 1 h of injection may increase the rate of absorption.
Massage of the injection site	Do not rub or vigorously massage injection sites within 1 h of injection.
Thermal modalities	Heat increases absorption, whereas cold decreases absorption. Avoid using thermal modalities for 1 to 3 h postinjection.
Insulin dose	Larger doses are associated with slower absorption rates.
Lipohypertrophy (accumulation of subcutaneous fatty lumps caused by repeated injections of insulin into the same spot)	Injection into lipohypertrophic sites delays absorption.

Diabetes Management Review Questions:

1. For the athletic trainer, what is the most important goal in managing an athlete with diabetes?

2. Explain the components of an athlete's diabetes care plan. In addition to this plan, list the supplies for treating diabetic-related emergencies that should be maintained in an athletic training kit and available during all practices and games. From this list, delineate the items athletic trainers should consider regularly maintaining in their athletic training kits whether or not they have identified any diabetic athletes under their care.

3. Explain how the signs, symptoms and treatment guidelines for mild and severe hypoglycemia differ from those of hyperglycemia.

4. As an athletic trainer, what recommendations can you make to an athlete with diabetes who has sustained trauma?

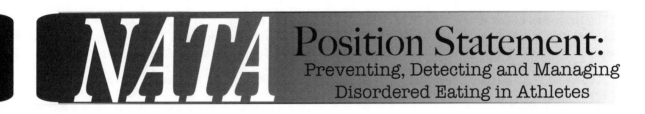

NATA Position Statement:
Preventing, Detecting and Managing Disordered Eating in Athletes

In This Section: As the intensity and demand of higher level sport training increases, cases of disordered eating are becoming more common. This position statement defines the different eating disorders, offers guidelines for building collaborative relationships and gives specific strategies for prevention and detection of disordered eating in athletes.

National Athletic Trainers' Association Position Statement: Preventing, Detecting, and Managing Disordered Eating in Athletes

Christine M. Bonci, MS, ATC*; Leslie J. Bonci, MPH, RD, LDN, CSSD†;
Lorita R. Granger, ATC‡; Craig L. Johnson, PhD§;
Robert M. Malina, PhD, FACSM*‖; Leslie W. Milne, MD¶; Randa R. Ryan, PhD*;
Erin M. Vanderbunt, MS, ATC#

*The University of Texas at Austin, Austin, TX; †The University of Pittsburgh Medical Center, Pittsburgh, PA; ‡University of California at Los Angeles, Los Angeles, CA; §Laureate Psychiatric Hospital, Tulsa, OK; ‖Tarleton State University, Stephenville, TX; ¶Massachusetts General Hospital, Boston, MA; #Paradise Valley Community College, Phoenix, AZ

Objective: To present recommendations for the prevention, detection, and comprehensive management of disordered eating (DE) in athletes.

Background: Athletes with DE rarely self-report their symptoms. They tend to deny the condition and are often resistant to referral and treatment. Thus, screenings and interventions must be handled skillfully by knowledgeable professionals to obtain desired outcomes. Certified athletic trainers have the capacity and responsibility to play active roles as integral members of the health care team. Their frequent daily interactions with athletes help to facilitate the level of medical surveillance necessary for early detection, timely referrals, treatment follow-through, and compliance.

Recommendations: These recommendations are intended to provide certified athletic trainers and others participating in the health maintenance and performance enhancement of athletes with specific knowledge and problem-solving skills to better prevent, detect, and manage DE. The individual biological, psychological, sociocultural, and familial factors for each athlete with DE result in widely different responses to intervention strategies, challenging the best that athletics programs have to offer in terms of resources and expertise. The complexity, time intensiveness, and expense of managing DE necessitate an interdisciplinary approach representing medicine, nutrition, mental health, athletic training, and athletics administration in order to facilitate early detection and treatment, make it easier for symptomatic athletes to ask for help, enhance the potential for full recovery, and satisfy medicolegal requirements. Of equal importance is establishing educational initiatives for preventing DE.

Key Words: eating disorders, anorexia nervosa, bulimia nervosa, subclinical eating disorders, pathogenic weight control behaviors, female athlete triad, body image

---

Disordered eating (DE) in athletes is characterized by a wide spectrum of maladaptive eating and weight control behaviors and attitudes. These include concerns about body weight and shape; poor nutrition or inadequate caloric intake, or both; binge eating; use of laxatives, diuretics, and diet pills; and extreme weight control methods, such as fasting, vomiting, and excessive exercise.[1–4] Susceptibility of athletes to DE is a serious concern because of increased physiologic demands imposed by high-intensity and high-volume sport training. Although the extent of DE in athletes is unclear due to methodologic limitations of existing studies (primarily the lack of standardized assessment tools and consistent criteria for defining DE), prevalence estimates have ranged as high as 62% among female athletes and 33% among male athletes.[5–16]

Disordered eating can lead to adverse effects on health and physical performance. In some cases, the condition can be fatal.[17,18] Consequences of DE upon health and performance depend on the athlete's immediate health status; the demands of sport-specific training; type, severity, and duration of the pathogenic weight control or eating behaviors; the degree of nutrient deficiency; the presence of comorbid physical and mental disorders; and the timing and quality of therapeutic interventions.[14,19,20]

PURPOSE

The purpose of this position statement is to provide recommendations to better prepare certified athletic trainers, other health care providers, sports management personnel, and coaches for the challenges of understanding and working with athletes who present with DE or who may be at risk. Special attention is given to addressing the physical and mental health needs of symptomatic and at-risk athletes through early detection and treatment, increased access to quality resources, and educational programs for prevention.

RECOMMENDATIONS

The National Athletic Trainers' Association (NATA) provides the following guidelines for creating the necessary team infrastructure, collaborative relationships, and strategies for preventing, detecting, and managing DE in athletes.

Immediate Action Items

1. Identify a team of qualified caregivers who have the requisite training for early case detection, treatment, and provision of other assistance as needed. Caregivers should represent multiple disciplines, including medicine, nutrition, mental health, and athletic training.[21-26] They should be readily accessible, understand their roles, and promote collaboration to facilitate a seamless continuum of care.

2. Reserve a place on the health care team for an athletics administrator.[27,28] Organizations are better prepared to handle complexities of DE management with an informed administrator who has authority to take action when unexpected events and worst-case scenarios challenge the scope of existing resources and expertise.

3. Assemble the health care team to formulate and implement a comprehensive management protocol complete with policies and procedures that facilitate early detection, accurate assessment, and treatment of athletes with DE (Figure).

4. Enlist the support and input of risk-management personnel and legal counsel in planning, developing, and implementing the management protocol. Certified athletic trainers, other caregivers, and athletics administrators should cooperate with these groups to determine what constitutes reasonable care to prevent foreseeable harm to participants and avoid potential liability for negligence.[29,30]

5. Establish a screening approach that recognizes signs and symptoms of the full spectrum of maladaptive eating and weight loss behaviors, as well as predisposing risk factors associated with their development. This is most effectively accomplished during the preparticipation examination (PPE) by compiling a thorough medical history with attention to the assessment of DE.[31-36]

6. Develop policies that clearly define the appropriate responses of coaches when dealing with athletes regarding body weight issues and performance. Coaches should not be allowed to disseminate improper weight loss advice, conduct mandatory weigh-ins, set target weights, or apply external pressure on athletes to lose weight.

7. Design mandatory structured educational and behavioral programs for all athletes, coaches, certified athletic trainers, administrators, and other support personnel to prevent DE.

Detecting Disordered Eating

Clinical Features and Behavioral Warning Signs

8. Early detection and treatment of DE should become a high priority for athletics programs. Disordered eating occurs along a continuum of severity. Mild symptoms that increase in frequency and severity may progress to 3 clinically diagnosable conditions identified in the *Diagnostic and Statistical Manual of Mental Disorders (DSM-IV)*[20] as anorexia nervosa (AN), bulimia nervosa (BN), and eating disorder not otherwise specified (EDNOS) (Tables 1, 2, and 3, respectively). Exclusive adherence to strict *DSM-IV* criteria without recognizing the subclinical precursors of eating disorders (EDs) may be a barrier to early detection and subsequently affect the timing and quality of therapeutic interventions.

9. Those supervising the health and performance of athletes should be alert to the most common behavioral and psychological characteristics that may indicate an athlete's impending lapse into a subclinical or full-syndrome ED in order to prevent or minimize problems (Table 4). The challenge is in determining whether the athlete's dietary and weight control behaviors are transient, safely managed behaviors associated with the physiologic demands of the sport or becoming increasingly unhealthy or persistent, which may signify a more serious problem.[37]

Signs, Symptoms, and Physical Complications

10. Signs and symptoms of EDs should be recognized at their earliest onset (Table 5). Medical complications associated with malnutrition and purging can affect multiple organ systems and progress to serious health consequences, including, but not limited to, cardiovascular, reproductive, and skeletal dysfunction and, in some cases, death.[17]

11. Given the possibility of sudden death resulting from cardiovascular complications, pulse rate and quality, blood pressure, orthostatic measurements, and body temperature should be serially recorded.[38] Clinical signs indicating possible physiologic instability include bradycardia (resting heart rate <50 beats/min during the day and <45 beats/min at night), hypotension (systolic pressure <90 mm Hg), orthostatic changes in pulse (>20 beats/min) or blood pressure (>10 mm Hg), and hypothermia (body temperature <96°F [35.56°C]).[18,39] The likelihood of cardiovascular problems depends upon the severity and/or chronicity of energy restriction, the amount, rate, and composition of weight loss, and electrolyte imbalances induced by purging.[27]

12. Recognizing that the reproductive system of female athletes is extremely sensitive to low energy availability and consequent menstrual cycle alterations (eg, amenorrhea)[40-42] and bone mineral disorders,[40-45] closely monitoring physically active girls and adolescents participating in a wide variety of sports is recommended. Female athletes presenting with amenorrhea should be evaluated within the first 3 months of onset.[46] Aggressive treatment should follow to reestablish normal menses and prevent progressive bone loss. This evaluation requires examining the athlete's eating and training regimens for adequate energy availability. If deficiencies exist, an increase in dietary intake or reduction in exercise intensity (or both) should be recommended. Consideration should also be given to calcium and vitamin D supplementation to achieve and maintain the recommended

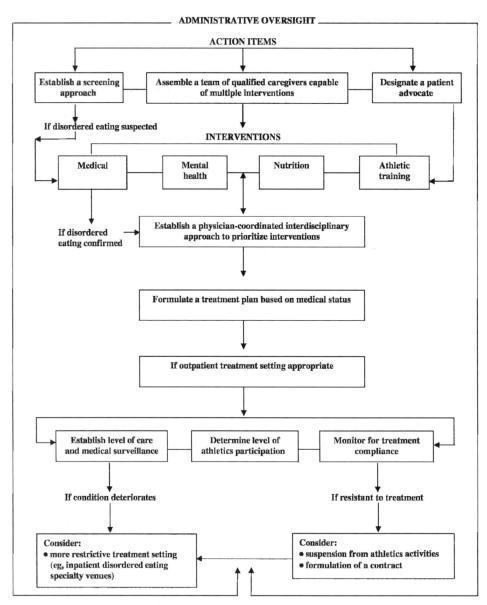

Figure. Disordered-eating management protocol: outpatient setting.

dietary intakes of 1000 to 1500 mg/d of calcium and 400 to 600 IU/d of vitamin D.[47–51] High doses of both supplements may be necessary to prevent or treat osteoporosis and minimize fracture risk or prevent fractures, especially in individuals who do not meet recommended dietary intakes.[45,50] Pharmacologic treatment administered in the form of hormone replacement therapy or the oral contraceptive pill[52–54] requires careful deliberation. The results of such treatment remain inconsistent in adequately restoring bone loss or correcting the metabolic abnormalities that compromise health and performance in amenorrheic athletes.[45] The reader is referred to the American College of Sports Medicine's revised position statement[45] on the female athlete triad for indications and contraindications for administration of these agents. In view of the potential irreversibility of bone loss despite some of these interventions,[45,53,54] prompt identification of early-onset low bone mineral density

through use of dual-energy x-ray absorptiometry (DXA) may contribute to reducing stress fracture incidence and future morbidity resulting from osteoporosis.[55,56]

13. The sequelae of reproductive and skeletal complications require familiarity with the revised description of the female athlete triad and its interrelationships among energy availability, menstrual function, and bone mineral density.[45] These triad components are now believed to exist along a continuum model of health and disease. At the pathologic end of the spectrum lies each component's clinical manifestations — low energy availability with or without eating disorder, functional hypothalamic amenorrhea, and osteoporosis. Although very few female athletes, whether elite, young adult, or adolescent, simultaneously possess all clinical manifestations of the triad,[14,57–59] clinicians need to be mindful of the interrelationship of triad components with respect to

Table 1. *Diagnostic and Statistical Manual of Mental Disorders* (4th edition) Criteria for Anorexia Nervosa[a]

Description
A. Refusal to maintain body weight at or above a minimally normal weight for age and height (eg, weight loss leading to maintenance of body weight less than 85% of that expected or failure to make expected weight gain during period of growth, leading to body weight less than 85% of that expected).
B. Intense fear of gaining weight or becoming fat, even though underweight.
C. Disturbance in the way in which one's body weight or shape is experienced, undue influence of body weight or shape on self-evaluation, or denial of the seriousness of the current low body weight.
D. In post-menarcheal females, amenorrhea, ie, the absence of at least three consecutive menstrual cycles. (A woman is considered to have amenorrhea if her periods occur only following hormone, eg, estrogen, administration.)

Specify Type

Restricting type: During the current episode of anorexia nervosa, the person has not regularly engaged in binge-eating or purging behavior (ie, self-induced vomiting or the misuse of laxatives, diuretics or enemas).

Binge-eating/purging: During the current episode of anorexia nervosa, the person has regularly engaged in binge-eating or purging behavior (ie, self-induced vomiting or the misuse of laxatives, diuretics or enemas).

[a]Reprinted with permission from the *Diagnostic and Statistical Manual of Mental Disorders*, Text Revision. © 2000:589. American Psychiatric Association.[20]

cause and pathogenesis. Individual disorders (alone or in combination) should be addressed as soon as they present to decrease the potential for irreversible health consequences.[45,59–61]

14. Equal attention should be paid to male athletes who exhibit signs and symptoms of EDs. Compared with female athletes, males have no diagnostic hallmark such as amenorrhea for detecting EDs.[62] Absent overt clinical signs coupled with the reluctance of males to openly discuss their eating problems because of feelings of shame and embarrassment over having a stereotypically "female" disorder could result in a delay in diagnosis and treatment.[63–66]

15. Because more commonalities than differences exist in the physical and psychological characteristics of EDs in young adult male and female athletes, similar strategies should be used to detect and treat the condition in both sexes.[63,67,68]

Predisposing Risk Factors

16. All certified athletic trainers should become knowledgeable about the most common predisposing risk factors for development of DE to understand its

complex causes and to minimize the possibility of missing crucial information that may have important implications for early detection and treatment. For purposes of DE prevention and containment, the focus of attention should be on those risk factors most amenable to alteration: in particular, the pressure on athletes to manipulate eating and weight for performance and appearance thinness, as well as the sociocultural and media-driven emphasis on appearance thinness.[27,69,70]

17. The index of suspicion for DE should be high in all types of sports. Current literature[59] challenges the perception that the prevalence of DE is greater in sports in which a low body weight or small physique is important for maximizing performance, subjective evaluation and aesthetic ideals coexist, or body weight restrictions apply.[8,10,14,71,72] Intensified pressure to attain or maintain an ideal body weight or body fat percentage is not necessarily inherent in the activity itself but in the athlete's perception of what is required for optimizing performance. It only follows that avoiding external pressure on athletes to lose weight is essential to avert a preoccupation with

Table 2. *Diagnostic and Statistical Manual of Mental Disorders* (4th edition) Criteria for Bulimia Nervosa[a]

Description
A. Recurrent episodes of binge eating. An episode of binge eating is characterized by both of the following:
1. Eating, in a discrete period of time (eg, within any two-hour period), an amount of food that is definitely larger than most people would eat during a similar period of time and under similar circumstances.
2. A sense of lack of control over eating during the episode (eg, a feeling that one cannot stop eating or control what or how much one is eating).
B. Recurrent inappropriate compensatory behavior in order to prevent weight gain, such as self-induced vomiting; misuse of laxatives, diuretics, enemas or other medications; fasting; or excessive exercise.
C. The binge eating and inappropriate compensatory behaviors both occur, on average, at least twice a week for three months.
D. Self-evaluation is unduly influenced by body shape and weight.
E. The disturbance does not occur exclusively during episodes of anorexia nervosa.

Specify Type

Purging type: During the current episode of bulimia nervosa, the person has regularly engaged in self-induced vomiting or the misuse of laxatives, diuretics or enemas.

Non-purging type: During the current episode of bulimia nervosa, the person has used other inappropriate compensatory behaviors, such as fasting or excessive exercise, but has not regularly engaged in self-induced vomiting or the misuse of laxatives, diuretics or enemas.

[a]Reprinted with permission from the *Diagnostic and Statistical Manual of Mental Disorders*, Text Revision. © 2000:594. American Psychiatric Association.[20]

Table 3. *Diagnostic and Statistical Manual of Mental Disorders* (4th edition) Criteria for Eating Disorder Not Otherwise Specified[a]

Description
A. For females, all of the criteria for anorexia nervosa are met except that the individual has regular menses.
B. All of the criteria for anorexia nervosa are met except that, despite significant weight loss, the individual's current weight is in the normal range.
C. All of the criteria for bulimia nervosa are met, except that the binge eating and inappropriate compensatory mechanisms occur at a frequency of less than twice a week or for a duration of less than three months.
D. The regular use of inappropriate compensatory behavior by an individual of normal body weight after eating small amounts of food (eg, self-induced vomiting after the consumption of two cookies).
E. Repeatedly chewing and spitting out, but not swallowing, large amounts of food.
F. Binge-eating disorder: recurrent episodes of binge eating in the absence of the regular use of inappropriate compensatory behaviors characteristic of bulimia nervosa.

[a]Reprinted with permission from the *Diagnostic and Statistical Manual of Mental Disorders*, Text Revision. © 2000:594–595. American Psychiatric Association.[20]

dieting, which is considered the number-one trigger for DE.[13,73–75]

Screening Methods

18. Because athletes with DE rarely self-identify due to secrecy, shame, denial, and fear of reprisal,[10,70,76] specific questionnaire items designed to assess DE behaviors and attitudes should be incorporated into the medical history portion of the PPE to facilitate the detection process (Tables 6a, 6b).

19. If suspicions of DE are raised from interpretation of questionnaire results, an in-depth personal interview by a member of the health care team should follow for a more accurate interpretation of circumstances.[14,77–80]

20. Practitioners should proceed with caution when considering the use of self-report psychometric questionnaires such as the Eating Disorders Inventory (EDI),[31] the Eating Disorders Examination (EDE-Q),[81] and the Eating Attitudes Test (EAT)[82] to screen for behavioral and cognitive characteristics of DE in athletes. Although the questionnaires have been widely used to screen athletes for DE, they have not been specifically tested for external validity with athletic populations and, consequently, may result in inaccurate information. If additional screening measures are desired to complement the medical history portion of the PPE, consideration should be given to using instruments designed specifically for athletes, as more information becomes available on their validity with larger sample sizes and with athletes in a variety of sports and sport settings and at various levels of performance (Table 7).

21. In addition to using questionnaires and interviews, certified athletic trainers, other health care providers, and coaches should become more skilled observers of an athlete's behavior (eg, inappropriate dieting, weight loss, suboptimal weight, fatigue, performance decrement, and excessive exercise),[37] which may provide the quickest means of detecting DE.

Physiologic Measurements

22. Pursuit of performance and appearance thinness in sport necessitates strategies that have the potential to

Table 4. Psychological and Behavioral Characteristics of Eating-Disordered Athletes[a]

Dieting (unnecessary for health, sports performance, or appearance)
Self-critical; especially concerning body weight, size and shape in addition to performance
Avoidance of eating and eating situations
Secretive eating
Ritualistic eating patterns
Claims of "feeling fat" despite being thin[b]
Resistance to weight gain or maintenance recommended by medical providers
Unusual weighing behavior (ie, excessive weighing, refusal to weigh for health or safety reasons, negative reaction to being weighed)
Compulsiveness and rigidity, especially regarding eating and exercising
Excessive or obligatory exercise beyond that recommended for training or performance
Exercising while injured despite medically prescribed activity restrictions
Restlessness; relaxing is difficult or impossible
Change in behavior from open, positive, and social to suspicious, untruthful, and sad
Social withdrawal
Depression and insomnia
Binge eating[c]
Agitation when binging is interrupted[c]
Evidence of vomiting unrelated to illness[c]
Excessive use of the restroom or "disappearing" after eating[c]
Use of laxatives or diuretics (or both) that is unsanctioned by medical providers[c]
Substance abuse, whether legal, illegal, prescribed, or over-the-counter drugs, medications, or other substances[c]

[a]Adapted from *The Female Athlete*, Mary Lloyd Ireland and Aurelia Nattiv (eds.), Jorunn Sundgot-Borgen, Disordered Eating, p. 243, 2002, with permission from Elsevier Science.[24]
[b]Indicates especially for anorexia nervosa.
[c]Indicates especially for bulimia nervosa.

Table 5. Physical Signs/Symptoms of Eating-Disordered Athletes[a]

Cardiovascular
- Bradycardia
- Hypotension
- Atrial and ventricular arrhythmias
- Electrocardiographic abnormalities
- Acrocyanosis

Endocrine
- Hypoglycemia
- Decreased testosterone levels in males
- Low female sex hormone levels
- Amenorrhea or menstrual dysfunction
- Reduced bone mineral density
- Stress fractures
- Delayed onset of puberty[b]
- Short stature/arrested skeletal growth[b]

Gastrointestinal
- Constipation, bloating, postprandial distress
- Abdominal pain
- Bowel irregularities

Fluids and Electrolytes
- Dehydration
- Electrolyte abnormalities
- Hypokalemia
- Muscle cramps
- Metabolic alkalosis
- Edema

Thermoregulation
- Hypothermia[b]

Hematologic
- Anemia

Dermatologic
- Hair loss[b]
- Dry skin, brittle hair and nails[b]
- Lanugo[b]
- Callus or abrasion on back of hand (from inducing vomiting)[c]

Oral/facial
- Dental decay
- Pain in pharynx
- Swollen parotid glands[c]

Others
- Significant weight loss (beyond that necessary for adequate sport performance)[b]
- Frequent and often extreme weight fluctuations[c]
- Low weight despite eating large volumes[c]
- Fatigue (beyond that normally expected in training or competition)
- Muscle weakness

[a]Adapted from *The Female Athlete*, Mary Lloyd Ireland and Aurelia Nattiv (eds.), Jorunn Sundgot-Borgen, Disordered Eating, p. 242, 2002, with permission from Elsevier Science.[24]
[b]Indicates especially for anorexia nervosa.
[c]Indicates especially for bulimia.

provide essential information for nutritional support and training status of athletes over and above the use of scale weight.[27,86] Consideration should be given to assessing body composition, with special reference to gradual changes in fat mass and fat-free mass and, if possible, the amount and quality of lean muscle mass instead of percentage of body fat. Calculating the body mass index (BMI) should also be considered to monitor

appropriateness of weight for height, which varies by age and sex.

a. **Assessing Body Composition.** Body composition should be monitored only under the following conditions: (1) A qualified individual, who is appropriately trained and proficient in assessing and interpreting results, has been designated to handle the process, (2) The same individual is available for serial measurements to minimize variation among assessments and technicians, and (3) A registered dietitian is available if results call for nutritional support. Additionally, the measurement process and data exchange should be handled in a manner that protects the privacy, confidentiality, and self-esteem of athletes. The following procedures will facilitate the process:

- Deemphasize the importance of an ideal body weight or body fat percentage. Individual differences in body weight and composition are considerable, so a range of normal variation among athletes in a given sport or event should be recognized.
- Emphasize changes in estimated fat mass or lean muscle mass in individual athletes during the season. Absolute estimates of fat mass or percentage of body fat have limited utility given the wide range of individual differences and potential measurement variability.
- Avoid public discussion of the results. Data should be confidential and shared only with the athlete in a private setting. Coaches should not be present during the measurement process or the data exchange. Depending on the health and training status of the athlete, it may be necessary to share results with coaches or close significant others (CSOs). This should be determined on an individual basis and only after receiving disclosure permission from the athlete.
- Establish an interval of at least 2 to 3 months between serial measurements, so that short-term fluctuations in body weight do not confound assessments or decisions.

b. **Calculating the Body Mass Index.** The body mass index (BMI) should be used as a screening tool to determine the appropriateness of an athlete's body weight for height, which varies with age and sex. For the measurement of height, the athlete should not be wearing shoes. Weight should be measured with the athlete wearing minimal clothing (shorts, T-shirt) and using a regularly calibrated scale. Accuracy of measurement is essential.

- A BMI <18.5 kg/m^2 has been recommended by the World Health Organization (1998) as indicative of being underweight in adults (≥ 18 years of age).[87] Although this level may

Table 6a. Medical History Review — Disordered Eating Questionnaire Items[a]

- Are you currently, or have you in the past year, followed a particular "diet"?___Yes___ No
- How many meals (ie, breakfast, lunch, dinner) do you eat each day? _____ How many snacks? _____
- Are there certain food groups that you refuse to eat (meat, breads, etc?) _____
- Do you ever limit food intake to control weight? ___Yes ___ No
    If yes, do you (circle below)...
        Decrease the amount of food you eat during the day / skip meals /
        limit carbohydrate intake / limit fat intake / cut out snack items /
        Other_____
- Do you ever feel out of control when eating or feel that you cannot stop eating? ___Yes ___ No
- Do you take vitamin supplements?___Yes___ No
    If yes, what type?_____ How often (daily, a few times a week)?_____
- Do you take nutritional supplements?___Yes ___ No
    If yes, what type?_____ How often (daily, a few times a week)?_____
- What do you currently weigh?_____ Are you happy with this weight?___Yes___ No
    If not, what would you like to weigh?_____
- What was the most you've weighed in the past year? _____
- What was the least you've weighed in the past year? _____
- Do you gain or lose weight regularly to meet demands of your sport?___Yes ___ No
- Has anyone recommended that you change your weight or eating habits?___Yes ___ No
    If yes, specify (coach, parent, friend) _____
- Has anyone ever set a target weight for you or subjected you to routine weigh-ins? ___Yes___ No
- Have you ever tried to lose weight by using any of the following methods? (circle below)
    Vomiting / laxatives / diuretics / diet pills / exercise
- Do you regularly exercise outside of your normal practice schedule? ___Yes ___ No
    If yes, describe your activities. _____
- Have you ever been diagnosed with an eating disorder? ___ Yes ___ No
- Do you think that you might have an eating disorder? ___Yes ___ No
- Have you ever been treated for a stress fracture? ___Yes ___ No
    If yes, how many have you had?____ What body part(s) was involved? ____When did the injury occur? _____
    How was the diagnosis made (X-ray, bone scan, MRI, CT)? _____

[a]Sample questionnaire items for recognition of disordered eating. Adapted from Agostini R et al: *Medical and Orthopedic Issues of Active and Athletic Women.* © 1994:39, with permission from Elsevier.

be somewhat arbitrary, it is widely used internationally and should be considered in context with other health indicators and history.

- No agreed-upon cut-off points exist for individuals <18 years of age. When evaluating the BMI of an adolescent athlete of high school age (approximately 14 to 18 years) in the context of being underweight, the 5th percentile of the Centers for Disease Control and Prevention growth charts (2002) may be used (http://www.cdc.gov/

Table 6b. Menstrual History Review — Sample Questionnaire Items[a]

- Have you ever had a menstrual period? ___Yes___ No
    If yes –
    - How old were you when you had your first menstrual period?_____
    - When was your last period?_____
    - How many days are there between your periods from the first day of your menstrual cycle to the first day of your next cycle?
        _____ 3 days _____ more than 3 – 10 days_____ more than 10 days
    - How many periods have you had in the past 12 months?_____ In the past 6 months?_____
    - Have you ever missed 3 or more consecutive months of your menstrual periods? ___ Yes ___ No
        If yes, how many consecutive months have you missed your period?_____
    - Does your menstrual cycle change with a change in the intensity, frequency or duration of training?
        ___ Yes ___ No
        If yes, does it become (circle below)...
            Lighter / Heavier / Shorter / Longer / Disappear
    - Do you ever have trouble with heavy bleeding? ___ Yes ___ No
    - Do you ever experience cramps during your period? ___ Yes ___ No
        If yes, how do you treat them? _____
    - Are you on birth control pills or hormones? ___ Yes ___ No
        If yes, were they prescribed for (circle below)...
            Irregular periods / No periods / Painful periods / Birth control
    - When was your last pelvic examination? _____
    - Have you ever had an abnormal Pap smear? ___Yes ___ No
    - Have you ever been treated for anemia (low hemoglobin or iron)? ___Yes ___ No
    - Is there any history of osteoporosis (thinning of the bones) in your family? ___Yes ___ No

[a]Adapted from Agostini R et al: *Medical and Orthopedic Issues of Active and Athletic Women.* © 1994:39, with permission from Elsevier.

Table 7. Representative Screening Instruments for Assessment of Disordered Eating in Athletes

Instrument	Description
Survey of Eating Disorders among Athletes (SEDA)[9]	Self-report: a 33-item questionnaire for identifying eating abnormalities in addition to factors specific to the athletics environment that may contribute to the onset or development of disordered eating. These factors include whether weight loss was required for performance thinness, appearance thinness, or to meet a lower weight classification, and/or triggered by comments or instructions by coaches or other athletics support personnel. It also examines whether the athlete was subjected to public weigh-ins and/or public scrutiny of the results.
Athletic Milieu Direct Questionnaire (AMDQ)[83]	Self-report: a 19-item screening instrument for identification of eating disorders/disordered eating in National Collegiate Athletic Association Division I female athletes. A variety of response categories are used, including a 4- to 6-point Likert scale as well as multiple and dichotomous responses.
Female Athlete Screening Tool (FAST)[84]	Self report: a 33-item screening instrument that examines atypical exercise and eating behaviors in female athletes. Respondents rate each item on a 4-point Likert scale.
College Health Related Information Survey (CHRIS)[85]	Self-report: a 32-item screening test designed to ascertain information relevant to college athletes in 4 areas – mental health problems, eating problems, risk behaviors, and performance pressure. The screen is appropriate for both male and female athletes.
The Physiologic Screening Test (PST)[79]	Self-report combined with physiologic measurements: An 18-item screening test consisting of 14 items that require self-report responses based on physiologic factors (instead of eating behaviors) and 4 items based on physiologic measurements. The following variables are assessed: standing diastolic blood pressure, waist:hip ratio, percentage of body fat, parotid gland enlargement, menstrual history and frequency, weight history and perceptions of body weight, exercise habits after practice, frequency of bowel movements and normalcy of stools, pain and bloating in the abdomen, and dizziness when rising quickly.
The Health, Weight, Dieting, and Menstrual History Questionnaire[59]	Self-report: a 53-item questionnaire divided into 4 categories for the assessment of disordered eating — general health (including menstrual function and bone health), body weight (including abnormally high or low body weight and/or weight fluctuations), dieting behaviors (including energy restriction, bingeing, and/or purging), and body image (including global and specific body part satisfaction/dissatisfaction). The questions were derived from 2 existing eating-disorder screening tools along with information gleaned from an extensive review of the literature pertaining to disordered eating in female athletes.

growthcharts/). An athlete with a BMI less than the sex-specific and age-specific 5th percentile may be underweight (allowing for individual differences in maturity status and, in particular, the timing and tempo of the adolescent growth spurt).

- A young adult athlete with a BMI <18.5 kg/m^2 or an adolescent athlete with a BMI less than the age-specific and sex-specific cut-off who experiences a decline in BMI should be monitored for a reasonable period and evaluated for eating behaviors, training practices, and potential stressors (eg, pressure from coaches). In the case of the adolescent athlete, the evaluation may require an assessment of maturity status.
- An interval of at least 2 to 3 months should be established between serial measurements of height and weight to evaluate short-term fluctuations in the BMI.
- An athlete with a persistently low or a declining BMI should be referred for medical evaluation.
- Preadolescent and early-adolescent athletes (generally <12 years of age) should not have the BMI evaluated routinely. Instead, attention should be focused on monitoring growth in height and weight, assessing maturity status if necessary, improving nutrition and physical activity behaviors, promoting self-acceptance, and developing attitudes related to healthy lifestyles.

Managing Athletes with Disordered Eating

Initial Contact

23. If DE is suspected, the initial intervention should be facilitated by an authority figure who has the best rapport with the athlete. The facilitator should be prepared to (1) approach the athlete with sensitivity and respect while adhering to disclosure regulations regarding patient confidentiality; (2) indicate specific observations of concern; (3) expect denial, anger, and/or resistance; and (4) have expertise readily accessible for consultation and/or timely referral.[88]

24. If suspicions of DE are confirmed, the athlete should be referred to the supervising physician for an initial evaluation, beginning with a thorough medical history review and physical examination (Table 8). Based on the findings of the evaluation, laboratory studies and electrocardiography may also be indicated to obtain a more accurate representation of the seriousness of the problem. Collaboration among all members of the health care team should follow to determine the most appropriate setting for treatment and to prioritize interventions.

Treatment Settings

25. Outpatient treatment settings should suffice for most athletes who have mild symptoms of brief duration; stable weight, cardiac, and metabolic function; absence of comorbid conditions; and cooperative fami-

lies.[24,25,27,76] Development of a treatment plan that includes medical surveillance, timely nutritional intervention, and a supportive environment may be all that is necessary to contain incipient problems and promote recovery.[18,76] More established cases require psychotherapy.[22,28,89] Although athletes undergoing outpatient treatment can remain in their homes or in residential campus settings, attend school, and participate in athletics, these advantages must be balanced against the risks of failure to progress in recovery.

26. More restrictive and intensive treatment settings, including inpatient hospitalization, residential centers specializing in EDs, or partial hospitalization, should be considered if weight, cardiac, and metabolic status destabilize or outpatient treatment is unsuccessful.[17,24,89]

Therapeutic Interventions

27. In an outpatient treatment setting, physician-coordinated interventions should first be aimed at enlisting the expertise of a registered dietitian to optimize calorie and nutrient intakes for energy homeostasis and, in more serious cases, to design and implement medical nutrition therapy protocols that address the biological and psychological effects of severe caloric deprivation.[90–92] Enlisting the services of a clinical psychotherapist may be necessary simultaneously to help interrupt pathogenic behaviors and resolve psychological, familial, social, and environmental issues contributing to their development and perpetuation.[22,89,93,94] Pharmacologic treatment may also be helpful, especially in patients with significant symptoms of depression, anxiety, or obsessions.[76,89]

28. All certified athletic trainers should be prepared to assume the role of informed patient advocates in the management of athletes with DE. Because of their frequent daily interactions with athletes and familiarity with their immediate and long-term health care needs, athletic trainers are in a unique position to assist with or supervise the myriad of anticipated tasks described in Table 9.

29. Certified athletic trainers should be mindful of their scope of practice limitations. Although they have the clinical knowledge and skills to identify signs and symptoms that indicate risk, confront athletes with suspicious behaviors, and provide assistance as needed to facilitate timely referrals and treatment compliance, diagnosis and treatment can only be managed by physicians and psychotherapists who specialize in EDs.[23]

30. Certified athletic trainers should resist pleas from athletes with DE to work individually with them in a subconscious attempt to avoid referral and comprehensive treatment.[23] The therapeutic alliance that often develops makes it tempting to accommodate the request.

31. Certified athletic trainers should be prepared to enforce limitations of physical workouts based on recommendations of caregivers and to intervene when training expectations are potentially dangerous or detrimental.

32. Certified athletic trainers should have knowledge of the psychotropic medications commonly prescribed to treat symptoms that accompany EDs, including their potential side effects. They should also be able to recognize symptoms of missed doses or overdose. The supervising physician, other caregivers, and family members should be contacted immediately if behavioral warning signs such as agitation, irritability, suicidal tendency, or unusual changes in behavior are observed.

33. Certified athletic trainers should work closely with athletics administrators, legal counsel, and coaches when handling health, safety, ethical, and procedural questions related to managing athletes with DE. Successful outcomes are highly dependent on skillful handling of issues that arise after DE identification and during the course of treatment and follow-up care.

Issues in Treatment and Follow-Up Care

34. It is reasonable for an athlete with DE to continue sport participation only if health risks are determined to be minimal and the athlete complies with all treatment components and training modifications, has a genuine interest in competing, and realizes treatment must always take precedence over sport participation.[69]

35. Consequences for athletes who are noncompliant with treatment recommendations should be appropriate. When treatment is resisted, suspending participation should be considered by the health care team until compliance is established.[25,69] However, caregivers should be mindful that suspension could result in potentially harmful consequences, as it represents a major setback in the athlete's ability to achieve training and competitive goals.[28]

36. A written contract, agreed upon and signed by the athlete and health care team coordinator or designate, may be helpful in some circumstances to promote treatment compliance.[27,93] Table 10 provides an example of a contract that can be easily modified to meet the situational needs of an athlete who is in the active phase of an ED.

37. At the outset, parental support should be obtained within disclosure regulations when discussing and implementing management strategies for symptomatic athletes. Engaging parents and CSOs early in the process helps to facilitate cooperation with the treatment protocol and acceptance of any changes in treatment settings or strategies that may be required if health destabilizes.

38. If an outpatient treatment setting is unsuccessful, caregivers should be prepared to handle issues that surface when transitioning the athlete's care to a more

Table 8. Components of the Initial Medical Evaluation

Medical History[a]
- Symptoms and screening results related to the diagnosis of disordered eating
- Eating patterns, weight history (lowest, highest, recent changes), and nutritional status with special reference to dietary and fluid restraint; growth and development in children and adolescents
- Details of previous and current treatment programs for disordered eating (ie, medications, psychological and nutritional interventions)
- Exercise/sports training history: duration and frequency of training per week; aerobic and anaerobic training volumes; time spent exercising outside of normal training regimen (eg, cycling, jogging, calisthenics)
- Prior or current bone stress injuries/reactions and chronic musculoskeletal injuries
- History and treatment of other conditions, including endocrine disorders, infections, chronic diseases, previous surgeries, and medications
- Family history, including weight history, disordered eating, and osteoporosis among family members and ages at menarche and menstrual problems of mothers and sisters
- Brief psycho-social history: life stressors (eg, social, academic, sports, family, or economic); conflict and support systems at home, at school, in social environment; coping skills and methods; history of depressive symptoms; physical or sexual abuse; general mood, body image satisfaction; and sources of self esteem
- Use of alcohol, tobacco, and/or controlled substances

Physical Examination[a]
- General physical examination: age (decimal age: date of measurement minus date of birth); height, weight, BMI; comparison with age- and sex-specific references for children and adolescents (http://www.cdc.gov/growthcharts/); note change/rate of change from prior measurements.
- Stage of sexual maturation (breasts, pubic hair in girls; genitals, pubic hair in boys — if appropriate to examine at the time); age at menarche
- Evaluation of vital signs; pulse by palpation, blood pressure with auscultation in both supine and standing, and temperature
- Cardiac examination
- Oral, salivary gland, and thyroid examination
- Skin, hand, and finger examination
- Consider pelvic examination in female athletes presenting with irregular or absent menses
- Consider differential diagnoses for an eating disorder: metabolic disease, malignancy, inflammatory bowel disease, achalasia (difficulty swallowing), infection

Laboratory Assessments[b]
- Basic Analyses: Consider for all patients.
  - Complex metabolic profile (CMP): electrolytes, blood urea nitrogen (BUN) level; creatinine level; liver function studies, glucose, calcium
  - Thyroid function (free T4, TSH)
  - Complete blood count (CBC)
  - Urinalysis (evaluate for pH, specific gravity, signs of infection)
- Additional Analyses: Consider for undernourished and severely symptomatic patients
  - Magnesium, phosphorus levels
- Osteopenia and Osteoporosis Assessments: Consider for patients underweight more than 6 months or amenorrheic for more than 3 months
  - Dual-energy X-ray absorptiometry (DXA)
  - Estradiol level in females; Testosterone level in males
- Nonroutine Assessments: Consider for specific unusual indications
  - Luteinizing hormone (LH) and follicle-stimulating hormone (FSH) levels: For persistent amenorrhea at normal weight
  - Brain magnetic resonance imaging (MRI) and computerized tomography (CT): For ventricular enlargement correlated with degree of undernutrition
  - Stool: For blood
  - Chest X-ray

Electrocardiography[a]
- Appropriate if resting, supine pulse is <50 beats/min, electrolyte abnormality is present, or if there is frequent purging, dehydration, or prolonged caloric restriction
- Note for findings of bradycardia, low voltage, low or inverted T-waves, QT dispersion, or prolonged QT interval

[a]Adapted from Agostini R et al: *Medical and Orthopaedic Issues of Active and Athletic Women.* © 1994:147, with permission from Elsevier.
[b]Adapted, by permission, from the American Psychiatric Association. Practice guideline for the treatment of patients with eating disorders (revision). *Am J Psychiatry.* 2000;157(suppl 1):1–39.

restrictive setting. Caregivers should continue to advocate for the athlete by facilitating referrals; maintaining open lines of communication with providers and CSOs to keep abreast of the patient's progress; and preparing the athlete and CSOs for the possibility that access to appropriate care may be delayed due to waiting lists or constrained by monetary or insurance difficulties.[95–97]

39. If the athlete responds favorably to outside treatment and is medically cleared to reengage in the previous environment with the goal of sport reentry, the organization's resources should be assessed for adequacy in handling the full complement of maintenance

care required to prevent potential relapse. The ultimate responsibility should rest with the organization's supervising physician, in consultation with other members of the DE health care team, after careful review of all pertinent medical records and completion of a comprehensive physical examination.

The Uniqueness of Adolescence: Special Considerations

40. Given the biological and behavioral changes occurring during adolescence and, importantly, their interactions, certified athletic trainers who work with adolescent athletes should have a firm understanding of the basic principles of physical growth (specifically

Table 9.   Anticipated Responsibilities of the Certified Athletic Trainer

- Intervene if an athlete is suspected of having disordered eating and make appropriate referrals when warranted;
- Prepare the athlete for referral and address any questions or concerns relevant to the referral;
- Arrange for treatment according to the caregivers' directives;
- Maintain open lines of communication on a regular basis with and among caregivers as individual treatment plans are formulated for the patient;
- Ensure that all caregivers are aware of the treatment plan in its entirety;
- Provide feedback to caregivers regarding the athlete's progress relative to training and performance, interpersonal issues, academics, and family factors;
- Assist in the coordination of ongoing medical surveillance plans characterized by periodic check-ups and serial health testing that helps caregivers monitor the progress of athletes and determine if treatment plans are in line with meeting their special medical needs;
- Monitor the athlete's compliance with the treatment plan by maintaining records of scheduled appointments, noting missed appointments, and charting changes in body weight, body composition, and sport-specific measures; share noncompliance issues with all caregivers;
- Assume the role as liaison among coaches and caregivers in circumstances where athletics participation may have to be modified or discontinued due to energy deficits, injury, or treatment noncompliance;
- Enforce limitations of workouts based on recommendations of caregivers and intervene when training expectations are potentially dangerous or detrimental;
- Intervene in a crisis situation when the immediate welfare and safety of the athlete is in jeopardy (eg, impending relapse, athlete is acutely suicidal) and arrange for appropriate referral;
- Field questions, concerns, observations, and criticisms from the athlete as well as coaches, teammates, parents, and close significant others (the latter group of individuals should be encouraged to share observations and concerns with the certified athletic trainer and other caregivers, being mindful of the patient's right to privacy);
- Remain sensitive to the athlete's preferences for staying connected with teammates in an effort to help ease the feelings of loneliness and alienation that are associated with participation restrictions;
- Adhere to disclosure regulations regarding patient confidentiality;
- Ensure that matters relative to insurance and expense coverage have been discussed and that the financial aspects of the treatment plan are manageable for the athlete and his/her family;
- Consult with athletics administrators on issues that can complicate care, in particular, coaches and support staff who trigger or perpetuate the problems and ignore suspicious behaviors, athletes who are resistant to referral or noncompliant with the treatment process; and parents or close significant others who are uncooperative.

Table 10.   Sample Contractual Agreement for Continued Athletic Participation in the Active Phase of an Eating Disorder (Noncompliance)[a]

Dear

As a representative of your health care team, I am pleased to inform you that your physical condition presently suggests no immediate health risk. However, it has been brought to my attention that you have not been complying fully with the treatment plan that has been formulated for you. I want to remind you how important it is to take the appropriate steps to care for yourself. Our health care team will do everything possible to assist you in this effort. To ensure that your health remains stable, your current athletics participation status for the remainder of the school year will be contingent on your compliance with the following:

1. Receive individual psychotherapy from _____ once a week so that you can address all issues and find healthy ways to cope with them;
2. See Dr. _____ for medical evaluation of your health status, including lab tests if necessary, every other week to ensure your physical well-being;
3. Participate in nutritional counseling sessions according to a schedule recommended by our registered dietitian, _____;
4. Maintain your body weight over _____ pounds (if applicable). Anticipate weekly monitoring of your weight if it falls below this level.
5. Sign and leave on file a release of information with _____ permitting our health care professionals to communicate openly and freely with each other, members of the coaching staff, your parents, and your caregivers at home.
6. See your home-based physician and therapist during the winter and summer breaks. Prior to your return to campus, your attending physician and therapist must send Dr. _____ a letter indicating the following: (a) you are ready to return to school; (b) you have been in treatment; (c) you are ready to take on the academic, training, performance, and social challenges for the semester; and (d) you are taking any medication recommended and prescribed by your psychotherapist. This letter should be in the possession of Dr. _____ prior to your arrival on campus in _____. Additionally, we would like you to talk with Dr. _____ in person or by phone to discuss your plans for the semester and confirm your ability to return. Upon your return to campus, you should anticipate meeting with Dr. _____ for a re-entry evaluation so that your medical status can be assessed, activity status determined, and further treatment options explored, if necessary.
7. Check-in routinely with your certified athletic trainer, _____, who will be available to assist you.
   (Athlete's Name), I am confident that you have the ability and support to address the health concerns that you are currently facing. It is our every expectation that you will comply with all necessary medical and personal advice to advance your recovery so that you can continue to flourish in this environment.

Please sign below verifying that you are prepared to comply with the stipulations outlined above.
Athlete's Signature _____Date _____
Sincerely,
(Athletics Administrator or Supervising Physician)

---

[a]Sample contractual disordered-eating agreement. Adapted with permission of author, D.C. Wood, J.D. (debra.wood@scrippscollege.edu, email), April 21, 2006.

the growth spurt), biological maturation (sexual, skeletal, and somatic), and behavioral development occurring at this critical stage in the life cycle.

41. Changes in size, physique, and body composition during adolescence may influence perceptions of self and specifically appearance. Some adolescent athletes may display dissatisfaction with, and anxiety over, body weight, size, and shape.[98–101] Certified athletic trainers should be aware of potential changes in self-perceptions and concerns for appearance, especially in aesthetic sports (eg, gymnastics, diving, figure skating) in which physical appearance may be a part of the judging process.

42. Potential biomedical complications of DE during adolescence, specifically prolonged energy deficiency, altered menstrual function, and impaired bone mineral accretion during this period of rapid physical growth and attainment of biological maturity, can have long-term effects.[18] In this context, the threshold for potential intervention with adolescent athletes at risk should be lower than that for adult athletes.[18]

43. Certified athletic trainers who work with adolescent athletes should be aware of the need for regular monitoring and recognition of potential problems in this age group and for prompt referral to medical staff as required.

44. Many athletics programs for adolescents have limited resources and may not have access to essential support staff when potential problems with athletes arise. In addition to the certified athletic trainer, it is essential that the family and relevant school authorities (eg, school nurses, guidance counselors) be involved in the process. It is also important to identify resources in the community such as psychotherapists and registered dietitians in anticipation of the need for additional assistance.

Preventing Disordered Eating

45. Mandatory educational programs for athletes, coaches, certified athletic trainers, and other athletics staff members should be implemented on an annual basis. Information focused on the most commonly asked questions about DE should be disseminated: Who is at risk? What are the barriers to identifying problems at an early stage? What are the signs, symptoms, and medical complications? What are the medical and performance consequences? What resources are available to help symptomatic athletes? How is treatment accessed? How should certified athletic trainers, coaches, teammates, and CSOs respond to an athlete suspected of having DE? What are the best preventive measures?

46. All athletes should be educated on the importance of optimal nutrition practices to reduce the risk of medical and performance problems associated with prolonged energy and nutrient deprivation.

47. Female athletes should be educated on the health and performance consequences of menstrual irregularities and the importance of seeking timely medical intervention at the first sign of abnormalities.

48. The educational program should be evaluated routinely to determine its effectiveness in changing the knowledge level, attitudes, and behaviors of athletes as well as those participating in their health maintenance and performance enhancement to better minimize, contain, manage, and prevent problems.

49. Certified athletic trainers should be familiar with reputable Web sites of organizations that provide factual information on DE, healthy eating, and safe weight-regulation practices (Table 11).

50. Certified athletic trainers should also be familiar with disreputable Web sites, such as pro-ana (anorexia) and pro-mia (bulimia), consisting of harmful information devoted to the continuation, promotion, and support of EDs that glamorize the deadly disorders.[18]

BACKGROUND AND LITERATURE REVIEW

Definitions and Diagnostic Criteria

Disordered eating is best conceptualized along a continuum of pathogenic eating and weight control behaviors encompassing a full spectrum of clinical and subclinical classifications.[1–4] For purposes of this discussion, *DE* is preferred when reference is made to the entire spectrum of abnormal behaviors, whereas *ED* is preferred when a definite clinical classification of abnormal behaviors is discussed. Classifications of particular importance include AN, BN, and EDNOS.

Anorexia and Bulimia Nervosa. Clinical or full-syndrome EDs are characterized by strict diagnostic criteria established by the American Psychiatric Association and identified in the *DSM-IV*.[20] The 2 most identifiable clinical EDs are AN and BN, which are complicated by dysfunction of multiple physiologic systems, nutritional deficiencies, and psychiatric diagnoses.[102]

Anorexia nervosa is distinguished as the extreme of restricting behavior and is manifested as a refusal to maintain normal body weight for age and height, whereas BN refers to a cycle of food restriction or fasting followed by binging and purging.[20] Although the disorders have typical clinical features for establishing the diagnoses (Tables 1 and 2),[20] both are characterized by body weight preoccupation, excessive self-evaluation of weight and shape, and an illusion of control gained by manipulating weight and dietary intake. These commonalities clarify why up to 50% of patients with AN develop bulimic symptoms and some patients who are initially bulimic develop anorexic symptoms.[103]

In the United States, it is estimated that AN and BN affect nearly 10 million females and 1 million males, primarily adolescents and young adults.[104,105] Although clinical EDs are more common in females than males, they have similar incidences of comorbid psychopathology and similar levels of core behaviors and attitudes when matched for current age, ED subtypes, and age at onset of the ED.[63] In adolescents, the incidence of clinical EDs has increased

Table 11. Useful Resources

Web Sites

Academy of Eating Disorders (www.aedweb.org)
National Eating Disorders Association
   (www.nationaleatingdisorders.org)
International Association of Eating Disorder Professionals
   (www.iaedp.com)
National Association of Anorexia Nervosa and Associated Disorders
   (www.anad.org)
Sports, Cardiovascular and Wellness Nutritionists (www.scandpg.org)
National Collegiate Athletic Association Web site on nutrition and
   performance
   (http://www1.ncaa.org/membership/ed_outreach/
   nutrition-performance/index.html)
Bloomington Center for Counseling and Human Development
   (www.bloomington-eating-disorders.com)

Position Statements

American Academy of Pediatrics (www.aap.org)
   (http://aappolicy.aappublications.org/cgi/content/full/pediatrics;111/1/
   204)
Society for Adolescent Medicine (www.adolescenthealth.org)
   (http://www.adolescenthealth.org/PositionPaper_Eating_Disorders_
   in_Adolescents.pdf)
American Psychiatric Association (www.psych.org)
   (http://www.psych.org/psych_pract/treatg/pg/EatingDisorders3ePG_
   04-28-06.pdf)
American College of Sports Medicine (www.acsm.org)
   (http://www.acsm-msse.org/pt/pt-core/template-journal/msse/media/
   0597.pdf)
American Dietetic Association (www.eatright.org)
   (http://www.eatright.org/cps/rde/xchg/ada/hs.xsl/index.html,
   http://www.eatright.org/ada/files/EDNP.pdf)
Female athlete triad (www.femaleathletetriad.org)
International Olympic Committee position stand on the female athlete triad
   (http://multimedia.olympic.org/pdf/en_report_917.pdf)

---

at an alarming rate over the past few decades; AN represents the third most common chronic illness among adolescent girls.[106] Its true prevalence may be even higher because it is undiagnosed in up to 50% of cases.[107]

Eating Disorders Not Otherwise Specified. Individuals who present with all but a few of the diagnostic criteria that distinguish AN or BN are classified as having atypical EDs defined by *DSM-IV*[20] criteria as EDNOS (Table 3). Nearly 50% of patients in the general population with EDs who present to tertiary care programs are diagnosed with EDNOS; moreover, the subsyndrome appears to be particularly common among adolescents.[89]

Subclinical Syndromes

The *DSM-IV*[20] clinical criteria for diagnosis of AN, BN, and EDNOS were developed for nonathletes and are distinguished by significant psychiatric morbidity. Athletes are more likely to present with less extreme behavioral indicators and psychological symptoms that represent subclinical variants of AN, BN, and EDNOS.[6,12–15,27,108–111] Maladaptive behaviors may begin simply as a means of enhancing performance by losing weight or, perhaps inadvertently, by failing to maintain adequate energy availability during high-intensity or high-volume sport training and not necessarily from psychopathology.[110,112] Athletes may also show evidence of some common psychological traits associated with clinical EDs, such as high achievement orientation, self-motivation, rigid self-discipline, and perfec-

tionism.[6,22,113–115] However, these traits also correlate with success in athletics and are important determinants in the drive for performance excellence.

Athletes comprise a unique population.[13] They are widely regarded as a special subgroup of healthy individuals with physically demanding lifestyles who are seemingly invincible and are often capable of extraordinary athletic feats.[116] Determining when behaviors and attitudes specific to diet and exercise are progressing to pathogenic levels consistent with EDs is challenging due to the influence of performance expectations, training demands, energy requirements, and personality characteristics.[10,89,117] Awareness of behavioral and psychological indicators of athletes with EDs may be helpful in determining an athlete's risk potential (Table 4).

Physical Signs, Symptoms, and Medical Complications

Recognizing physical signs and symptoms associated with EDs is critical to prevention and early treatment of a wide range of medical complications secondary to malnutrition or purging (Table 5). Some complications are relatively benign, whereas others are potentially life threatening. In some cases, the athlete may only present with vague medical complaints, generalized muscle fatigue, or dehydration.[14,19] The fact that ED behaviors are well concealed further complicates the scenario in terms of recognition. Therefore, the degree of physiologic compromise is best understood with an examination of signs, symptoms, and potentially serious complications that can manifest with full-syndrome EDs.

Anorexia nervosa has the highest mortality rate of any psychiatric illness, estimated at 10% within 10 years of diagnosis.[118] Death is secondary to cardiac arrest, starvation, other medical complications, and suicide.[89] The mortality rate in BN is lower, approximately 1% within 10 years of diagnosis.[119] However, these figures may be deceiving,[102] as patients frequently move between diagnostic categories over the course of their illness. As previously mentioned, up to 50% of patients with AN develop bulimic symptoms[103] but still carry the primary diagnosis of AN.

Physiologic effects of EDs are widespread, and no organ system is spared.[17] Malnutrition decreases metabolic rate and causes abnormalities in the cardiovascular, reproductive, skeletal, thermoregulatory, gastrointestinal, and other systems. The resultant abnormalities can be particularly dangerous and especially problematic for athletes who continue to train intensively in an energy-deficient or nutrient-deficient state.

Cardiovascular complications include sudden cardiac death due to arrhythmias, electrolyte abnormalities, and ipecac-induced cardiomyopathy.[120–122] The signs of cardiovascular abnormalities secondary to chronic caloric and fluid deprivation can include severe sinus bradycardia (resting heart rate <50 beats/min during the day and <45 beats/min at night), hypotension (<80/50 mm Hg), orthostatic changes in pulse (>20 beats/min) or blood pressure (>10 mm Hg), decreased myocardial contractility, valvular dysfunction, impaired left ventricular function, delayed capillary refill, and acrocyanosis (bluish color of the distal extremities or lips).[17,18,120,123–125] Electrocardiographic changes can be present[126] and manifest as ventricular arrhythmias[124] and abnormal QT intervals.[127,128] A prolonged QT interval is associated with sudden death and may be aggravated by bradycardia or electrolyte disturbance but can also occur in the presence of normal serum electrolytes.[127,128]

Bradycardia (resting heart rate between 40 and 60 beats/min)[129] is not only a clinical feature of individuals with AN but also of healthy, well-conditioned athletes who participate in dynamic physical activities such as distance running, cycling, swimming, or rowing.[116] Quite often, athletes with bradycardia are considered to have athletic heart syndrome. This benign syndrome is characterized by an increase in cardiac mass and represents normal adaptations to exercise in the anatomy and physiology of the cardiovascular system.[116] As a result of the cardiac changes, resting heart rates as low as 45 beats/min have been reported.[130] In a study of 1299 athletes representing endurance events, ball games, strength sports, and gymnastics, average heart rates were 62.5 ±12.5 beats/min in males and 65.2 ±12.7 beats/min in females.[131] Heart rates of less than 50 beats/min were reported in 18.7% of athletic males and 10.2% of athletic females. Therefore, in bradycardic athletes, resting heart rates of less than 50 beats/min during the day and less than 45 beats/min at night may not always indicate cardiac fitness and may instead represent physiologic instability in athletes with EDs.[18]

Reproductive complications in female athletes, characterized by menstrual cycle alterations (particularly amenorrhea) merit special attention. Amenorrhea is a clinical feature of AN and of exercise training.[37] The cause of amenorrhea in athletes has been theorized as low energy availability resulting from a decrease in caloric intake either to lose weight or maintain a low body weight, an increase in exercise volume without a concomitant increase in consumption of calories, or a combination of both.[40,45] Because amenorrhea is common in female athletes,[37] it is all too often characterized and unfortunately disregarded as a convenient byproduct of intense physical exercise. Ascribing menstrual cycle variations to exercise without proper clinical evaluation to rule out other medical problems underlying cessation of menses is a dangerous practice.[132] The onset of amenorrhea is accompanied by rapid bone loss,[21,37,133,134] and timely interventions are necessary to prevent low bone mass[43,135–137] and increased susceptibility to stress fractures.[44,45,138,139] Considering that it is statistically uncommon for girls and adolescents to remain amenorrheic for more than 90 days between periods, evaluation within the first 3 months of onset may be beneficial.[46]

The consequences of bone loss are considerable, and many different treatment strategies have been recommended to minimize their severity. These include maximizing energy availability, defined as the amount of dietary energy remaining for other body functions after exercise training.[45] To address low energy availability, the mainstays of treatment are increasing the athlete's caloric intake to meet exercise energy requirements or reducing exercise training volume and intensity (or both).[40–42,45] Another important treatment strategy is the administration of bone building nutrients, such as calcium and vitamin D, to maximize skeletal health.[49–51] However, it has been estimated that only about 25% of boys and 10% of girls

ages 9 to 17 years meet the recommended dietary intake of calcium at 1300 mg/d.[51] It is estimated that 50% to 60% of adults meet the recommended calcium intake at 1000 to 1500 mg/d.[51] Adequate intake of vitamin D is estimated at 400 to 600 IU/d; however, this amount may represent the minimum.[50,51] Insufficient vitamin D prevents children from attaining genetically programmed peak bone mass and contributes to osteoporosis in adults.[50] In individuals who fail to meet dietary intakes, restrict calories, show signs of bone loss, or are osteoporotic, the dosages for both supplements may need to be higher.[45,50,41] From the standpoint of calcium supplementation and stress fracture prevention, a recent study conducted on female navy recruits during 8 weeks of basic training showed that taking 2000 mg/d of calcium and 800 IU of vitamin D supplements significantly reduced stress fracture incidence compared with those receiving placebo pills.[140] As further investigations confirm the findings of this promising research, future consideration may be given to increasing dosages of these supplements, especially in physically active individuals. The last treatment strategy focuses on the administration of hormone replacement therapy or the oral contraceptive pill.[37,52–54] However, these pharmacologic agents have not been sufficient in reversing loss of bone mineral density or correcting the metabolic abnormalities that lead to deterioration in health and performance of amenorrheic athletes with or without eating disorders.[45]

The aforementioned reproductive and skeletal complications were introduced in the scientific literature in 1997 as 3 interrelated medical conditions — DE, amenorrhea, and osteoporosis — referred to collectively as the *female athlete triad*.[21] Severe physiologic and psychological consequences were theorized to result from the synergistic effect of all 3 components. Over the past decade, scientific investigations into the prevalence, causes, prevention, and treatment of the triad have led to a revised description. The female athlete triad now refers to the interrelationships among energy availability, menstrual function, and bone mineral density.[45] Compared with the original description, low energy availability is the key disorder underlying the other components of the triad. Additionally, a spectrum of severity exists for each of the components, ranging from health to disease. Low energy availability with or without an ED, functional hypothalamic amenorrhea, and osteoporosis now represent the pathologic end of the spectrum and not the focal point of the triad. The first study to directly examine the combined prevalence of the triad components in a heterogeneous sample of United States collegiate athletes was published in 2006.[59] A study of high school athletes followed shortly thereafter.[58] In both studies, the number of athletes reported to suffer from all 3 clinical conditions was small. However, a significant number suffered from individual disorders (eg, DE or amenorrhea, or both), underscoring the need to recognize and treat each individual component as it presents, so that potentially irreversible consequences are prevented.[45,59]

From a general perspective, researchers have emphasized that more similarities than differences exist between young adult males and females in the signs and symptoms[67] and medical complications[141] characterizing AN. Of the noted differences, attention has focused on the severity of medical complications in males compared with their female counterparts due to delays in diagnosis and treatment.[64,65]

Additionally, males have no overt signs of malnutrition, such as amenorrhea, which serves as a recognizable clinical feature for diagnosis of EDs in females.[62]

These known medical consequences have been examined and reviewed primarily from the perspective of adult-onset AN. Generalizations to adolescents are limited by the range of variation among individuals in the timing and tempo of the growth spurt, sexual (pubertal) maturation, and associated hormonal changes.[86,107] Chronic maladaptive eating and weight control behaviors during adolescence may be associated with linear growth retardation (if the behaviors persist before closure of the epiphyseal growth plates) and arrested sexual maturation; impaired acquisition of peak bone mass, which may increase fracture risk; severe bradycardia, with heart rates as low as 40 beats/min; and blood pressure changes.[18]

Physical complications associated with BN are less extensive than those of AN. Unfortunately, physical indicators of BN are not easily recognized, and early intervention strategies to prevent potential medical complications and facilitate eventual recovery are often delayed.[89] Delay in referral and subsequent treatment is due in part to the near normalcy of body weight evidenced. Bulimic patients often recognize their disorder, yet pursuit of early treatment is frequently overridden by shame and guilt.

The binge-eating aspect of bulimia rarely causes significant physical problems with the uncommon exception of gastric rupture.[142] Most serious medical complications stem from self-induced vomiting, which is the most common form of purging, reported in more than 75% of patients with BN.[143,144] This form of purging is also found in patients with AN and EDNOS.

Frequent vomiting can cause swelling of the parotid glands, lacerations of the mouth and throat stemming from the use of foreign objects to induce regurgitation, calluses on the dorsum of the hand (Russell sign), irritation of the esophagus or pharynx, and dental erosion due to contact of the teeth with gastric acids.[17,89] Other complaints include constipation or diarrhea, menstrual irregularities, sore throat, chest pain, and facial edema.[17]

Excessive loss of fluids during vomiting can disrupt the electrolyte and acid-base balance of the body, leading to depletions in hydrogen chloride, potassium, sodium, and magnesium, which are all necessary for nerve and muscle function.[17] Effects of dehydration and electrolyte imbalances may be experienced for as long as 1 week after an episode of binge-purge behavior.[145] Frequent binge-purge episodes may result in transient periods of dehydration characterized by fatigue, irritability, muscle spasms, dizziness or even fainting, generalized bloating, swelling of hands and feet, heart palpitations, and a decrease in balance and coordination. More severe complications such as paresthesia, tetany, seizures, and cardiac arrhythmias may result and warrant immediate referral and care.[142] It is important for clinicians to be mindful of maladaptive purging behaviors other than vomiting, such as ipecac abuse, which can cause irreversible cardiac abnormalities and fatal cardiomyopathies due to its accumulation in cardiac tissue.[123]

Although adolescent male and female patients with BN reportedly have similar physical signs such as dental enamel erosion, parotid gland swelling, esophagitis, and electrolyte disturbances, a significant delay between the onset of symptoms and the age of first treatment has been described in males but not in females.[66] It has been suggested that the lag time may result from reluctance of males to openly discuss their eating problems because of feelings of shame and embarrassment in having a stereotypically "female" disorder.[66]

Risk Factors

Several non–sport-related risk factors that are biopsychosocial in nature have consistently been associated with DE development in adolescents and young adults. These include biological factors such as pubertal status, pubertal timing, and the BMI[142–148]; psychological factors such as body image dissatisfaction,[73,149,150] negative affect (mood states such as depression, stress, shame, inadequacy, guilt, and helplessness),[151] low self-esteem,[152,153] and perfectionism[115,154,155]; and sociocultural factors such as perceived pressure to conform to an unrealistic standard of thinness.[156,157] Athletes are vulnerable to these factors and to others that are sport specific.

Type of Sport Participation. Athletes participating in sports that emphasize appearance, a thin body build, or low body weight or that require weight classifications have historically displayed a significantly higher prevalence of subclinical and clinically diagnosed EDs than athletes in other sports.[12,14,73] However, the perception and association of DE primarily with lean-build sports is slowly diminishing. Authors[59] of a recent investigation of the prevalence of DE in collegiate female athletes participating in lean-build and non–lean-build sports found they were susceptible to DE, regardless of the type of sport participation.

Susceptibility of male athletes to DE has garnered much interest, particularly those participating in sports such as distance running,[158] wrestling,[15,73,159,160] body building,[161,162] lightweight football,[163] horseracing,[164] rowing,[15] and ski jumping.[165] Moreover, authors[72] of a meta-analysis of 17 studies involving adolescent and adult male athletes reported more DE than comparison groups across all categories of sport but particularly among aesthetic and weight class-dependent sports.

Serious competitors in aesthetic sports often begin intensive training at relatively early ages, usually before puberty. Puberty is characterized by major changes in hormonal levels and other physiologic indicators; body size, proportion, and composition; and behaviors.[86,166] A primary concern is often the increase in absolute and relative fat mass associated with puberty, which may negatively influence performance.[167–169] From early to late adolescence, about 11 to 18 years, girls gain an estimated 17.3 kg (38.1 lb) in fat-free mass and 7.1 kg (15.7 lb) in fat mass, while boys gain an estimated 32.5 kg (71.6 lb) in fat-free mass and 3.2 kg (7.1 lb) in fat mass.[86] The weight gain in boys is predominantly due to an increase in lean tissue, specifically muscle, whereas about one third of the gain in girls is fat tissue.[170] Consequently, young girls may struggle more than boys in adapting to physical changes of puberty and may try to prevent or counter normal changes associated with growth and maturation through the use of maladaptive eating behaviors.[167]

Increasing preoccupation with meeting unrealistic body weight goals for performance enhancement is also evident in endurance sports such as distance running, swimming, and cross-country skiing. Elite endurance athletes are reportedly able to maintain a high level of performance with exceptionally low energy expenditure due to increased metabolic efficiency.[40,171] As fitness improves with training, metabolism becomes more efficient, so fewer calories are needed to accomplish the same amount of work. If the energy cost of training exceeds caloric intake, an energy deficit results. In female athletes, biochemical consequences of chronic caloric (energy) deprivation are theorized to induce menstrual cycle alterations (eg, amenorrhea).[40–42] Researchers[171,172] of the metabolic, hormonal, and body composition status of distance runners concluded that amenorrheic runners maintained body weight on substantially fewer calories, about 60% to 70%, of expected. These results suggest that an athlete's ability to perform at a high level despite chronic undernutrition presents a challenging scenario for clinicians from the standpoint of early identification of DE in athletes. If the imbalance between caloric intake and energy expenditure goes unrecognized, severe and/or chronic energy deficit may result and play an important role in the pathogenesis of an ED.

In sports requiring weight restrictions, athletes routinely experience frequent periods of restrictive dieting or weight cycling. Wrestling is the extreme and drew considerable national attention in the fall of 1997, when 3 collegiate wrestlers died within 33 days from intentionally using extreme and unsafe methods to rapidly "cut" weight to gain a competitive advantage.[173] Shortly after these deaths, the National Collegiate Athletic Association (NCAA) established new rules and procedures that appear promising in minimizing potentially life-threatening practices.[174]

Body Image Dissatisfaction. A positive body image is often associated with physical activity.[175] However, subgroups of physically active people have been targeted as possessing body image concerns and DE.[73,175–180] The issue of body image in athletes is not only negatively influenced by socioculturally driven pressures to achieve and maintain an unrealistic body shape and size but also by demands to be thin for maximizing performance.[10,13,75,181] Although female athletes face stronger sociocultural pressure to be thin, male athletes may be subject to pressure from within their sport to conform to an ideal body shape or weight for performance and aesthetic reasons. Thus, male athletes may be more susceptible to DE than previously believed.[15,72] Sociocultural pressure to be thin, coupled with performance anxiety or negative performance appraisal, may predispose athletes to body dissatisfaction, which often mediates the development of DE attitudes and behaviors.[69,74,182,183]

Attitudes reflecting dissatisfaction and anxiety with body size, shape, and weight are common concerns for children and adolescents[4,98–101] and are connected with puberty and the growth spurt.[184,185] At this time, the degree of satisfaction with one's own body is a significant predictor of eating disturbances,[186] self-esteem,[187] and depression.[184,188] Additionally, recurrent peer, parental, and media messages that equate desirability with appearance thinness play a central role in creating and intensifying the phenomenon of body dissatisfaction.[150,189–191] The indoctrination for appearance thinness begins as early as 6 years of age[192,193] and can trigger unhealthy body image attitudes and associated eating concerns that can become established and difficult to reverse by 11 to 14 years of age.[101]

Internalization of the thin ideal and body dissatisfaction is more of a problem with adolescent girls than boys.[101,147,194,195] In boys, body dissatisfaction is more likely to be associated with pursuit of muscularity.[196] Some boys long for a larger and more muscular physique, whereas others express a desire to lose body fat and develop a leaner and more muscular body.[197] It has been suggested that several risk factors and underlying mechanisms that may lead adolescent boys to pursue muscularity are similar to those that trigger development of DE.[63,71]

Detection

The National Institute of Clinical Excellence,[198] the American Academy of Pediatrics,[39] the Society for Adolescent Medicine,[18] the American Psychiatric Association,[20] the American College of Sports Medicine,[21] and the NCAA,[10] among others, have stressed the importance of early recognition in the management of DE. Because DE self-reporting is rare among athletes due to secrecy, shame, denial, and fear of reprisal,[10,70,76] early detection requires the development and implementation of a confidential and accessible screening program. Some screening methods, including the PPE, standardized self-report psychometric questionnaires, individual interviews, and direct observation are more useful than others in identifying athletes in need of treatment and those who would benefit from preventive strategies.

Preparticipation Physical Examination. The PPE affords clinicians an ideal opportunity to screen for eating and body weight disturbances. The most sensitive and productive screening component is the medical history questionnaire. Compiling a useful medical history for both male and female athletes depends on the inclusion of specific questionnaire items that solicit information on dietary restraint, body weight fluctuations, weight control behaviors, body weight and shape satisfaction or dissatisfaction, nutritional beliefs and practices, typical eating patterns, exercise habits, and musculoskeletal injuries with special reference to bone stress injuries.[32–34,77] In female athletes, ancillary questions are necessary to screen for menstrual dysfunction.[32,35,36,134] A comprehensive menstrual history survey includes questions pertaining to age of menarche, length and frequency (number of cycles per year) of periods, regularity of periods since menarche, date of last menstrual period, amount of flow, frequency and duration of amenorrhea, and oral contraceptive use and its purpose.[32,35,36,134] Specific questionnaire items to screen for DE and menstrual dysfunction are listed in Table 6a and 6b.

Although experts have recommended use of the PPE to screen for DE, such an approach is underutilized.[77,90–92,199] A survey of the nature, scope, and perceived effectiveness of screening in select Division I schools for DE in addition to menstrual dysfunction in female athletes indicated major shortcomings.[77] Screening for DE during the PPE was reported by 60% of the schools. Self-developed questionnaires or more indirect measures of assessing eating disturbances (eg, weight-for-height standards, weight-loss history, and excessive injuries) were used. Fewer than 6% of the schools used standardized, self-report psychometric questionnaires to screen for DE. However, questionnaires of this nature are not entirely satisfactory when used in an athletic population, and clinicians must be mindful of factors that can compromise their effectiveness. These factors will be discussed in the next section.

Of schools that incorporated specific questions to screen for menstrual dysfunction, only 24% reported using a comprehensive menstrual history survey. The screening consisted of only 1 or 2 questions, which would not have provided sufficient information for most experts.[32,35,61]

Screening for DE and menstrual dysfunction in high school athletes is essential, particularly because adolescence is a vulnerable time for development of DE and a critical period for optimizing bone mineral accrual.[58] However, many PPEs are reported to be inadequate due to lack of a comprehensive medical history questionnaire.[200] A survey completed at the high school level involving 34 athletics programs demonstrated the lack of effectiveness of the medical history questionnaire in screening for DE and menstrual dysfunction.[200] A total of 22% of schools reported screening female athletes for DE via weight-for-height measurements, weight loss history, or reports from coaches and teammates. Screening for menstrual dysfunction was reported by 33% of the schools; however, the questionnaires were inadequate for soliciting useful information.

Unfortunately, even if the medical history questionnaire is adequate for gathering concise information, clinicians rarely take advantage of the information as a means of health maintenance and optimization.[33] This omission is particularly damaging to some adolescent athletes, whose only opportunity for routine health care may be the annual PPE.[201] Therefore, the adequacy of the PPE, particularly in terms of the medical history review, cannot be underestimated as a preventive approach in identifying high-risk athletes in this age group.[202]

Standardized, Self-Report Screening Questionnaires. The most widely used standardized, self-report screening questionnaires in athletes include the Eating Disorders Inventory (EDI),[31] the Eating Disorder Examination (EDE-Q),[81] and the Eating Attitudes Test (EAT).[82] Although these psychometric instruments have been validated in the general population, they have not been specifically tested for sensitivity or validity with athletes. Hence, the resultant information may not be accurate.[78,203,204] If identified as having DE, athletes are often fearful that their positions on the team will be jeopardized or their careers will suffer adverse consequences. Even when anonymity is assured, some athletes fear their coaches will be able to distinguish individual responses. A fake profile may emerge that results in underreporting DE.[6,8,10,13,205] In addition to incongruities noted between an athlete's reported and actual behavior, some instruments are fairly intrusive or time consuming. The utility of screening large numbers of athletes with lengthy surveys that often require psychometric expertise for administration and data interpretation is seldom practical in most athletics settings.[80]

The need for psychometrically valid and clinically useful instruments for screening for eating and weight disturbances in athletes has provided the impetus for further study. As a result, numerous screening instruments have been designed specifically for athletes: the Survey of Eating Disorders among Athletes (SEDA),[9] the Athletic Milieu Direct Questionnaire (AMDQ),[83] the Female Athlete Screening Tool (FAST),[84] the College Health Related Information Survey (CHRIS-73),[85] the Physiological Screening Test,[79] and the Health, Weight, Dieting, and Menstrual History Questionnaire.[59] Table 7 describes these instruments.

As a group, the screening instruments developed for athletes have shown promise in initial applications. Their concurrent validity has been established with other standardized psychometric instruments developed for the general population. As more investigations surface on internal validity, content and criterion validity, and response bias with larger sample sizes and with athletes in a variety of sports and sport settings and at various performance levels, the generalizability of screening measures will increase.[79,80]

In-Depth Personal Interviews. Self-report questionnaires should be complemented with other information-gathering tools. One option that has the potential to provide a more accurate representation of the problem is in-depth personal interviews.[14,77–80] Personal interviews allow athletes to converse about their thoughts and feelings without judgment from coaches or teammates. Accuracy of the information exchange depends upon how comfortable the athlete feels in providing candid and unsolicited comments regarding concerns about body weight, shape, and appearance. Accuracy also depends on how secure the athlete feels about divulging information on whether he or she has been subjected to public weigh-ins, public scrutiny of results, remarks concerning the need for weight loss, or coercion to lose weight in accordance with the desired ideal of a coach or CSO.[80] Therefore, the individual who facilitates the interview must have professional and personal qualities that promote a secure and nonthreatening environment; otherwise, fear of reprisal, shame, and denial and secrecy associated with the disorders will continue as barriers to identification. The facilitator should be knowledgeable of DE, understand the language and demands of sport, emanate confidence in handling the information exchange, display excellent listening skills, possess the ability to remain objective, and refrain from disapproval or criticism.[70]

Despite the use of self-report questionnaires and personal interviews, information obtained simply from observing the behavior of individual athletes cannot be underestimated.[70] A knowledgeable observer of the team, such as a certified athletic trainer, coach, teammate, or other athletic staff member, often provides the quickest means of identifying a problem.

Physiologic Measurements. Athletes need specialized guidance to attain and maintain reasonable body weight goals, regardless of whether weight reduction is motivated by physiologic or aesthetic reasons or out of necessity to compete in weight-class events. However, pursuit of a reasonable weight is often complicated by an erroneous and overemphasized belief held by coaches and athletes that an ideal body weight or body fat percentage exists for optimal performance in a given sport. An ideal target weight or percentage of body fat is very difficult to define and even harder for an athlete to achieve without triggering harmful weight loss practices.[6,70] Moreover, weight loss recommendations without proper guidance, particularly from coaches, have been reported as a risk factor for development of maladaptive weight loss behaviors.[13,206]

Many coaches lack the formal education necessary to properly supervise athletes during periods of weight loss.[13,207,208] An assessment of the mental health of elite female student-athletes on a university campus revealed that they were particularly disturbed about how their coaches handled body weight issues.[28] Athlete concerns were triggered and perpetuated by mandatory weekly weigh-ins, assignment of target weights, perceived subtle psychological pressure to lose weight, and feelings that their coaches were generally uncomfortable about issues pertaining to body weight and eating. Undue emphasis on appearance and performance thinness necessitates methods to monitor the nutritional and training status of the athlete over and above the measurement of scale weight. Assessing body composition is one option.

Assessing Body Composition. Body composition pertains to the amount and distribution of fat mass, as well as lean (fat-free) body mass. Studies of body composition attempt to partition body mass into its major components. The component of body composition that has generally received most attention is relative fatness, expressed as percentage of body fat.[160] Diet and physical activity habits readily influence fat mass. Increases in fat mass and percentage of body fat are generally perceived as having a negative influence on functional performance capacity and detracting from appearance in aesthetic sports.[167] In young athletes, body composition is influenced by both growth and individual differences in the timing and tempo of the adolescent growth spurt and sexual maturation.[86]

Athletes often increase muscle mass and decrease fat mass during intensive training, especially during preseason conditioning and resistance training. They feel leaner and stronger, and their clothes fit more loosely. Yet they are confused as to why the scale frequently indicates an increase in body weight. Muscle tissue, which produces the force necessary for performance, is denser, takes up less space, and weighs more than fat tissue. Without access to an accurate estimate of body composition, athletes may not understand how training influences these changes and, more importantly, which ranges of values are acceptable from a health and safety standpoint.

Body composition can be estimated through measurement of skinfold thicknesses, hydrostatic weighing, air displacement plethysmography (BOD POD; Life Measurement, Inc, Concord, CA), bioelectric impedance, and DXA, among others.[86] With the exception of DXA, most methods provide a 2-component model of assessing body composition (ie, fat mass and fat-free mass). The DXA is based on a 3-component model (fat mass, fat-free mass, and bone) derived from different X-ray attenuation properties of soft tissue and bone mineral.[55,56] The DXA is advantageous in not only providing a precise measurement of body composition but also in evaluating bone density, which is an invaluable tool in determining stress fracture susceptibility in female athletes.[55,56] However, the instrument is costly and requires skilled technicians to administer the scan and interpret the data output.[209]

In general, all techniques provide estimates of body composition and all have potential sources of error. The techniques are based upon different theoretic models and assumptions for estimating body composition; consequently, values derived from the different methods are not directly comparable. Therefore, methodologic issues and assumptions underlying each technique and associated errors of estimation should be recognized and appreciated, so the risk of misinterpretation is minimized, especially in the hands of relative novices in the field.

Problems associated with the assessment of body composition and interpretation of data may trigger DE.[21,210] In response to this scenario, one organization, The Canadian Academy of Sport Medicine has recommended eliminating body composition assessment to reduce DE risk potential.[211] However, this approach may not be reasonable in many sport settings.[27,86] Changes in body composition may reflect subtle alterations in energy balance not readily apparent in scale weight and may provide essential information for the nutritional support and training status of the athlete.[27,86] Serial measurements of body composition can assist in determining the efficacy of a given training program, identifying unhealthy weight fluctuations, and evaluating whether a particular course of remedial action (eg, dietary recommendations) is in line with meeting the athlete's special health care needs.[27] In young athletes, it can be an important complement to the evaluation of physical growth and maturity status,[167,212] especially when changes in size, physique, and muscle mass are anticipated in the transition from childhood to adolescence and from adolescence to young adulthood (ie, from high school into college).[86,167]

Calculating the Body Mass Index. Appropriateness of body weight for height at a given age in either sex varies considerably. It can be assessed by calculating the BMI.[17] The BMI is used internationally as a simple indicator of heaviness and lightness, specifically at the extremes of the distribution: that is, overweight/obesity and underweight. The BMI expresses weight for height: $BMI = weight/height^2$, where weight is in kilograms and height is in meters squared (kg/m^2).[80] Therefore, accurate measurements of height and weight are essential. The BMI is correlated with total body fat and percentage of fat in heterogeneous samples but is also related to fat-free mass; thus, it has limitations.[212] Correlations between BMI and fat and lean components of body composition, respectively, vary among children, adolescents, and young adults, and at many ages, correlations between BMI and fat mass and fat-free mass are reasonably similar.[213–216] Moreover, caution is advised in interpreting estimates of normal weight and overweight based on the BMI in both athletes and nonathletes.[217]

Associations between the BMI and components of body composition in several samples indicate a wide range of variability. Individuals with the same BMI can differ considerably in percentage of fat and fat mass, which limits use of the BMI as an indicator of fatness. Interpreting the BMI calls for consideration of both fat and lean components of body composition.

Interpretation of the BMI in adolescents and young adults, and especially active individuals, as an indicator of fatness needs to be addressed carefully. It is more appropriately an index of heaviness and not necessarily fatness. As a group, athletes tend to be leaner and have less fat than nonathletes, so a higher BMI is more likely indicative of the greater muscle development in active athletes.[218,219] Nevertheless, concern for a low BMI in some athletes may be necessary. The World Health Organization[87] classifies individuals 18 years of age or older (adults) with a BMI less than 18.5 kg/m^2 as underweight. For individuals younger than 18 years of age, no agreed cut-offs exist. However, a BMI that is less than the age-specific and sex-specific 5th percentile of a nationally representative sample of United States children and adolescents derived from the Centers for Disease Control and Prevention growth charts (2002) can be used as an indicator of being underweight. These growth charts can be accessed at http://www.cdc.gov/growthcharts/. Note, however, that the BMI of children and adolescents is influenced by individual differences in growth and maturity status, especially the timing and tempo of the adolescent growth spurt and sexual maturation.[86]

Management

Repeatedly cited in the literature is the statement that athletes with DE require medical care from a physician-coordinated team of experts representing nutrition, mental health, and athletic training.[21-26] Because the similarities between males and females with DE are more notable than the differences in terms of clinical features,[64,220,221] similar strategies for identification and treatment are recommended for both sexes.[63]

If DE is suspected, the initial contact has been recommended to come from an authority figure — one whom the athlete knows and trusts to ensure that the intervention is facilitated with sensitivity and compassion.[88,113,222] The initial conversation should be straightforward, disclosing evidence of DE and balancing concerns for the athlete's health and well being.[88,113] There should be no hint of disapproval or criticism.

If DE suspicions are confirmed after the initial confrontation, the most pressing referral is to the supervising physician for a detailed medical history review and physical examination.[89,93] A positive evaluation requires classifying the athlete, detecting the presence or absence of physical complications, formulating an interdisciplinary management plan, providing for continuing care and surveillance,[223] and determining the extent of sport or exercise participation.[93] If the diagnosis has already been established, the evaluation should review the past and present degree of symptoms, assess the athlete's degree of compliance with past and current treatment protocols, and ascertain an anticipated level of continued care and athletic participation. Laboratory tests and an electrocardiographic evaluation may be required[89,93]; the comprehensiveness of the tests will be dictated by symptoms and clinical findings.

The components of the initial evaluation, including the medical history review, physical examination, laboratory studies, and electrocardiography, are described in Table 8. A focus on these components will assist the health care team in determining the appropriate setting for treatment and ensure optimal management of the athlete from an interdisciplinary standpoint.

Treatment Settings. Accurate assessment of health risks is essential to determine the appropriate setting for treatment, which may include hospitalization, intensive inpatient specialty venues or residential programs, partial hospitalization, and various levels of outpatient care. Outpatient treatment settings suffice for most athletes[24,25] who are carefully monitored and have a high level of motivation to comply with treatment recommendations, cooperative families, brief symptom duration, and stable weight, cardiac, and metabolic status.[89] A more restrictive setting is necessary with a rapid or persistent decline in oral food intake, rapid weight loss despite nutritional intervention, severe electrolyte imbalances, severe or intractable purging, cardiac arrhythmias, comorbid psychiatric problems, unresponsiveness to adequate outpatient care, and environmental considerations no longer conducive to healing.[17,24,89]

Therapeutic Interventions. The desired goals of intervention strategies include (1) the athlete's acceptance of the problem; (2) modifying maladaptive thoughts, attitudes, feelings, and habits that perpetuate the condition; (3) identifying and resolving psychosocial triggers; (4) stabilizing medical conditions; (5) reestablishing healthy eating patterns; (6) enlisting family support when appropriate; and (7) preventing relapse.[17,22,25] Because of the complexity of issues involved in working with athletes who present with DE, optimal management requires an organized, systematic approach to the development and implementation of interventions specific to nutrition, mental health, and athletic training. Administrative support is also necessary to define what constitutes reasonable care within the confines of the organization's resources and budgetary considerations.

Nutrition. The main goal of dietary counseling and management is to help athletes maintain adequate energy availability.[224] In more severe cases of persistent energy drain and marked weight loss, the primary focus is reestablishment of healthy target weights. Achieving this goal is essential for patients who present with reproductive and endocrine abnormalities, specifically female patients with irregular menses and abnormal ovulation, male patients with abnormal hormonal levels, and children and adolescents with abnormal patterns of physical and sexual growth and maturation.[89] Even if weight is within the normal range, as in most cases of BN, nutritional counseling is important to monitor binge eating and purging behaviors and address nutritional deficiencies.

The individual most qualified to provide this type of nutritional counseling is a registered dietitian, credentialed by the American Dietetic Association, who is knowledgeable in DE and understands the demands of sport. The American Dietetic Association has exceptional educational resources targeted to enhance the nutritional management of patients with EDs. These include a position statement entitled "Nutrition Intervention in the Treatment of Anorexia Nervosa, Bulimia Nervosa, and Eating Disorders Not Otherwise Specified"[225] as well as medical nutrition therapy (MNT) protocols that provide the framework for identifying appropriate interventions and expected outcomes.[90,91]

The role of the registered dietitian is to optimize nutritional status through the use of MNT protocols. The following treatment components are included in MNT: (1) a nutrition assessment to evaluate the athlete's food intake, metabolic status, lifestyle, and readiness to make changes; (2) dietary instruction and evaluation; (3) nutrition protocols for weight management; and (4) goal setting.[223] The registered dietitian is also instrumental in determining safe body weight and composition values in addition to helping the athlete establish and maintain a pattern of regular and healthful eating by involving caregivers, parents, and CSOs in meal planning.

The use of MNT protocols with athletes was first documented in 2001.[92] As more information becomes available, the protocols will serve to delineate both specific nutritional interventions and outcomes to advance the recovery of athletes with EDs and the most effective methods to reach those goals.

Mental Health. At least at the university level, athletes have been reported to underutilize mental health services.[28,226] Many athletes are also particularly sensitive to, and fearful of, psychological evaluation and treatment. Possible explanations include reluctance to admit personal weakness, desire to maintain autonomy, receipt of social support from teammates, and fear of derogation.[227,228] Consequently, athletes who present for therapy show a continuum of readiness. Some will be determined to change, whereas others will be reluctant or even hostile.[76] Regardless of where they fall along the continuum, motivation is essential to effect behavior change. It is the role of the therapist to assess and enhance the athlete's level of motivation for change and to identify the best treatment approach for meeting the following desired goals: (1) increasing the athlete's motivation to participate in treatment and enhancing cooperation to restore healthy eating patterns; (2) correcting core maladaptive thoughts, attitudes, and feelings related to DE, particularly how an athlete's chosen sport or athletic participation may be contributing to perpetuating the condition; (3) addressing themes that may underlie DE, such as developmental issues, identity formation, body image concern, and self-esteem; (4) identifying and addressing additional stressors, both in and out of sport, including academic pressure, relationships with teammates and coaches, social contacts, and family; (5) treating associated comorbid conditions, particularly mood disorders that can manifest as a decrease in energy, motivation, and arousal and depression, increased perception of effort, suicidal ideation, and impaired cognitive function; (6) encouraging the athlete to be open and to ask for support from family, friends, coaches, and teammates; (7) enlisting family support and providing counseling to immediate family members and CSOs when appropriate; and (8) preventing relapse.[22,89,93,94] The format for attaining these goals can include individual, group, and family counseling.[27,229]

The success of mental health interventions is highly dependent on identifying an appropriate psychotherapist. A licensed clinical psychologist or other licensed mental health professional who has an understanding of sport culture and expertise in treating DE is the clinician of choice to manage psychopathological conditions and to promote the healthy coping behaviors, self-esteem, and assertiveness skills necessary for athletes to achieve desired treatment goals.[230] Athletes are often referred to performance enhancement psychologists to deal with the complexity of issues associated with DE. However, it is important to recognize that performance enhancement psychologists generally lack the background and requisite training to address the needs of athletes who present with psychopathologic conditions.[230]

Pharmacologic agents may be necessary to treat patients.[89] Psychotropic medications such as the selective serotonin reuptake inhibitors (eg, fluoxetine, sertraline, citalopram, paroxetine) are commonly used in patients with BN to alleviate symptoms of depression.[76,89] It is important to note that presently only fluoxetine has Food and Drug Administration approval for treatment of BN. Although there are presently no Food and Drug Admin-

istration-approved medications for AN, some evidence suggests that a variety of medications, including antidepressants, anticonvulsants, mood stabilizers, lithium, and antipsychotics, have shown promise in treating some anorexic patients with anxiety, obsessions, and psychosis.[89,231] The use of any of these classes of medications for treatment of symptoms that accompany EDs is not without side effects. Therefore, caregivers and others serving in a supervisory capacity should be educated accordingly.

Certified Athletic Trainers. Certified athletic trainers, by virtue of their close working relationships with athletes, are in the best position to detect DE. They also have the capability and generally the responsibility to intervene and establish their role as integral members of the health care team.[29,232,233]

Certified athletic trainers are often considered informed patient advocates in the management of DE cases. Generally, the athletic trainer's duties include confronting an athlete who is suspected of DE and assisting with the logistics involved in referral and treatment follow-through as well as issues related to communication, confidentiality, health status, athletic participation status, treatment noncompliance, and billing and insurance (Table 9). Although certified athletic trainers have the necessary background and education to assist in the care of athletes with DE, they must be cognizant of their scope of practice limitations with regard to diagnosis and treatment. These aspects of case management must be relegated to physicians and psychotherapists who specialize in DE.[23] Substandard conduct of certified athletic trainers in managing athletes with DE can result in liability exposure for themselves and subject employers to legal ramifications.[29,232,233]

Issues in Treatment and Follow-Up Care

Treatment Noncompliance. Although one of the most challenging issues at the outset is persuading an ambivalent athlete to undergo an initial medical evaluation,[93] an even greater challenge may be convincing the athlete to follow through with treatment recommendations.[234] Resistance to treatment has been reported among athletes with DE[25,69] and is no less a problem with individuals presenting with DE in the general population.[199]

One of the objectives of the first National Eating Disorders Screening Program (NEDSP)[199] held on collegiate campuses was to assess the level of an individual's adherence in following through on treatment recommendations. Although the subjects reported an increased awareness of the dangers of EDs and the availability of treatment, enhanced knowledge in these areas did not greatly affect the actual number of participants who sought treatment. Furthermore, nonpursuit of treatment was marked in a group of respondents who had been sufficiently motivated to attend an educational and screening program, presumably had access to health care services, and reported enhanced awareness of the need for treatment and the availability of treatment resources. These findings underscore the level of vigilance required on the part of caregivers to convince patients of the necessity for treatment follow-through and compliance.

In an athletic population, resistance to consultation or treatment is a challenging problem and may necessitate restricting training and competition until compliance is established.[25,69] When an athlete has been cleared to train and compete while undergoing treatment, suspension may be necessary with signs of continual weight loss, noncompliance with treatment recommendations, and manifestation of resistant behaviors within treatment sessions, such as interrupting, arguing, sidetracking, and defensiveness. Although suspension is advantageous in such circumstances, it may result in several potentially harmful consequences, as it represents a major setback in achieving athletic goals.[25,69]

Stress induced by curtailing participation may become an unmanageable situation for athletes whose identity is based on receiving recognition for participation and success in sport.[28] The athlete's identity may be thrown into chaos, and self-esteem and self-acceptance may deteriorate further. The process is compounded by feelings of loneliness and alienation as coaches and teammates are no longer readily available for support. The athlete may resort to fewer coping mechanisms, which may worsen an already volatile situation. Moreover, with the sport connection severed, no other outlet may be available for physical and emotional release, and the athlete may continue to train on his or her own. This is a dangerous scenario, as it becomes more difficult to maintain the level of medical surveillance appropriate to safeguard the athlete's health and safety. However, suspension may not be needed if health risks are determined to be minimal based on the severity and chronicity of the problem, type of sport, training schedule and conditions, immediate health status, presence of complications or other medical conditions, and eating patterns.[94]

A written contract, agreed upon and signed by the athlete and the health care team's coordinator or designate, may be necessary to promote patient compliance with the recommended treatment protocol.[27,93] Under such a contractual agreement, the patient is expected to meet certain health maintenance criteria to continue athletic participation or resume participation after suspension (Table 10). The contract should include information that details the type, frequency, and location of treatments; the caregivers who will be supervising the various treatment components, their contact information and procedures for after-hour emergencies; the type and level of training permitted with special reference to intensity, duration and frequency of workouts; and body weight allowances with emphasis on expected rates of controlled weight gain, if applicable. If any condition of the contract is breached, the consequences must be explicitly spelled out. Any changes to the initial contract in terms of expectations must be documented accordingly.

The confidential handling of an athlete's medical information, according to disclosure regulations mandated by the Family Equal Rights and Privacy Act[215] and/or the Health Insurance, Portability, and Accountability Act[235] is crucial to fostering a caregiver-patient relationship based on trust and mutual respect. To communicate appropriately, guard against a breach in confidentiality, and comply with disclosure regulations, the health care team's coordinator or designate must obtain written authorization from the patient indicating who will have access to the medical information and to what extent the information may be disclosed.

Maintaining confidentiality can be difficult. The team environment fosters close working relationships among teammates, coaches, certified athletic trainers, and other sport management personnel. Most athletes will agree to share medical information with their coaches or CSOs on a limited basis as long as it focuses on treatment progress rather than on personal issues relating to their medical condition.[70]

Transitional Care. If athletes with DE are in their early stages and maladaptive behaviors occur less frequently than with full-syndrome disorders, an ongoing medical surveillance plan and nutritional education may be the only intervention needed to keep the athletes emotionally stable and physically capable of functioning at a high level.[76] However, more severe and long-standing cases have the potential to drain existing resources and manpower, resulting in compromised treatment effectiveness. Recovery is further jeopardized when the environment is no longer conducive to healing.

Athletes typically function in an environment beset with stressors related to performance, rigors of academic coursework, personal development, and social adjustment.[76] The physical and emotional consequences of EDs superimposed on these stressors may complicate recovery. Also, the pathogenic eating and weight loss behaviors associated with the condition can cause stress and anxiety, as well as discomfort for teammates, coaches, and others who come in close contact with the symptomatic athlete.[70,236] This situation is especially problematic when the athlete is clearly underweight, restricting dietary intake, or vomiting frequently.[236] Caregivers may have no recourse but to curtail athletic participation, remove the athlete from persons and circumstances aggravating the condition, and consider a more restrictive setting for treatment. For young adult athletes who reside in residential campus settings, this action often requires a shift in the supervision of care from the organization to parents or guardians.

The transition of care from organizational to parental accountability must be approached with forethought. Many parents, guardians, or CSOs may not have an adequate level of understanding about the seriousness of the conditions to make medically responsible decisions. Even with adequate information, the emotional and financial repercussions can be overwhelming and present obstacles to accessing quality care.[95–97]

Access to appropriate care may be constrained by monetary or insurance difficulties.[95] Out-of-pocket expenses for care are often high, but insurance benefits can be the equalizer. However, many companies do not provide benefits for mental health care and those that do often exclude treatment for EDs.[96] For patients who have coverage, a limit to the type and extent of resources available exists. For example, if hospitalization or residential treatment is required, the allowable length of stay is often too short to prevent relapse. Before managed care contracts proliferated, patients in 1 residential facility solely dedicated to the treatment of EDs had an average length of stay of 50 days, with a return rate of under 10%.[97] Now, the average stay is closer to 15 days, with a return rate of 33%.[97] Additionally, insurance companies may restrict the number of outpatient visits per year, establish lifetime caps on coverage, and preclude payment to some medical practitioners.[18] Accessing the appropriate care for adolescents may also have challenges. Adolescents may not satisfy the age requirements at treatment institutions able to provide the most appropriate care.[18] Moreover, qualified professionals may not be available to care for teenagers and young adults with EDs because of low reimbursement rates for psychosocial services common among insurers.[18]

Administrative Support. As a general rule, an organization must take reasonable care in administering its athletic program to prevent foreseeable harm to its participants and avoid potential liability for negligence.[30,232] This includes optimizing sports medicine services to adequately protect the health and safety of athletes. The NATA[237] and the NCAA[238] have established health and safety initiatives and guidelines to assist organizations in identifying practices to potentially reduce individual risk and institutional liability. However, lacking are specific legal standards on what is obligatory, particularly in nonemergent situations.[30] Therefore, organizations must thoroughly examine both the benefits to their athletes and the financial implications to their sports medicine programs in ascertaining how to satisfy the legal duty of reasonable care.[29,30] An appropriate response plan must start at the top, with administrators sending clear signals about what must be done and to what extent to prevent, minimize, contain, and manage problems.

Prevention

The design and implementation of mandatory, structured educational and behavioral programs for all athletes, coaches, certified athletic trainers, administrators, and other support staff are key to preventing DE in athletic settings.[21,23,69,74,77,182,239–242] However, fewer than 41% of Division I athletics programs make such education a requirement.[77] Similarly, a study conducted at the high school level revealed that 33% of schools provided educational programs; however, fewer than 9% required student attendance and only 15% of the schools made education a requirement for coaches.[243]

Educational programs have been recommended by The American College of Sports Medicine[21] and the NCAA.[244] Additionally, a number of unique educational initiatives have been developed and implemented by national governing bodies of sports and high school associations in response to the need to limit the seriousness of DE or, preferably, prevent its development.[245–247]

Seminars, guest speakers, written material, audiovisual presentations, and use of the Internet are all viable options for disseminating educational information. The content of information exchange varies depending on the needs of the targeted population and anticipated outcomes.

Athletes. First and foremost, athletes require information that destigmatizes DE through open, truthful, and factual discussions. Fear associated with talking about the condition must be allayed as well as the social stigma, shame, and guilt that prevent athletes from seeking help.[70] Accomplishing this goal requires increased awareness of EDs as conditions for which treatment is available and effective.[199] This helps break down presumed barriers to accessing care that stem from lack of information relative to the seriousness of the disorders, referral resources, and treatment options.[199]

Second, athletes should be educated on the harmful effects of pathogenic weight control methods, which some players consider necessary for performance.[88,206,248] This factor alone underscores the necessity for athletes to receive quality information from knowledgeable professionals and other reputable sources. The Internet is one information source that can be helpful (Table 11).[249,250] However, those who supervise athletes should also be alert to the existence of harmful Internet sites, such as pro-ana (anorexia) and pro-mia (bulimia) sites, devoted to the continuance, promotion, and support of EDs and glamorizing the unhealthy behaviors.[18,251] Although these Web sites have been in existence for quite some time, they are becoming more prevalent on social networking sites.[252] This is a disturbing trend considering that the information is presently reaching a much wider audience.

Third, it is important that athletes become knowledgeable about sound nutritional practices so they are better equipped to scrutinize their eating habits to a level that ensures adequate energy availability. It is a challenge for most athletes to maintain a positive energy balance over long periods of training with adequate amounts of food and nutrients, particularly with a coexisting goal of body weight control.[41] For example, the daily energy intake reported by many female athletes is often below the estimated energy expenditure of their training regimens,[41,42,250] particularly some endurance-based programs that have a predicted energy expenditure of 700 to 1000 kcal/d.[41] Athletes participating in less aerobically demanding sports such as gymnastics and figure skating have reduced total energy requirements and may increase dependency on energy deprivation to control or manipulate body weight.[254] To prevent an imbalance between energy expenditure and dietary intake, athletes must make appropriate food choices that will provide adequate macronutrients and micronutrients so that metabolic fuels are readily available. Athletes with more nutrition knowledge are inclined to make better food choices, resulting in improved health status and enhanced athletic performance.[254–256] However, numerous investigators have identified problems and deficiencies in the athlete's diet, especially as it relates to adequate consumption of macronutrients[257–260] and micronutrients.[261]

Lastly, although educating young adults about DE and related nutritional problems has been effective in prevention, an important question is whether this educational approach works for children.[262] From a general perspective, researchers and organizations have emphasized the need for developing and implementing educational programs that challenge the definition of thinness and promote self-acceptance, healthy eating, and reasonable physical activity among children and youth.[98,263] In a study of 222 boys and girls in the 4th and 6th grades, short-term outcomes of a school-based curriculum program for developing healthy body image and preventing DE resulted in increased knowledge, positive attitudes, and healthful intentions related to body image, hazards of weight loss dieting, and unrealistic media-driven messages.[98]

Coaches. Coaches are in a unique position to denounce unhealthy attitudes and behaviors that may trigger DE. However, they also juggle a combination of role demands and conflicts that are not always consistent with making decisions in the best interest of their athletes' health.[264–266] Good decision making is further complicated by the fact that many coaches lack formal training in sport science disciplines known to favorably affect health and performance, specifically sports psychology, physiology of exercise, nutrition, and sports medicine.[264,267] When demands and stressors of coaching combine with less-than-adequate educational preparation, coaches are more vulnerable to careless comments, misinformation, and inappropriate actions that may jeopardize the health and safety of their athletes and constitute a liability exposure for themselves and their employers.[268,269]

Evidence suggests that collegiate coaches could benefit from comprehensive education in all domains related to knowledge of DE,[241] as well as strategies to properly communicate with their athletes about body weight issues.[70] For example, competitive female gymnasts who were told by their coaches to lose weight resorted to pathogenic weight control methods.[206,270] Among 131 lightweight football players, 42% showed evidence of DE and reported that their "teacher/coach" was perceived to be the individual who most encouraged dieting practices.[163]

The more enlightened coaches are about nutritional issues, the more apt they are to follow nutritional guidelines, emphasize healthy eating habits rather than weight standards, and have a better understanding of why weight is such a sensitive and personal issue for athletes, particularly women.[271] Similarly, educated coaches also realize the best way to interact with symptomatic athletes is to be specific about their suspicions, encourage medical care, and reassure the athlete that his or her position on the team will not be jeopardized.[94] Only through mandatory, formal education programs can coaches promote healthy exercise and nutrition alternatives that have the potential to counteract development of DE.

Certified Athletic Trainers. Unlike coaches, certified athletic trainers have clearly defined, standardized educational competencies established by the NATA that can help guide their work with athletes in the areas of DE, nutrition, and weight management.[272] The knowledge gleaned from mastering the educational competencies coupled with exposure in working with athletes who present with DE increases the certified athletic trainer's overall effectiveness and confidence in dealing with the complexities of this condition.

In one survey of head certified athletic trainers at NCAA Division IA and IAA institutions, most felt their role was to identify (78%) and help (97%) athletes with EDs, but only 27% felt confident in their ability to identify an athlete with an ED, and only 38% felt confident confronting an athlete suspected of having an ED.[273] Among certified athletic trainers, females felt significantly more confident than males in identifying athletes with the conditions. Access to ongoing educational preservice and inservice programs is critical to enhancing knowledge and awareness of EDs among all certified athletic trainers. Similarly, developing a management protocol to handle problems should they occur is essential to improving confidence levels.[23] However, few schools have established a formal treatment protocol.[77,273] For example, 1 in 4 certified athletic trainers (25%) reportedly worked at collegiate institutions that did not have a management protocol in place.[274] In a survey completed in 2005 at the high school level, only 18% of schools reported having a standard treatment protocol for confirmed cases of EDs.[200]

CONCLUSIONS

A comprehensive array of interventions and educational strategies is imperative to meet the challenges in understanding and working with athletes who present with DE or may be at risk. The key is to establish a network of qualified and knowledgeable professionals who can skillfully handle interventions, provide a seamless continuum of care, institute screening measures for early detection, and develop educational initiatives for prevention. The management of athletes is complex and requires interdisciplinary collaboration among physicians, dietitians, psychotherapists, certified athletic trainers, administrators, coaches, and CSOs to obtain desired outcomes. The certified athletic trainer is in a unique position to play a significant role as a caregiver, informed patient advocate, and educator and should be prepared to act accordingly.

ACKNOWLEDGMENTS

We gratefully acknowledge the efforts of Michael E. Brunet II, PhD, ATC; Edward P. Tyson, MD; Jayd M. Grossman, MEd, ATC; Jeanne F. Nichols, PhD, FACSM; and the Pronouncements Committee in the preparation of this document.

DISCLAIMER

The NATA publishes its position statements as a service to promote the awareness of certain issues to its members. The information contained in the position statement is neither exhaustive not exclusive to all circumstances or individuals. Variables such as institutional human resource guidelines, state or federal statutes, rules, or regulations, as well as regional environmental conditions, may impact the relevance and implementation of these recommendations. The NATA advises its members and others to carefully and independently consider each of the recommendations (including the applicability of same to any particular circumstance or individual). The position statement should not be relied upon as an independent basis for care but rather as a resource available to NATA members or others. Moreover, no opinion is expressed herein regarding the quality of care that adheres to or differs from NATA's position statements. The NATA reserves the right to rescind or modify its position statements at any time.

REFERENCES

1. Dancyger IF, Garfinkel PE. The relationship of partial syndrome eating disorders to anorexia nervosa and bulimia nervosa. *Psychol Med.* 1995;25(5):1019–1025.
2. Johnson CL, Stuckey MK, Lewis LD, Schwartz DM. Bulimia: a descriptive survey of 316 cases. *Int J Eat Disord.* 1982;2(1):3–16.
3. Lowe MR, Gleaves DH, DiSimone-Weiss RT, et al. Restraint, dieting, and the continuum model of bulimia nervosa. *J Abnorm Psychol.* 1996;105(4):508–517.
4. Shisslak CM, Crago M, Estes LS. The spectrum of eating disturbances. *Int J Eat Disord.* 1995;18(3):209–219.
5. Byrne S, McLean N. Eating disorders in athletes: a review of the literature. *J Sci Med Sport.* 2001;4(2):145–159.
6. Wilmore JH. Eating and weight disorders in the female athlete. *Int J Sport Nutr.* 1991;1(2):104–117.
7. Beals KA, Manore MM. The prevalence and consequences of subclinical eating disorders in female athletes. *Int J Sport Nutr.* 1994;4(2):175–195.

8. Brownell KD, Rodin J. Prevalence of eating disorders in athletes. In: Brownell KD, Rodin J, Wilmore JH, eds. *Eating, Body Weight, and Performance in Athletes: Disorders of Modern Society.* Philadelphia, PA: Lea & Febiger; 1992:128–143.

9. Guthrie SR. Prevalence of eating disorders among intercollegiate athletes: contributing factors and preventive measures. In: Black DR, ed. *Eating Disorders Among Athletes: Theory, Issues, and Research.* Reston, VA: Association for Girls and Women in Sport, Associations for Health, Physical Education, Recreation, and Dance; 1991:43–66.

10. Johnson C, Powers PS, Dick R. Athletes and eating disorders: the National Collegiate Athletic Association study. *Int J Eat Disord.* 1999;26(2):179–188.

11. Reinking MF, Alexander LE. Prevalence of disordered-eating behaviors in undergraduate female collegiate athletes and nonathletes. *J Athl Train.* 2005;40(1):47–51.

12. Smolack L, Murnen SK, Ruble AE. Female athletes and eating problems: a meta-analysis. *Int J Eat Disord.* 2000;27(4):371–380.

13. Sundgot-Borgen J. Risk and trigger factors for the development of eating disorders in female elite athletes. *Med Sci Sports Exerc.* 1994;26(4):414–419.

14. Sundgot-Borgen J, Torstveit MK. Prevalence of eating disorders in elite athletes is higher than in the general population. *Clin J Sport Med.* 2004;14(1):25–32.

15. Thiel A, Gottfried H, Hesse FW. Subclinical eating disorders in male athletes: a study of the low weight category in rowers and wrestlers. *Acta Psychiatr Scand.* 1993;88(4):259–265.

16. Warren BJ, Stanton AL, Blessing DL. Disordered eating patterns in competitive female athletes. *Int J Eat Disord.* 1990;9(4):565–569.

17. Becker AE, Grinspoon SK, Klibanski A, Herzog DB. Eating disorders. *N Engl J Med.* 1999;340(14):1092–1098.

18. Golden NH, Katzman DK, Kreipe RE, et al. Eating disorders in adolescents: position paper of the Society for Adolescent Medicine. *J Adolesc Health.* 2003;33(6):496–503.

19. Stephenson JD. Medical consequences and complications of anorexia nervosa and bulimia nervosa in female athletes. *Athl Train J Natl Athl Train Assoc.* 1991;26(2):130–135.

20. American Psychiatric Association. Eating Disorders. In: *Diagnostic and Statistical Manual of Mental Disorders.* 4th ed, Text Revision. Washington, DC: American Psychiatric Association; 2000:583–595.

21. Otis CL, Drinkwater B, Johnson M, Loucks A, Wilmore J. American College of Sports Medicine position stand: the female athlete triad. *Med Sci Sports Exerc.* 1997;29(5):i–ix.

22. Johnson C, Tobin DL. The diagnosis and treatment of anorexia nervosa and bulimia among athletes. *Athl Train J Natl Athl Train Assoc.* 1991;26(2):119–128.

23. Grandjean AC. Eating disorders: the role of the athletic trainer. *Athl Train, J Natl Athl Train Assoc.* 1991;26(2):105–112.

24. Nattiv A, Callahan LR, Kelman-Sherstinsky A. The female athlete triad. In: Ireland ML, Nattiv A, eds. *The Female Athlete.* Philadelphia, PA: WB Saunders; 2002:223–235.

25. Sundgot-Borgen J. Disordered eating. In: Ireland ML, Nattiv A, eds. *The Female Athlete.* Philadelphia, PA: WB Saunders; 2002:237–247.

26. Tobin D, Johnson C, Franke K. Clinical treatment of eating disorders. In: Brownell KD, Rodin J, Wilmore JH, eds. *Eating, Body Weight, and Performance in Athletes: Disorders of Modern Society.* Philadelphia, PA: Lea & Febiger; 1992:330–343.

27. Beals KA. *Disordered Eating Among Athletes: A Comprehensive Guide for Health Professionals.* Champaign, IL: Human Kinetics; 2004:87, 97–98,105–109,133–141,167–173.

28. Ryan R, Lopiano D, Tharinger D, Starke K. *The Mental Health of Female College Student-Athletes: Research and Interventions on a University Campus: A Report to the Hogg Foundation for Mental Health and RGK Foundation.* Austin, TX: Intercollegiate Athletics, Department of Academics and Student Affairs, The University of Texas at Austin; 1994:13–18,56–60,74–80,120–121,132–133.

29. West SA, Ciccolella ME. Issues in the standard of care for certified athletic trainers. *J Leg Aspects Sport.* 2004;14(1):63–74.

30. Mitten MJ. Medical care guidelines not legally bound. 2000. The NCAA News Comment. http://www.ncaa.org/wps/portal/newsdetail? WCM_GLOBAL_CONTEXT=/wps/wcm/connect/NCAA/NCAA+ News/NCAA+News+Online/2000/Editorial/Medical+care+guidelines+ not+legally+bound+-+8-28-00. Accessed November 12, 2005.

31. Garner DM, Olmsted MP, Polivy J. *The Eating Disorders Inventory: A Measure of Cognitive-Behavioral Dimensions of Anorexia Nervosa and Bulimia. Anorexia Nervosa: Recent Developments in Research.* New York, NY: Alan R. Liss; 1983:173–184.

32. Johnson MD. Tailoring the preparticipation exam to female athletes. *Physician Sportsmed.* 1992;20(7):61–72.

33. Peltz JE, Haskell WL, Matheson GO. A comprehensive and cost-effective preparticipation exam implemented on the World Wide Web. *Med Sci Sports Exerc.* 1999;31(12):1727–1740.

34. Walsh JM, Wheat ME, Freund K. Detection, evaluation, and treatment of eating disorders the role of the primary care physician. *J Gen Intern Med.* 2000;15(8):577–590.

35. American Academy of Pediatrics. Committee on Sports Medicine and Fitness. Medical concerns in the female athlete. *Pediatrics.* 2000;106(3):610–613.

36. Tanner SM. Preparticipation examination targeted for the female athlete. *Clin Sports Med.* 1994;13(2):337–353.

37. Drinkwater BL, Loucks A, Sherman RT, Sundgot-Borgen J, Thompson RA. International Olympic Committee (IOC) consensus statement on the female athlete triad. 2005. http://multimedia.olympic. org/pdf/en_report_917.pdf. Accessed November 14, 2005.

38. Silber TJ. Anorexia nervosa among children and adolescents. *Adv Pediatr.* 2005;52:49–76.

39. American Academy of Pediatrics. Committee on Adolescence. Identifying and treating eating disorders. *Pediatrics.* 2003;111(1):204–211.

40. Loucks AB, Mortola JF, Girton L, Yen SS. Alterations in the hypothalamic-pituitary-ovarian and the hypothalamic-pituitary-adrenal axes in athletic women. *J Clin Endocrinol Metab.* 1989;68(2):402–411.

41. Harber VJ. Menstrual dysfunction in athletes: an energetic challenge. *Exerc Sport Sci Rev.* 2000;28(1):19–23.

42. Dueck CA, Manore MM, Matt KS. Role of energy balance in athletic menstrual dysfunction. *Int J Sport Nutr.* 1996;6(2):165–190.

43. Drinkwater BL, Bruemner B, Chesnut CH III. Menstrual history as a determinant of current bone density in young athletes. *JAMA.* 1990;263(4):545–548.

44. Myburgh KH, Hutchins J, Fataar AB, Hough SF, Noakes TD. Low bone density is an etiologic factor for stress fractures in athletes. *Ann Intern Med.* 1990;113(10):754–759.

45. Nattiv A, Loucks AB, Manore MM, Sanborn CF, Sundgot-Borgen J, Warren MP. Position stand: the female athlete triad. *Med Sci Sports Exerc.* 2007;39(10):1–9.

46. American Academy of Pediatrics Committee on Adolescence, American College of Obstetricians and Gynecologists Committee on Adolescent Health Care, Diaz A, Laufer MR, Breech LL. Menstruation in girls and adolescents: using the menstrual cycle as a vital sign. *Pediatrics.* 2006;118(5):2245–2250.

47. United States Food and Drug Administration Web site. Reference daily intakes, recommended dietary allowances. http://www.fda.gov/fdac. Accessed March 22, 2007.

48. Opinion on the tolerable upper intake level of Vitamin D. Scientific Committee on Food. http://www.imace.org/nutrition/pdf/poster.pdf. Accessed March 22, 2007.

49. Greer FR, Krebs NF. Optimizing bone health and calcium intakes of infants, children, and adolescents. *Pediatrics.* 2006;117(2):578–585.

50. Holick MF. High prevalence of vitamin D inadequacy and implications for health. *Mayo Clin Proc.* 2006;81(3):353–373.

51. National Institutes of Health Consensus Development Panel. Osteoporosis prevention, diagnosis, and therapy. *JAMA.* 2001;285(6):785–795.

52. Akin JW. Hormonal disorders. In: Ireland ML, Nattiv A, eds. *The Female Athlete.* Philadelphia, PA: WB Saunders; 2002:141–147.

53. Warren MP, Shantha S. The female athlete. *Baillieres Best Pract Res Clin Endocrinol Metab.* 2000;14(1):37–53.

54. Weaver CM, Teegarden D, Lyle RM, et al. Impact of exercise on bone health and contraindication of oral contraceptive use in young women. *Med Sci Sports Exerc*. 2001;33(6):873–880.

55. Marx RG, Saint-Phard D, Callahan LR, Chu J, Hannafin JA. Stress fracture sites related to underlying bone health in athletic females. *Clin J Sport Med*. 2001;11(2):73–76.

56. Lukaski HC. Soft tissue composition and bone mineral status: evaluation by dual-energy X-ray absorptiometry. *J Nutr*. 1993; 123(suppl 2):438–443.

57. Torstveit MK, Sundgot-Borgen J. The female athlete triad exists in both elite athletes and controls. *Med Sci Sports Exerc*. 2005;37(9): 1449–1459.

58. Nichols JF, Rauh MJ, Lawson MJ, Ji M, Barkai HS. Prevalence of the female athlete triad syndrome among high school athletes. *Arch Pediatr Adolesc Med*. 2006;160(2):137–142.

59. Beals KA, Hill AK. The prevalence of disordered eating, menstrual dysfunction, and low bone mineral density among US collegiate athletes. *Int J Sport Nutr Exerc Metab*. 2006;16(1):1–23.

60. Beals KA, Manore MM. Disorders of the female athlete triad among collegiate athletes. *Int J Sport Nutr Exerc Metab*. 2002;12(3): 281–293.

61. Nattiv A, Lynch L. The female athlete triad: managing an acute risk to long-term health. *Physician Sportsmed*. 1994;22(1):60–68.

62. Farrow JA. The adolescent male with an eating disorder. *Pediatr Ann*. 1992;21(11):769–774.

63. Braun DL, Sunday SR, Huang A, Halmi KA. More males seek treatment for eating disorders. *Int J Eat Disord*. 1999;25(4):415–424.

64. Andersen AE, Holman JE. Males with eating disorders: challenges for treatment and research. *Psychopharmacol Bull*. 1997;33(3):391–397.

65. Siegel JH, Hardoff D, Golden NH, Shenker IR. Medical complications in male adolescents with anorexia nervosa. *J Adolesc Health*. 1995;16(6):448–453.

66. Carlat DJ, Camargo CA Jr, Herzog DB. Eating disorders in males: a report on 135 patients. *Am J Psychiatry*. 1997;154(8):1127–1132.

67. Kreipe RE, Birndorf SA. Eating disorders in adolescents and young adults. *Med Clin North Am*. 2000;84(4):1027–1049, viii–ix.

68. Woodside DB, Garfinkel PE, Lin E, et al. Comparisons of men with full or partial eating disorders, men without eating disorders, and women with eating disorders in the community. *Am J Psychiatry*. 2001;158(4):570–574.

69. Thompson RA, Sherman RT. *Helping Athletes with Eating Disorders*. Champaign, IL: Human Kinetics; 1993:123–146.

70. Ryan R. Management of eating problems in athletic settings. In: Brownell KD, Rodin J, Wilmore JH, eds. *Eating, Body Weight, and Performance in Athletes: Disorders of Modern Society*. Philadelphia, PA: Lea & Febiger; 1992:344–362.

71. Ricciardelli LA, McCabe MP. A biopsychosocial model of disordered eating and the pursuit of muscularity in adolescent boys. *Psychol Bull*. 2004;130(2):179–205.

72. Hausenblas HA, Carron AV. Eating disorder indices and athletes: an integration. *J Sport Exerc Psychol*. 1999;21(3):230–258.

73. Engel SG, Johnson C, Powers PS, et al. Predictors of disordered eating in a sample of elite Division I college athletes. *Eat Behav*. 2003;4(4):333–343.

74. Powers P, Johnson C. Small victories: prevention of eating disorders among elite athletes. *Eat Disord*. 1996;4(4):364–377.

75. Byrne S, McLean N. Elite athletes: effects of the pressure to be thin. *J Sci Med Sport*. 2002;5(2):80–94.

76. Currie A, Morse ED. Eating disorders in athletes: managing the risks. *Clin Sports Med*. 2005;24(4):871–883,ix.

77. Beals KA. Eating disorder and menstrual dysfunction screening, education, and treatment programs: survey results from NCAA Division I schools. *Physician Sportsmed*. 2003;31(7):33–38.

78. Fairburn CG, Beglin SJ. Assessment of eating disorders: interview or self-report questionnaire? *Int J Eat Disord*. 1994;16(4):363–370.

79. Black DR, Larkin LJ, Coster DC, Leverenz LJ, Abood DA. Physiologic screening test for eating disorders/disordered eating among female collegiate athletes. *J Athl Train*. 2003;38(4):286–297.

80. DePalma MT, Koszewski WM, Romani W, Case JG, Zuiderhof NJ, McCoy PM. Identifying college athletes at risk for pathogenic eating. *Br J Sports Med*. 2002;36(1):45–50.

81. Fairburn CG, Cooper Z. The eating disorder examination. In: Fairburn CG, Wilson GT, eds. *Binge Eating: Nature, Assessment, and Treatment*. New York, NY: Guilford Press; 1993:317–360.

82. Garner DM, Garfinkel PE. The eating attitudes test: an index of the symptoms of anorexia nervosa. *Psychol Med*. 1979;9(2):273–279.

83. Nagel DL, Black DR, Leverenz LJ, Coster DC. Evaluation of a screening test for female college athletes with eating disorders and disordered eating. *J Athl Train*. 2000;35(4):431–440.

84. McNulty KY, Adams CH, Anderson JM, Affenito SG. Development and validation of a screening tool to identify eating disorders in female athletes. *J Am Diet Assoc*. 2001;101(8):886–892.

85. Steiner H, Pyle RP, Brassington GS, Matheson G, King M. The College Health Related Information Survey (C.H.R.I.S.-73): a screen for college student athletes. *Child Psychiatry Hum Dev*. 2003;34(2): 97–109.

86. Malina RM, Bouchard C, Bar-Or O. *Growth, Maturation, and Physical Activity*. 2nd ed. Champaign, IL: Human Kinetics; 1994.

87. World Health Organization. *Obesity: Preventing and Managing the Global Epidemic. Report of a WHO Consultation on Obesity*. Geneva, Switzerland: World Health Organization; 1998.

88. Rosen LW, McKeag DB, Hough DO, Curley V. Pathogenic weight-control behavior in female athletes. *Physician Sportsmed*. 1986; 14(1):79–86.

89. American Psychiatric Association. Practice guideline for the treatment of patients with eating disorders. 3rd ed. American Psychiatric Association Work Group on Eating Disorders. *Am J Psychiatry*. 2006;163(suppl 7):4–54.

90. American Dietetic Association. *Medical Nutrition Therapy Across the Continuum of Care. Anorexia and Bulimia Nervosa (Pediatric, Adolescent, and Adult)*. Chicago, IL: American Dietetic Association and Morrison Healthcare; 1998:(suppl 1):1–16.

91. American Dietetic Association. Medical nutrition therapy protocols: an introduction. *J Am Diet Assoc*. 1999;99(3):351.

92. Skinner P, Kopecky L, Seburg S, Roth T, Eich J, Lewis NM. Development of a medical nutrition therapy protocol for female collegiate athletes. *J Am Diet Assoc*. 2001;101(8):914–917.

93. Johnson MD. Disordered eating. In: Agostini R, Titus S, eds. *Medical and Orthopedic Issues of Active and Athletic Women*. Philadelphia, PA: Hanley & Belfus, Inc; 1994:141–151.

94. Sundgot-Borgen J, Bahr R. Eating disorders in athletes. In: Harries M, Williams C, Stanish WD, Micheli LJ, eds. *Oxford Textbook of Sports Medicine*. New York, NY: Oxford University Press; 1998: 138–152.

95. Eating Disorders Coalition for Research, Policy & Action. Policy Recommendations. http://www.eatingdisorderscoalition.org/reports/policyrecs.html. Accessed April 13, 2005.

96. Herzog D, Smeltzer D, Smeltzer T, Honan D, Weinstein M, Menaged S. The dangers of eating disorders and the need for health care reform. Briefing presented at: the House of Representatives; April 24 2001; Washington, D.C. http://www.eatingdisorderscoalition.org/congbriefings/042401/housebriefing042401.thml#herzog. Accessed August 13, 2005.

97. Herzog D, Smeltzer D, Smeltzer T, Honan D, Weinstein M, Menaged S. Removing the obstacles to accessing care. Briefing presented at: the House of Representatives; April 24 2001; Washington, D.C. http://www.eatingdisorderscoalition.org/congbriefings /042401/housebriefing042401.html#menaged. Accessed August 13, 2005.

98. Kater KJ, Rohwer J, Levine MP. An elementary school project for developing healthy body image and reducing risk factors for unhealthy and disordered eating. *J Treat Prev Eating Disord*. 2000(1);8:3–16.

99. Kostanski M, Gullone E. Dieting and body image in the child's world: conceptualization and behavior. *J Genet Psychol*. 1999; 160(4):488–499.

100. Smolack L, Levine MP. Adolescent transitions and the development of eating problems. In: Smolack L, Levine MP, Striegel-Moore R,

eds. *The Developmental Psychopathology of Eating Disorders*. Mahwah, NJ: Lawrence Erlbaum; 1996:207–234.

101. Thelen M, Powell A, Lawrence C, Kuhnert M. Eating and body image concerns among children. *J Clin Child Psychol*. 1992;21(1):41–46.

102. Patrick L. Eating disorders: a review of the literature with emphasis on medical complications and clinical nutrition. *Altern Med Rev*. 2002;7(3):184–202.

103. Bulik CM, Sullivan PF, Fear J, Pickering A. Predictors of the development of bulimia nervosa in women with anorexia nervosa. *J Nerv Ment Dis*. 1997;185(11):704–707.

104. Fairburn CG, Hay PJ, Welch SL. Binge eating and bulima nervosa: distribution and determinants. In: Fairburn CG, Wilson GT, eds. *Binge Eating: Nature, Assessment, and Treatment*. New York: Guilford; 1993:123–143.

105. Hoek HW. The distribution of eating disorders. In: Brownell KD, Fairburn CG, eds. *Eating Disorders and Obesity: A Comprehensive Handbook*. New York, NY: Guilford; 1995:207–211.

106. Lucas AR, Beard CM, O'Fallon WM, Kurland LT. 50-Year trends in the incidence of anorexia nervosa in Rochester, Minn.: a population-based study *Am J Psychiatry*. 1991;148(7):917–922.

107. Misra M, Aggarwal A, Miller KK, et al. Effects of anorexia nervosa on clinical, hematologic, biochemical, and bone density parameters in community-dwelling adolescent girls. *Pediatrics*. 2004;114(6): 1574–1583.

108. Sudi K, Ottl K, Payerl D, Baumgartl P, Tauschmann K, Muller W. Anorexia athletica. *Nutrition*. 2004;20(7–8):657–661.

109. DiGioacchino DeBate R, Wethington H, Sargent R. Sub-clinical eating disorder characteristics among male and female triathletes. *Eat Weight Disord*. 2002;7(3):210–220.

110. Smith NJ. Excessive weight loss and food aversion in athletes simulating anorexia nervosa. *Pediatrics*. 1980;66(1):139–142.

111. Sundgot-Borgen J. Prevalence of eating disorders in elite female athletes. *Int J Sport Nutr*. 1993;3(1):29–40.

112. Rumball JS, Lebrun CM. Preparticipation physical examination: selected issues for the female athlete. *Clin J Sport Med*. 2004;14(3): 153–160.

113. Johnson MD. Disordered eating in active and athletic women. *Clin Sports Med*. 1994;13(2):355–369.

114. Fulkerson JA, Keel PK, Leon GR, Dorr T. Eating-disordered behaviors and personality characteristics of high school athletes and nonathletes. *Int J Eat Disord*. 1999;26(1):73–79.

115. Hopkinson RA, Lock J. Athletics, perfectionism, and disordered eating. *Eat Weight Disord*. 2004;9(2):99–106.

116. Maron BJ, Pelliccia A. The heart of trained athletes: cardiac remodeling and the risks of sports, including sudden death. *Circulation*. 2006;114(15):1633–1644.

117. Hadigan CM, Anderson EJ, Miller KK, et al. Assessment of macronutrient and micronutrient intake in women with anorexia nervosa. *Int J Eat Disord*. 2000;28(3):284–292.

118. Sullivan P. Course and outcome of anorexia nervosa and bulimia nervosa. In: Fairburn CG, Brownell KD, eds. *Eating Disorders and Obesity*. New York, NY: Guilford; 2002:226–232.

119. Sullivan PF. Mortality in anorexia nervosa. *Am J Psychiatry*. 1995;152(7):1073–1074.

120. Garcia-Rubira JC, Hidalgo R, Gomez-Barrado JJ, Romero D, Cruz Fernandez JM. Anorexia nervosa and myocardial infarction. *Int J Cardiol*. 1994;45(2):138–140.

121. Isner JM, Roberts WC, Heymsfield SB, Yager J. Anorexia nervosa and sudden death. *Ann Intern Med*. 1985;102(1):49–52.

122. Joy E. Cardiac concerns. In: Ireland ML, Nattiv A, eds. *The Female Athlete*. Philadelphia, PA: WB Saunders; 2002:271–281.

123. Pomeroy C, Mitchell J. Medial issues in eating disorders. In: Brownell K, Rodin J, Wilmore JH, eds. *Eating, Body Weight, and Performance in Athletes*. Philadelphia, PA: Lea & Febiger; 1992:202–221.

124. de Simone G, Scalfi L, Galderisi M, et al. Cardiac abnormalities in young women with anorexia nervosa. *Br Heart J*. 1994;71(3):287–292.

125. Kreipe RE, Harris JP. Myocardial impairment resulting from eating disorders. *Pediatr Ann*. 1992;21(11):760–768.

126. Harris RT. Bulimarexia and related serious eating disorders with medical complications. *Ann Intern Med*. 1983;99(6):800–807.

127. Cooke RA, Chambers JB, Singh R, et al. QT interval in anorexia nervosa. *Br Heart J*. 1994;72(1):69–73.

128. Galetta F, Franzoni F, Cupisti A, Belliti D, Prattichizzo F, Rolla M. QT interval dispersion in young women with anorexia nervosa. *J Pediatr*. 2002;140(4):456–460.

129. Rich BS, Havens SA. The athletic heart syndrome. *Curr Sports Med Rep*. 2004;3(2):84–88.

130. Abdulla A. The athletic heart syndrome: when, why and how? *Perspect Cardiol*. 2005;22(10):29–31.

131. Bjornstad H, Storstein L, Dyre Meen H, Hals O. Electrocardiographic findings according to level of fitness and sport activity. *Cardiology*. 1993;83(1):268–279.

132. Apgar B. Diagnosis and management of amenorrhea. *Clin Fam Pract*. 2002;4(3):643.

133. Otis CL. Exercise-associated amenorrhea. *Clin Sports Med*. 1992; 11(2):351–362.

134. Shangold M, Rebar RW, Wentz AC, Schiff I. Evaluation and management of menstrual dysfunction in athletes. *JAMA*. 1990; 263(12):1665–1669.

135. Drinkwater BL, Nilson K, Chesnut CH III, Bremner WJ, Shainholtz S, Southworth MB. Bone mineral content of amenorrheic and eumenorrheic athletes. *N Engl J Med*. 1984;311(5):277–281.

136. Lindberg JS, Fears WB, Hunt MM, Powell MR, Boll D, Wade CE. Exercise-induced amenorrhea and bone density. *Ann Intern Med*. 1984;101(5):647–648.

137. Marcus R, Cann C, Madvig P, et al. Menstrual function and bone mass in elite women distance runners: endocrine and metabolic features. *Ann Intern Med*. 1985;102(2):158–163.

138. Nattiv A. Stress fractures and bone health in track and field athletes. *J Sci Med Sport*. 2000;3(3):268–279.

139. Nattiv A, Puffer JC, Casper J, et al. Stress fracture risk factors, incidence and distribution: a 3-year prospective study in collegiate runners. *Med Sci Sports Exerc*. 2000;32(suppl 5):S347.

140. Cullen D, Becker R, Thompson K, Ahif R. Calcium and vitamin D supplements reduce stress fractures in Navy recruits. Paper presented at: 53rd Annual Orthopaedic Research Society meeting; February 11, 2007; San Diego, CA.

141. Fisher M, Golden NH, Katzman DK, et al. Eating disorders in adolescents: a background paper. *J Adolesc Health*. 1995;16(6):420–437.

142. Sansone RA, Sansone LA. Bulimia nervosa: medical complications. In: Alexander-Mott L, Lumsden DB, eds. *Understanding Eating Disorders: Anorexia Nervosa, Bulimia Nervosa, and Obesity*. Washington, DC: Taylor & Francis; 1994:181–201.

143. Fairburn CG. *Overcoming Binge Eating*. New York, NY: Guilford; 1995:48–52.

144. Mcgilley BM, Pryor TL. Assessment and treatment of bulimia nervosa. *Am Fam Physician*. 1998;57(11):2743–2750.

145. Otis C, Goldingay R. *Campus Health Guide: The College Student's Handbook for Healthy Living*. New York, NY: College Board; 1989.

146. Rodriguez-Tome H, Bariaud F, Zardi MF, Delmas C, Jeanvoine B, Szylagyi P. The effects of pubertal changes on body image and relations with peers of the opposite sex in adolescence. *J Adolesc*. 1993;16(4):421–438.

147. Stice E. Risk and maintenance factors for eating pathology: a meta-analytic review. *Psychol Bull*. 2002;128(5):825–848.

148. Yates A. Biologic considerations in the etiology of eating disorders. *Pediatr Ann*. 1992;21(11):739–744.

149. Furnham A, Badmin N, Sneade I. Body image dissatisfaction: gender differences in eating attitudes, self-esteem, and reasons for exercise. *J Psychol*. 2002;136(6):581–596.

150. Presnell K, Bearman SK, Stice E. Risk factors for body dissatisfaction in adolescent boys and girls: a prospective study. *Int J Eat Disord*. 2004;36(4):389–401.

151. Watson D, Clark LA, Tellegen A. Development and validation of brief measures of positive and negative affect: the PANAS scales. *J Pers Soc Psychol*. 1988;54(6):1063–1070.

152. Cooper PJ. Eating disorders and their relationship to mood and anxiety disorders. In: Brownell KD, Fairburn CG, eds. *Eating Disorders and Obesity: A Comprehensive Handbook*. New York, NY: Guilford; 1995:159–164.

153. Johnson C, Maddi KL. The etiology of bulimia nervosa: biopsychosocial perspectives. *Adolesc Psychiatry*. 1986;13:253–273.

154. Chang EC. Perfectionism as a predictor of positive and negative psychological outcomes: examining a mediation model in younger and older adults. *J Couns Psychol*. 2000;47(1):18–26.

155. Halmi KA, Sunday SR, Strober M, et al. Perfectionism in anorexia nervosa: variation by clinical subtype, obsessionality, and pathological eating behavior. *Am J Psychiatry*. 2000;157(11): 1799–1805.

156. Brownell KD. Dieting and the search for the perfect body: where physiology and culture collide. *Behav Ther*. 1991(1) 22:1–12.

157. Killen JD, Taylor CB, Hayward C, et al. Pursuit of thinness and onset of eating disorder symptoms in a community sample of adolescent girls: a three-year prospective analysis. *Int J Eat Disord*. 1994;16(3):227–238.

158. Parks PS, Read MH. Adolescent male athletes: body image, diet, and exercise. *Adolescence*. 1997;32(127):593–602.

159. Kiningham RB, Gorenflo DW. Weight loss methods of high school wrestlers. *Med Sci Sports Exerc*. 2001;33(5):810–813.

160. Oppliger RA, Landry GL, Foster SW, Lambrecht AC. Bulimic behaviors among interscholastic wrestlers: a statewide survey. *Pediatrics*. 1993;91(4):826–831.

161. Andersen RE, Barlett SJ, Morgan GD, Brownell KD. Weight loss, psychological, and nutritional patterns in competitive male body builders. *Int J Eat Disord*. 1995;18(1):49–57.

162. Blouin AG, Goldfield GS. Body image and steroid use in male bodybuilders. *Int J Eat Disord*. 1995;18(2):159–165.

163. DePalma MT, Koszewski WM, Case JG, Barile RJ, DePalma BF, Oliaro SM. Weight control practices of lightweight football players. *Med Sci Sports Exerc*. 1993;25(6):694–701.

164. King MB, Mezey G. Eating behaviour of male racing jockeys. *Psychol Med*. 1987;17(1):249–253.

165. Rankinen T, Lyytikainen S, Vanninen E, Penttila I, Rauramaa R, Uusitupa M. Nutritional status of the Finnish elite ski jumpers. *Med Sci Sports Exerc*. 1998;30(11):1592–1597.

166. Yu L, Smith AD. Figure skating. In: Ireland ML, Nattiv A, eds. *The Female Athlete*. Philadelphia, PA: WB Saunders; 2002:653.

167. Malina RM. Performance in the context of growth and maturation. In: Ireland ML, Nattiv A, eds. *The Female Athlete*. Philadelphia, PA: WB Saunders; 2002:48–65.

168. Slaughter MH, Lohman TG, Misner JE. Relationship of somatotype and body composition to physical performance in 7- to 12-year-old boys. *Res Q*. 1977;48(4):159–168.

169. Slaughter MH, Lohman TG, Misner JE. Association of somatotype and body composition to physical performance in 7–12 year-old-girls. *J Sports Med Phys Fitness*. 1980;20(2):189–198.

170. Rodin J. *Body Traps: Breaking the Binds that Keep You from Feeling Good About Your Body*. New York, NY: William Morrow & Co; 1992:58–65.

171. Brownell KD, Steen SN, Wilmore JH. Weight regulation practices in athletes: analysis of metabolic and health effects. *Med Sci Sports Exerc*. 1987;19(6):546–556.

172. Wilmore JH, Wambsgans KC, Brenner M, et al. Is there energy conservation in amenorrheic compared with eumenorrheic distance runners? *J Appl Physiol*. 1992;72(1):15–22.

173. Centers for Disease Control and Prevention. Hyperthermia and dehydration-related death associated with intentional rapid weight loss in three collegiate wrestlers: North Carolina, Wisconsin, and Michigan, November-December 1997. *JAMA*. 1998;279(11):824–825.

174. Oppliger RA, Utter AC, Scott JR, Dick RW, Klossner D. NCAA rule change improves weight loss among national championship wrestlers. *Med Sci Sports Exerc*. 2006;38(5):963–970.

175. Sonstroem RJ. Physical self-concept: assessment and external validity. *Exerc Sport Sci Rev*. 1998;26(1):133–164.

176. Davis C, Kennedy SH, Ravelski E, Dionne M. The role of physical activity in the development and maintenance of eating disorders. *Psychol Med*. 1994;24(4):957–967.

177. Johnson C, Crosby R, Engel S, et al. Gender, ethnicity, self-esteem and disordered eating among college athletes. *Eat Behav*. 2004; 5(2):147–156.

178. Pasman L, Thompson JK. Body image and eating disturbance in obligatory runners, obligatory weightlifters and sedentary individuals. *Int J Eat Disord*. 1988;7(6):759–769.

179. Rodin J. Cultural and psychosocial determinants of weight concerns. *Ann Intern Med*. 1993;119(7 part 2):643–645.

180. Rucinski A. Relationship of body image and dietary intake of competitive ice skaters. *J Am Diet Assoc*. 1989;89(1):98–100.

181. Rodin J, Larson L. Social factors and the ideal body shape. In: Brownell KD, Rodin J, Wilmore JH, eds. *Eating, Body Weight, and Performance in Athletes: Disorders of Modern Society*. Philadelphia, PA: Lea & Febiger; 1992:146–158.

182. Sanborn CF, Horea M, Siemers BJ, Dieringer KI. Disordered eating and the female athlete triad. *Clin Sports Med*. 2000;19(2):199–213.

183. Williamson DA, Netemeyer RG, Jackman LP, Anderson DA, Funsch CL, Rabalais JY. Structural equation modeling of risk factors for the development of eating disorder symptoms in female athletes. *Int J Eat Disord*. 1995;17(4):387–393.

184. Fabian LJ, Thompson JK. Body image and eating disturbance in young females. *Int J Eat Disord*. 1989;8:63–74.

185. Faust J. Correlates of the drive for thinness in young female adolescents. *J Clin Child Psychol*. 1987;16:313–319.

186. Cattarin J, Thompson JK. A three year longitudinal study of body image and eating disturbance in adolescent females. *Eating Disord*. 1999;2:114–125.

187. Verkuyten M. Self-esteem and the evaluation of ethnic identity among Turkish and Dutch adolescents in the Netherlands. *J Soc Psychol*. 1990;130(3):285–297.

188. Rierdan J, Koff E, Stubbs ML. Gender, depression, and body image in early adolescents. *J Early Adolesc*. 1988;8:109–117.

189. Anderson A, DiDeomenico L. Diet vs. shape content of popular male and female magazines: a dose-response relationship to the incidence of eating disorders? *Int J Eat Disord*. 1992;11: 283–287.

190. Field AE, Camargo CA Jr, Taylor CB, Berkey CS, Roberts SB, Colditz GA. Peer, parent, and media influences on the development of weight concerns and frequent dieting among preadolescent and adolescent girls and boys. *Pediatrics*. 2001;107(1):54–60.

191. Morris AM, Katzman DK. The impact of the media on eating disorders in children and adolescents. *J Paediatr Child Health*. 2003;8:287–289.

192. Lerner RM, Gellert E. Body build identification, preference, and aversion in kindergarten children. *Dev Psychol*. 1969;5:456–462.

193. Thelen MH, Lawrence CM, Powell AL. Body image, weight control, and eating disorders among children. In: Crowther JH, Tennenbaum DL, Hobfoll SE, Stephens MAP, eds. *The Etiology of Bulimia Nervosa: The Individual and Familial Context*. Washington, DC: Hemisphere Publishing Corp; 1992:81–101.

194. Mendelson BK, White DR. Relation between body-esteem and self-esteem of obese and normal children. *Percept Mot Skills*. 1982;54(3):899–905.

195. Rolland K, Farnill D, Griffiths RA. Children's perceptions of their current and ideal body sizes and body mass index. *Percept Mot Skills*. 1996;82(2):651–656.

196. McCabe MP, Ricciardelli LA. Body image dissatisfaction among males across the lifespan: a review of past literature. *J Psychosom Res*. 2004;56(6):675–685.

197. Middleman AB, Vazquez I, Durant RH. Eating patterns, physical activity, and attempts to change weight among adolescents. *J Adolesc Health*. 1998;22(1):37–42.

198. *Eating Disorders: Core Interventions in the Treatment and Management of Anorexia Nervosa, Bulimia Nervosa, and Related Eating Disorders*. London, United Kingdom: National Institute for Clinical Excellence; 2004.

199. Becker AE, Franko DL, Nussbaum K, Herzog DB. Secondary prevention for eating disorders: the impact of education, screening, and referral in a college-based screening program. *Int J Eat Disord.* 2004;36(2):157–162.

200. De La Torre DM, Snell BJ. Use of the preparticipation physical exam in screening for the female athlete triad among high school athletes. *J Sch Nurs.* 2005;21(6):340–345.

201. Athletic preparticipation examinations for adolescents: report of the Board of Trustees. Group on Science and Technology, American Medical Association. *Arch Pediatr Adolesc Med.* 1994;148(1):93–98.

202. Nichols JF, Rauh MJ, Lawson MJ, Ji M, Barkai HS. Prevalence of the female athlete triad syndrome among high school athletes. *Arch Pediatr Adolesc Med.* 2006;160(2):137–142.

203. Kashubeck-West S, Mintz LB, Saundersm KJ. Assessment of eating disorders in women. *Counsel Psychol.* 2002;29:662–694.

204. Lindeman AK. Self-esteem: its application to eating disorders and athletes. *Int J Sport Nutr.* 1994;4(3):237–252.

205. O'Connor PJ, Lewis RD, Kirchner EM. Eating disorder symptoms in female college gymnasts. *Med Sci Sports Exerc.* 1995;27(4):550–555.

206. Rosen LW, Hough DO. Pathogenic weight-control behaviors female college gymnasts. *Physician Sportsmed.* 1988;16(9):141–144.

207. Sundgot-Borgen J. Nutrient intake of female elite athletes suffering from eating disorders. *Int J Sport Nutr.* 1993;3(4):431–442.

208. Parr RB, Porter MA, Hodgson SC. Nutrient knowledge and practice of coaches, trainers, and athletes. *Physician Sportsmed.* 1984;12(3):127–138.

209. Modlesky CM, Lewis RD. Assessment of body size and composition. In: Rosenbloom CA, ed. *Sports Nutrition: A Guide for the Professional Working with Active People.* Chicago, IL: The American Dietetic Association; 2000:185–222.

210. Skinner R, Grooms A. Body composition assessment: a tool for use not abuse. *SCAN's PULSE.* 2002;21:9–11.

211. Carson JD, Bridges E, Canadian Academy of Sport Medicine. Abandoning routine body composition assessment: a strategy to reduce disordered eating among female athletes and dancers. *Clin J Sport Med.* 2001;11(4):280.

212. Goran MI, Allison DB, Poehlman ET. Issues relating to normalization of body fat content in men and women. *Int J Obes Relat Metab Disord.* 1995;19(9):638–643.

213. Wellens RI, Roche AF, Khamis HJ, Jackson AS, Pollock ML, Siervogel RM. Relationships between the body mass index and body composition. *Obes Res.* 1996;4(1):35–44.

214. Maynard LM, Wisemandle W, Roche AF, Chumlea WC, Guo SS, Siervogel RM. Childhood body composition in relation to body mass index. *Pediatrics.* 2001;107(2):344–350.

215. Pietrobelli A, Faith MS, Allison DB, Gallagher D, Chiumello G, Heymsfield SB. Body mass index as a measure of adiposity among children and adolescents: a validation study. *J Pediatr.* 1998;132(2):204–210.

216. Malina RM, Katzmarzyk PT. Validity of the body mass index as an indicator of the risk and presence of overweight in adolescents. *Am J Clin Nutr.* 1999;70(1):131S–136S.

217. Ode J, Pivarnik JM, Reeves MJ, Knous JL. Body mass index as a predictor of percent fat in college athletes and nonathletes. *Med Sci Sports Exerc.* 2007;39(3):403–409.

218. Wilmore JH. Body composition and sports medicine: research considerations. In: Roche AF, ed. *Body Composition Assessments in Youth and Adults.* Columbus, OH: Ross Laboratories; 1985:78–82.

219. Sinning WE. Body composition in athletes. In: Roche AF, Heymsfield SB, Lohman TG, eds. *Human Body Composition.* Champaign, IL: Human Kinetics; 1996:257–273.

220. Crisp AH, Burns T, Bhat AV. Primary anorexia nervosa in the male and female: a comparison of clinical features and prognosis. *Br J Med Psychol.* 1986;59(part 2):123–132.

221. Geist R, Heinmaa M, Katzman D, Stephens D. A comparison of male and female adolescents referred to an eating disorder program. *Can J Psychiatry.* 1999;44(4):374–378.

222. Garner DM, Rosen LW, Barry D. Eating disorders among athletes: research and recommendations. *Child Adolesc Psychiatr Clin N Am.* 1998;7(4):839–857.

223. American Diabetes Association. Standards of medical care for patients with diabetes mellitus. *Diabetes Care.* 2003;26(suppl 1):S33–S50.

224. Manore M, Thompson J. Nutrition and the active female. *Sport Nutrition for Health and Performance.* Champaign, IL: Human Kinetics; 2000:409–435.

225. Position of the American Dietetic Association. Nutrition intervention in the treatment of anorexia nervosa, bulimia nervosa, and eating disorders not otherwise specified (EDNOS). *J Am Diet Assoc.* 2001;101(7):810–819.

226. Bergandi T, Witting A. Availability of and attitudes toward counseling services for the collegiate athlete. *J Coll Stud Personnel.* 1984;25:557–558.

227. Linder DE, Brewer BW, Van Raalte JL, DeLange N. A negative halo for athletes who consult sport psychologists: replication and extension. *J Sport Exerc Psychol.* 1991;13(2):133–148.

228. Pinkerton RS, Hinz LD, Barrow JC. The college student-athlete: psychological considerations and interventions. *J Am Coll Health.* 1989;37(5):218–226.

229. Sim LA, Sadowski CM, Whiteside SP, Wells LA. Family-based therapy for adolescents with anorexia nervosa. *Mayo Clin Proc.* 2004;79(10):1305–1308.

230. Andersen MB, Denson EL, Brewer BW, Van Raalte JL. Disorders of personality and mood in athletes: recognition and referral. *J Appl Sport Psychol.* 1994;6(2):168–184.

231. Muscari M. Effective management of adolescents with anorexia and bulimia. *J Psychosoc Nurs Ment Health Serv.* 2002;40(2):22–31.

232. Bickford B. The legal duty of a college athletics department to athletes with eating disorder: a risk management perspective. *Marquette Sports Law Rev.* 1999;10(1):87–116.

233. National Athletic Trainers' Association. Code of ethics. http://www.nata.org/codeofethics/index.htm. Accessed November 14, 2005.

234. Clark N. How to help the athlete with bulimia: practical tips and a case study. *Int J Sport Nutr.* 1993;3(4):450–460.

235. Bates CR. Information systems security and privacy: regulatory and contractual privacy and security compliance obligations, resources, and insurance information. In: The wired university: legal issues at the copyright, computer law and Internet intersection. National Association of College and University Attorneys: Arlington, VA. http://www.nacua.org/meetings/virtualseminars/march2006/Documents/03%20Bates.doc. Accessed October 9, 2006.

236. Sherman R, Thompson R. *Managing the Female Athlete Triad: NCAA Coaches Handbook.* Indianapolis, IN: National Collegiate Athletic Association; 2005:21–26.

237. The National Athletic Trainers' Association support statement: recommendations and guidelines for appropriate medical coverage of intercollegiate athletics (AMCIA). http://www.NATA.org/employers/ss/AMCIARecs%20andguidesrevised.pdf. Accessed October 31, 2005.

238. The National Collegiate Athletic Association. Sports medicine handbook, 2005–2006. http://www.ncaa.org/health-safety. Accessed November 4, 2005.

239. Baer JT, Walker WF, Grossman JM. A disordered eating response team's effect on nutrition practices in college athletes. *J Athl Train.* 1995;30(4):315–317.

240. Sundgot-Borgen J. Eating disorders in female athletes. *Sports Med.* 1994;17(3):176–188.

241. Turk JC, Prentice WE, Chapell S, Shields EW. Collegiate coaches' knowledge of eating disorders. *J Athl Train.* 1999;34(1):19–24.

242. Yeager KK, Agostini R, Nattiv A, Drinkwater B. The female athlete triad: disordered eating, amenorrhea, osteoporosis. *Med Sci Sports Exerc.* 1993;25(7):775–777.

243. De La Torre DM, Snell BJ. Use of the preparticipation physical exam in screening for the female athlete triad among high school athletes. *J Sch Nurs.* 2005;21(6):340–345.

244. Dick RW. Eating disorders in NCAA athletic programs: Replication study of a 1990 study. *NCAA Sport Sciences Education Newsletter.* April 1993(suppl 1):3,4.

245. Sundgot-Borgen J, Klungland M. The female athlete triad and the effect of preventative work. *Med Sci Sports Exerc.* 1998;30(suppl 5):S181.

246. The National Wrestling Coaches Association. Optimal performance calculator. http://www.nwcaonline.com. Accessed November 4, 2005.

247. Elliot DL, Goldberg L, Moe EL, DeFrancesco CA, Durham MB, Hix-Small H. Preventing substance use and disordered eating: initial outcomes of the ATHENA (Athletes Targeting Healthy Exercise and Nutrition Alternatives) program. *Arch Pediatr Adolesc Med.* 2004;158(11):1043–1049.

248. Martin M, Schlabach G, Shibinski K. The use of nonprescription weight loss products among female basketball, softball, and volleyball athletes from NCAA Division I institutions: issues and concerns. *J Athl Train.* 1998;33(1):41–44.

249. National Collegiate Athletic Association. Nutrition and performance. http://www1.ncaa.org/membership/ed_outreach/nutrition-performance/index.html. Accessed December 9, 2005.

250. Sports, Cardiovascular and Wellness Nutritionists (SCAN). www.scandpg.org. Accessed December 9, 2005.

251. Boyles S. Internet: a refuge for those with eating disorders. WebMD Medical News. http://www.webmd.com/content/article/34/1728_85382.htm. Accessed March, 2002.

252. Head J. Seeking 'thinspiration.' http://news.bbc.co.uk/go/pr/fr/-/2/hi/uk_news/magazine/6935768.stm. Accessed August 10, 2007.

253. Houtkooper LB. Exercise and eating disorders. In: Lamb DR, Murray R, eds. *Perspectives in Exercise Science and Sports Medicine.* Carmel, IN: Cooper Publishing Group; 1998:151–197.

254. Grandjean AC. Diets of elite athletes: has the discipline of sports nutrition made an impact? *J Nutr.* 1997;127(suppl 5):874S–877S.

255. Werblow JA, Fox HM, Henneman A. Nutritional knowledge, attitudes, and food patterns of women athletes. *J Am Diet Assoc.* 1978;73(3):242–245.

256. Wiita BG, Stombaugh IA. Nutrition knowledge, eating practices, and health of adolescent female runners: a 3-year longitudinal study. *Int J Sport Nutr.* 1996;6(4):414–425.

257. Cole CR, Salvaterra GF, Davis JE Jr, et al. Evaluation of dietary practices of National Collegiate Athletic Association Division I football players. *J Strength Cond Res.* 2005;19(3):490–494.

258. Jacobson BH, Gemmell HA. Nutrition information sources of college varsity athletes. *J Appl Sport Sci Res.* 1991;5(4):204–207.

259. Jonnalagadda SS, Rosenbloom CA, Skinner R. Dietary practices, attitudes, and physiological status of collegiate freshman football players. *J Strength Cond Res.* 2001;15(4):507–513.

260. McMurray RG. Laboratory methods for determining energy expenditure of athletes. In: Driskell JA, Wolinsky I, eds. *Nutritional Assessment of Athletes.* Boca Raton, FL: CRC Press; 2002:203–224.

261. Beals KA, Manore MM. Nutritional status of female athletes with subclinical eating disorders. *J Am Diet Assoc.* 1998;98(4):419–425.

262. Rosenvinge JH, Gresko RB. Do we need a prevention model for eating disorders? Recent developments in the Norwegian school-based prevention model. *Eat Disord J Treatm Prevent.* 1997;5(2):110–118.

263. Killen JD. Development and evaluation of a school-based eating disorder symptoms prevention program. In: Smolak L, Levine MP, Striegel-Moore RH, eds. *The Developmental Psychopathology of Eating Disorders: Implications of Research, Prevention, and Treatment.* Mahwah, NJ: Lawrence Erlbaum Assoc; 1996:313–339.

264. Clark M. Who's coaching the coaches? In: Gerdy J, ed. *Sports in School: The Future of an Institution.* New York, NY: Teachers College Press; 2000:55–61.

265. Stapleton KL, Tomlinson CM, Shepard KF, Coon VA. High school coaches' perceptions of their responsibilities in managing their athletes' injuries. *J Orthop Sports Phys Ther.* 1984;5:253–260.

266. Vergeer I, Hogg JM. Coaches' decision policies about the participation of injured athletes in competition. *Sport Psychol.* 1990;13(1):42–56.

267. Stewart CC, Sweet L. Professional preparation of high school coaches: the problem continues. *J Phys Educ Recr Dance.* 1992;63(6):75–79.

268. Knorr J. The need to rethink coaching certification. *Scholastic Coach Athl Director.* 1996;65(1):4–6.

269. Mills BD, Dunleavy SM. Coaching certification: what's out there and what needs to be done? *Int J Phys Educ.* 1997;34(1):17–26.

270. Harris MB, Greco DO. Weight control and weight concern in competitive female gymnasts. *J Sport Exerc Psychol.* 1990;12(4):427–433.

271. Gill DL. Psychological, sociological and cultural issues concerning the athletic female. In: Pearl AJ, ed. *The Athletic Female.* Champaign, IL: Human Kinetics; 1993:19–40.

272. National Athletic Trainers' Association. *Athletic Training Educational Competencies.* Dallas, TX: National Athletic Trainers' Association; 2006.

273. Vaughan JL, King KA, Cottrell RR. Collegiate athletic trainers' confidence in helping female athletes with eating disorders. *J Athl Train.* 2004;39(1):71–76.

Christine M. Bonci, MS, ATC; Leslie J. Bonci, MPH, RD; Lorita Granger, ATC; Craig Johnson, PhD; Robert M. Malina, PhD, FACSM; Leslie W. Milne, MD; Randa R. Ryan, PhD; and Erin Vanderbunt, MS, ATC, contributed to conception and design; acquisition and analysis and interpretation of the data; and drafting, critical revision, and final approval of the article.

Disordered Eating Review Questions:

1. What are the possible behaviors included under the term *disordered eating?*
2. This position statement lists seven immediate action items that can serve as the first steps to building the infrastructure required for developing a comprehensive program to work with athletes who present with disordered eating or who may be at risk. After reviewing these seven items, determine those actions your institution or place of employment has already taken and those yet to be taken. Explain the roadblocks athletic trainers may encounter in the process of taking each of these seven actions and possible means of overcoming these potential roadblocks.
3. Explain the potential roles of the athletic trainer in managing athletes with disordered eating. How might these roles change based on the athletic trainer's employment setting? For example, an athletic trainer who is employed as the sole athletic trainer at a very large high school as compared to an athletic trainer employed by a professional sports team.

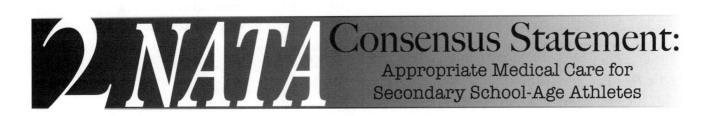

2 NATA Consensus Statement:
Appropriate Medical Care for
Secondary School-Age Athletes

In This Section: The following consensus statement gives guidelines on the proper
medical care for athletes in a secondary school setting.

Consensus Statement *NATA*

Appropriate Medical Care for Secondary School-Age Athletes

MISSION STATEMENT

Establish recommendations for the prevention, care and appropriate management of athletic-related injury and illness specific to the secondary school-age individual.

CONSENSUS STATEMENT

Athletic Health Care Team

The athletic health care team may be comprised of appropriate health care professionals in consultation with administrators, coaches, parents and participants. Appropriate health care professionals could be: certified athletic trainers, team physicians, consulting physicians, school nurses, physical therapists, emergency medical services (EMS) personnel, dentists and other allied health care professionals.

Recommendations for Appropriate Medical Care

Appropriate medical care of the secondary school-age individual involves more than basic emergency care during s ports participation. It encompasses the provision of many other health care services. While emergency medical care and event coverage are critical, appropriate medical care also includes activities of ongoing daily athletic health care.

Education

Designated athletic health care providers shall maintain expertise through continuing education and professional development.

All coaches should be trained in first aid, CPR and AED, utilization of athletic health care team professionals, injury prevention and modification of training in response to injury and illness.

The athletic health care team should have a designated athletic health care provider(s) who is educated and qualified to:

1. Determine the individual's readiness to participate.
2. Promote safe and appropriate practice, competition and treatment facilities.
3. Advise on the selection, fit, function and maintenance of athletic equipment.
4. Develop and implement a comprehensive emergency action plan.
5. Establish protocols regarding environmental conditions.
6. Develop injury and illness prevention strategies.
7. Provide for on-site recognition, evaluation and immediate treatment of injury and illness, with appropriate referrals.
8. Facilitate rehabilitation and reconditioning.
9. Provide for psychosocial consultation and referral.
10. Provide scientifically sound nutritional counseling and education.
11. Participate in the development and implementation of a comprehensive athletic health care administrative system (e.g. personal health information, policies, procedures, insurance, referrals).

The provision of appropriate medical care should be based on local needs and resources, with consideration of available personnel, state and local statutes, risk and type of activity.

Certified Athletic Trainer: An allied health professional who, upon graduation from an accredited college or university, and after successfully passing the NATABOC certification exam, is qualified and appropriately credentialed according to state regulations to work with individuals engaged in physical activity in the prevention of injuries and illnesses, the recognition, evaluation and immediate care of injuries and illnesses, the rehabilitation and reconditioning of injuries and illnesses and the administration of this health care system. This individual must have current certification in CPR and be qualified in first aid and blood borne pathogens. Other health care professionals with equivalent certification and/or licensure would also meet this standard.

Team Physician: The team physician must have an unrestricted medical license and be an MD or a DO who is responsible for treating and coordinating the medical care of athletic team members. The principal responsibility of the team physician is to provide for the well-being of individual athletes, enabling each to realize his or her full potential. The team physician should possess special proficiency in the care of musculoskeletal injuries and medical conditions encountered in sports. The team physician also must actively integrate medical expertise with other health care providers, including medical specialists, athletic trainers and allied health professionals. The team physician must ultimately assume responsibility within the team structure for making medical decisions that affect the athlete's safe participation.

PARTICIPANTS

CHAIR
Jon Almquist, ATC (NATA)

American Academy of Family Physicians
Robert Pallay, MD

American Academy of Orthopaedic Surgeons
Clarence Shields, Jr., MD

American Academy of Pediatrics
Keith Loud, MD, FAAP

American Medical Society for Sports Medicine
Dave Jenkinson, DO

American Orthopaedic Society for Sports Medicine
Robert Hunter, MD

American Osteopathic Academy of Sports Medicine
Angela Cavanna, DO
Michele Gilsenan, DO, FAOASM

American Physical Therapy Association
Erin Barill, PT, ATC

American Public Health Association
Andrew Lincoln, ScD, MS

Emergency Medical Services
Robb Rehberg, MS, ATC, NREMT

International Academy for Sports Dentistry
Leslie Rye, DDS

National Association of School Nurses

Elizabeth Mattey, MSN, RN, NCSN

National Association of Secondary School Principals
David Vodila

National Athletic Trainers' Association
Glenn Beachy, MS, ATC
Lorrie Howe, ATC, CAA
Roger Kalisiak, MS, ATC
Bart Peterson, MS, ATC
Craig Portwood, ATC
John Reynolds, MS, ATC
Brian Robinson, MS, ATC
Sandra Shultz, PhD, ATC, CSCS
Tom Woods, LAT, ATC

National Federation of State High School Associations
Jerry Diehl

National Interscholastic Athletic Administrators' Association
Alan Mallanda

National Safety Council
Barbara Caracci, MS

The President's Council on Physical Fitness and Sports
Christine G. Spain, MA

ADVISORY MEMBERS
Glen Cooper, ATC (NATA)
Perry Denehy, MEd, ATC, EMT-I (NATA)
Tony Fitzpatrick, MA, ATC (NATA)

NATA BOARD OF DIRECTORS LIAISON
Joe Iezzi, ATC

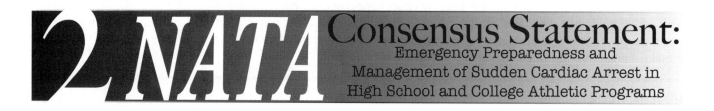

2 NATA Consensus Statement:
Emergency Preparedness and Management of Sudden Cardiac Arrest in High School and College Athletic Programs

In This Section: The following statement explains sudden cardiac arrest (SCA) and details how athletic trainers should prepare for and respond to an SCA situation. Included is background information as well as survival factors and guidelines for an SCA emergency action plan.

Consensus Statement *NATA*

Sudden Cardiac Arrest and Emergency Planning

Introduction

Sudden cardiac arrest (SCA) is the leading cause of death in young athletes.[1,2] Athletes are considered the healthiest members of our society, and their unexpected death during training or competition is a catastrophic event that stimulates debate regarding both pre-participation screening evaluations and appropriate emergency planning for athletic events.

Despite pre-participation screening, healthy-appearing competitive athletes may harbor unsuspected cardiovascular diseases with the potential to cause sudden death.[3] With the increasing availability of automated external defibrillators (AEDs) at athletic events, there is potential for effective secondary prevention of sudden cardiac death (SCD). The presence and timely access of AEDs at sporting venues provide a means of early defibrillation not only for athletes but also for spectators, coaches, officials, event staff, and other attendees on campus in the case of an unexpected SCA.

Many health-related organizations have guidelines for managing SCA during athletic practices and competitions. However, these guidelines have not directly linked emergency planning and SCA management in athletics. The National Athletic Trainers' Association (NATA) convened an Inter Association Task Force in Atlanta, Georgia, on April 24, 2006, to develop consensus recommendations on emergency preparedness and management of SCA in high school and college athletic programs.

The task force included representatives from 15 national organizations with special interest in SCA in young athletes and a multidisciplinary group of health care professionals from athletic training, cardiology, electrophysiology, emergency medicine, emergency medical technicians, family medicine, orthopaedics, paramedics, pediatrics, physical therapy, and sports medicine (Appendix).

The goal of this statement is to assist those in high school and college athletic programs to prepare for and respond to an unexpected SCA by summarizing the essential elements of SCA in young athletes and outlining the necessary elements for emergency preparedness and standardized treatment protocols in the management of SCA. Management guidelines are focused on basic life support measures for SCA that can be provided by both bystanders and health care professionals before the arrival of emergency medical services (EMS) personnel.

All recommendations in this statement are in agreement with the 2005 American Heart Association (AHA) guidelines for cardiopulmonary resuscitation (CPR) and emergency cardiovascular care (ECC),[4] the AHA scientific statement on response to cardiac arrest and selected life-threatening medical emergencies and the medical emergency response plan for schools,[5] and the NATA position statement on emergency planning in athletics.[6] Recommendations are directed toward the athletic health care team, including athletic trainers, team physicians, coaches, school administrators, and other potential first responders. This statement is intended for high school and college athletic programs and institutions, although the recommendations may be applicable in other settings.

BACKGROUND
Causes of Sudden Cardiac Death in Young Athletes

The underlying cardiac anomaly in young athletes with SCD is usually a structural cardiac abnormality. Hypertrophic cardiomyopathy and coronary artery anomalies represent approximately 25% and 14% of cases, respectively, in the United States.[1]

Commotio cordis is caused by a blunt, nonpenetrating blow to the chest that induces a ventricular arrhythmia in an otherwise

151

structurally normal heart and accounts for approximately 20% of SCD in young athletes.[1] A variety of other structural cardiac anomalies account for most of the remaining causes of SCD in athletes. These include conditions such as myocarditis, arrhythmogenic right ventricular dysplasia, Marfan syndrome, valvular heart disease, dilated cardiomyopathy, and atherosclerotic coronary artery disease. In about 2% of sudden deaths in young athletes, postmortem examination fails to identify a structural cardiac cause of death.[1,9,10] These deaths may be due to inherited arrhythmia syndromes and ion channel disorders such as long QT or short QT syndrome, Brugada syndrome, or familial catecholaminergic polymorphic ventricular tachycardia (VT).

Vigorous exercise appears to be a trigger for lethal arrhythmias in athletes with occult heart disease.[1] Authors of the best available studies estimate the incidence of SCD in high school athletes to be 1:100 000 to 1:200 000.[2,3] The estimated incidence of SCD in college-aged athletes is slightly higher, ranging from 1:65,000 to 1:69,000.[2,11] However, with no mandatory national reporting or surveillance system, the true incidence of SCA/SCD in athletes is unknown, and prior reports may have underestimated the actual occurrence of SCA/SCD in young athletes. More recently, Maron et al[12] reported on the frequency of sudden death in young competitive athletes and documented approximately 110 deaths per year, or about 1 death every 3 days in the United States.

Limitations of Cardiovascular Screening

A comprehensive discussion of pre-participation cardiovascular screening in athletes is beyond the scope of this task force. However, recognizing the limitations of current pre-participation screening strategies in detecting potentially lethal cardiac abnormalities in young athletes is critical to understanding the need for emergency preparedness and management protocols to prevent SCD.

Healthy-appearing athletes may harbor unsuspected cardiovascular disease with the potential to cause SCD.[3] In approximately 55% to 80% of cases of SCD, the athlete is asymptomatic until the cardiac arrest, with death representing the sentinel event of otherwise silent cardiovascular disease.[3,13] The task force supports the AHA recommendations

for cardiovascular screening in athletes,[14] as well as the use of a standardized questionnaire to guide examiners, such as the widely accepted monograph Pre-participation Physical Evaluation, 3rd edition.[15]

At this time, cardiovascular screening of asymptomatic athletes with electrocardiography or echocardiography is not recommended by the AHA in the United States because of the poor sensitivity, high false-positive rate, poor cost-effectiveness, and total cost of implementation.[14,16] Detection of premonitory cardiovascular symptoms such as a history of exertional syncope or chest pain should be improved by the use of standardized history forms and requires a careful and thorough cardiovascular evaluation to exclude underlying heart disease. Improved education for athletes, coaches, and health care professionals is needed regarding symptoms that may precede SCA.

Resuscitation Pathophysiology

About 40% of out-of-hospital cardiac arrest victims demonstrate ventricular fibrillation (VF) on first rhythm analysis.[17]

Ventricular fibrillation is characterized by chaotic rapid depolarizations and repolarizations, which cause the heart muscle to quiver and lose its ability to pump blood effectively. It is likely that a larger percentage of victims has VF or rapid VT at the time of collapse, but the rhythm has already deteriorated to asystole before the first rhythm analysis. The probability of successful defibrillation for VF SCA diminishes rapidly over time, with survival rates declining 7% to 10% per minute for every minute that defibrillation is delayed.[18,19] Defibrillation through deployment of electric energy terminates VF and allows the normal cardiac pacemakers to resume firing and produce an effective rhythm if the heart tissue is still viable. Survival after SCA is unlikely once VF has deteriorated to asystole.

Cardiopulmonary resuscitation is important both before and after defibrillation; it provides a small but critical amount of blood flow to the heart and brain and increases the likelihood that defibrillation will restore a normal rhythm in time to prevent neurologic damage. Chest compressions create blood flow by increasing intrathoracic pressure and directly compressing the heart. When bystander CPR is initiated, survival declines only 3% to 4% per minute for every minute defibrillation is delayed.[18,20] Thus, CPR can greatly improve survival from witnessed

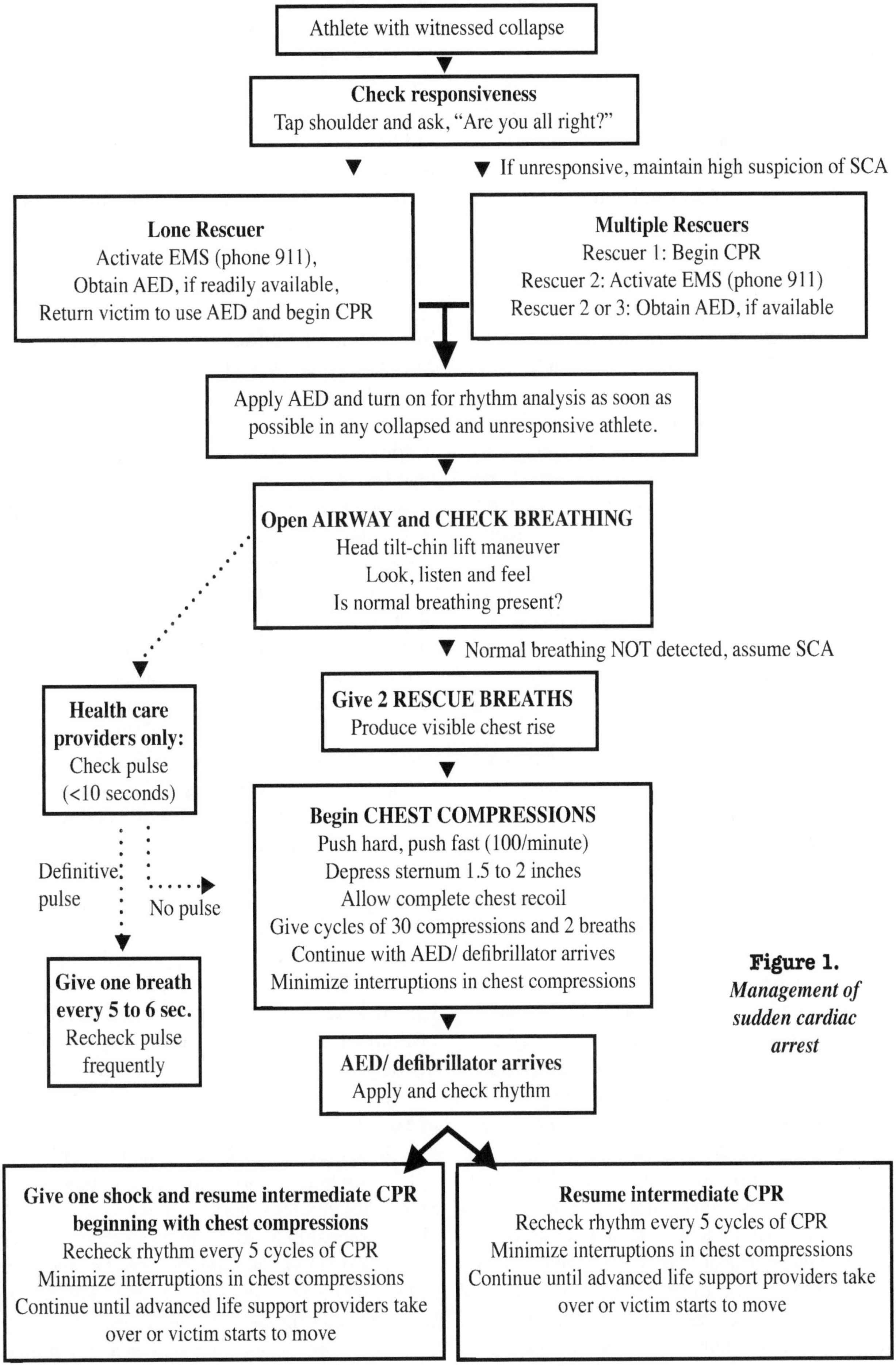

Athlete with witnessed collapse

Check responsiveness
Tap shoulder and ask, "Are you all right?"

▼ If unresponsive, maintain high suspicion of SCA

Lone Rescuer
Activate EMS (phone 911),
Obtain AED, if readily available,
Return victim to use AED and begin CPR

Multiple Rescuers
Rescuer 1: Begin CPR
Rescuer 2: Activate EMS (phone 911)
Rescuer 2 or 3: Obtain AED, if available

Apply AED and turn on for rhythm analysis as soon as possible in any collapsed and unresponsive athlete.

Open AIRWAY and CHECK BREATHING
Head tilt-chin lift maneuver
Look, listen and feel
Is normal breathing present?

▼ Normal breathing NOT detected, assume SCA

Health care providers only:
Check pulse
(<10 seconds)

Definitive pulse   No pulse

Give 2 RESCUE BREATHS
Produce visible chest rise

Begin CHEST COMPRESSIONS
Push hard, push fast (100/minute)
Depress sternum 1.5 to 2 inches
Allow complete chest recoil
Give cycles of 30 compressions and 2 breaths
Continue with AED/ defibrillator arrives
Minimize interruptions in chest compressions

Give one breath every 5 to 6 sec.
Recheck pulse frequently

Figure 1.
Management of sudden cardiac arrest

AED/ defibrillator arrives
Apply and check rhythm

Give one shock and resume intermediate CPR beginning with chest compressions
Recheck rhythm every 5 cycles of CPR
Minimize interruptions in chest compressions
Continue until advanced life support providers take over or victim starts to move

Resume intermediate CPR
Recheck rhythm every 5 cycles of CPR
Minimize interruptions in chest compressions
Continue until advanced life support providers take over or victim starts to move

SCA for any given time interval to defibrillation.

Resuming CPR immediately after shock delivery is also critical. Many victims are in pulseless electric activity or asystole for several minutes after defibrillation, and CPR is needed to provide perfusion.[21-23] Unfortunately, bystander CPR is initiated in less than one third of cases of witnessed SCA,[24,25] and, if initiated, more than 40% of chest compressions are of insufficient quality.[26] These deficiencies illustrate the tremendous need for increased public education and training in CPR.

Automated external defibrillators are computerized devices that analyze a victim's rhythm, determine if a shock is needed, charge to an appropriate shock dose, and use audio and visual instructions to guide the rescuer. These devices are easy to use and extremely accurate in recommending a shock only when VF or rapid VT is present.[27] In one study, AEDs were safely and successfully operated by untrained sixth graders almost as quickly as trained paramedics in a simulated resuscitation, with only a 23-second difference in mean time to defibrillation.

Weisfeldt and Becker[29] described a 3-phase model of resuscitation to account for the changes in cardiac arrest pathophysiology that occur with time. The model emphasizes phase-specific treatments based on the time interval from collapse and includes the following: (1) the electric phase, which extends from the time of cardiac arrest to approximately four minutes after cardiac arrest; (2) the circulatory phase, from approximately four minutes to 10 minutes after cardiac arrest; and (3) the metabolic phase, extending beyond 10 minutes from cardiac arrest.[29] The most critical intervention during the electric phase is early defibrillation, and CPR should be provided until an AED or a manual defibrillator is available.

After 4 to 5 minutes of untreated VF (circulatory phase), some authors suggest that outcomes may be better if shock delivery is preceded by a brief period of CPR to deliver blood to the heart and brain. In animals, outcomes improved for prolonged untreated VF when CPR was initiated before defibrillation compared with immediate defibrillation.[30,31] In some clinical studies,[32,33] survival was improved when CPR was initiated before defibrillation in cases of untreated VF lasting longer than 3 to 5 minutes. Thus, as the duration of cardiac arrest increases, initial chest compressions and oxygen delivery to vital tissues may take priority over defibrillation in some patients, with delay of shock delivery until 1 to 2 minutes of CPR has been completed.[29,32,33]

After approximately 10 minutes of cardiac arrest (metabolic phase), additional tissue injury can occur from global ischemia and with resumption of blood flow from reperfusion injury. Cellular protection from reperfusion injury may be augmented by hypothermia-mediated therapies to attenuate the rapid oxidant burst caused by restoring oxygen and substrates to ischemic tissues, although these therapies are not widely available.

Survival after Sudden Cardiac Arrest

The single greatest factor affecting survival after out-of-hospital cardiac arrest is the time interval from arrest to defibrillation.[19] Survival after out-of-hospital cardiac arrest has been greatly improved by lay rescuer and public access defibrillation programs designed to shorten the time interval from SCA to shock delivery. These programs train lay rescuers and first responders in CPR and AED use and place AEDs in high-risk public locations for SCA. Studies of rapid defibrillation using AEDs with nontraditional first responders and trained or untrained laypersons in high-risk locations such as casinos, airlines, and airports have demonstrated survival rates from 41% to 74% if bystander CPR is provided and defibrillation occurs within 3 to 5 minutes of collapse.[11,35-43] Key elements to the success of these programs include training of motivated responders in CPR and AED use, a structured and practiced response, and short response times.

Although SCA is a rare but catastrophic event in young athletes, it is more common in an older population, with an estimated annual frequency of 1 in 1000 persons aged 35 years or older in the United States.[19] The presence of AEDs in schools and institutions provides a means of early defibrillation, not only for young athletes but also for other individuals on campus who may experience an unexpected cardiac arrest.

Jones et al[44] found a 2.1% annual probability of SCA on high school campuses, mainly due to SCA among older school employees, spectators, and visitors on campus. At National Collegiate Athletic Association Division I universities, Drezner et al[11] found that older nonstudents, such as spectators, coaches, and officials, accounted for 77% of SCA cases at collegiate sporting venues and that placement of AEDs at these venues provided a significant survival benefit for older nonstudents, with a 54% overall immediate resuscitation rate.

Limited research is available regarding the survival rate in young athletes after SCA. Initially, authors[11,45] investigating AED use in the college athletic setting did not identify a survival benefit in a small number of collegiate athletes with SCA. Drezner and Rogers[46] later investigated the timing and details of resuscitation in 9 collegiate athletes with SCA. All athletes had a witnessed arrest, and most received immediate assessment by an athletic trainer skilled in basic life support and CPR. Seven athletes received defibrillation, with an average time from cardiac arrest to defibrillation of 3.1 minutes. Despite a witnessed collapse, timely CPR, and prompt defibrillation in most cases, only 1 of 9 (11%) athletes in this cohort survived—an unexpected finding given the young age, otherwise good health and physical conditioning of the athletes, and early reported defibrillation.[46]

Other groups[47,48] have also found the survival rate after SCA in young athletes to be lower than expected. Maron et al[47] analyzed 128 cases from the United States Commotio Cordis Registry and found an overall survival rate of 16%. Cardiopulmonary resuscitation was performed in 106 cases and defibrillation in 41 cases, with 19 of 41 (46%) of the individuals who received defibrillation surviving. Successful resuscitations using AEDs have been reported in the public media and in case reports[49,50] and demonstrate the lifesaving potential of public access defibrillation on the athletic field. Overall, the available studies on SCA in young athletes raise concern regarding the low survival rate and highlight the need for improved and more uniform resuscitation strategies for SCA in young athletes.

Factors Affecting Survival in Young Athletes
Several factors may contribute to a lower resuscitation rate in young athletes. Structural heart disease is consistently found in most cases of SCD in young athletes. Ventricular arrhythmias in the presence of structural heart disease, especially cardiomyopathies, may be more resistant to even short delays in defibrillation than SCA in the setting of a structurally normal heart. Berger et al[51] documented 18 episodes of unexpected SCA in previously asymptomatic children and adolescents

aged 12 to 25 years in Wisconsin from 1999 to 2003. Survival was poor in cases of structural heart disease: 1 of 9 survived with hypertrophic cardiomyopathy, 1 of 3 survived with an anomalous origin of the left coronary artery, and 0 of 1 survived with arrhythmogenic right ventricular dysplasia. In contrast, 5 of 6 patients with long QT syndrome and no structural heart disease survived.[51]

In patients with hypertrophic cardiomyopathy, immediate defibrillation within 10 seconds using implantable cardioverter defibrillators is almost always effective in terminating potentially lethal ventricular arrhythmias.[52,53] However, in athletes with hypertrophic cardiomyopathy, even a brief delay in defibrillation may cause a steep decline in survival.[46] In commotio cordis or primary electric disturbances, survival rates more closely follow the traditional decline of 7% to 10% per minute for every minute defibrillation is delayed.[54] In an animal model using juvenile swine, Link et al[54] demonstrated that successful resuscitation after commotio cordis was possible and highly dependent on the time interval to defibrillation.

After induction of VF via blunt chest impact using a baseball, defibrillation was performed after 1, 2, 4, and 6 minutes, with survival rates of 100%, 92%, 46%, and 25%, respectively.[54]

Other factors may also contribute to the apparently lower survival rate in young athletes after SCA. The overall incidence of SCA in athletes is relatively rare, and delayed recognition of cardiac arrest by first responders may lead to delay in initiating CPR and defibrillation. Rescuers may mistake agonal or occasional gasping for normal breathing or falsely identify the presence of a pulse. Sudden cardiac arrest may also be misdiagnosed as a seizure because of the presence of myoclonic activity after collapse. Thus, a high suspicion of SCA must be maintained for any collapsed and unresponsive athlete. Other potential factors affecting survival in young athletes include the duration and intensity of exercise before arrest, higher catecholamine levels produced during exercise, potential for oxygen debt and ischemia from exercise, metabolic and physiologic adaptations during exercise, and vascular changes such as decreased systemic vascular resistance.

Key changes from the 2005 AHA guidelines for CPR and ECC may positively affect survival in young athletes.[4] The new guidelines recommend that one attempted defibrillation be followed by immediate CPR, beginning with chest compressions.[7] The initiation of immediate CPR after defibrillation creates blood flow until the heart can generate adequate contractions for perfusion. This is particularly important when defibrillation is followed by pulseless electric activity or recurrent VF requiring multiple shocks. Of 9 cases reported in collegiate athletes, pulseless electric activity followed defibrillation in 2 patients and multiple shocks were deployed in 4.[46]

Thus, incorporating changes in CPR protocol and assisting perfusion in the early moments after defibrillation may have a significant effect on survival by limiting interruptions in blood flow and the need for repeat defibrillation.

EMERGENCY PREPAREDNESS
The "Chain of Survival"
Public access to defibrillators and first-responder AED programs improve survival from SCA by increasing the likelihood that SCA victims will receive bystander CPR and early defibrillation. These programs require an organized and practiced response with rescuers trained and equipped to recognize SCA, activate the EMS system, provide CPR, and use an AED.[36] The AHA describes 4 links in a "chain of survival" to emphasize the time-sensitive interventions for victims of SCA[19]:

• Early recognition of the emergency and activation of the EMS or local emergency response system: "phone 911"
• Early bystander CPR: immediate CPR can double or triple the victim's chance of survival from VF SCA[18,20]
• Early delivery of a shock with a defibrillator: CPR plus defibrillation within 3 to 5 minutes of collapse can produce survival rates as high as 49% to 75%[35,37–39,42,55]
• Early advanced life support followed by postresuscitation care delivered by health care providers

Establishing an Emergency Action Plan
Every institution or organization that sponsors athletic activities should have a written EAP.[6] The EAP should be specific to each athletic venue and encompass emergency communication, personnel,

equipment, and transportation. Core elements to an effective EAP include the following: (1) establishing an efficient communication system, (2) training of likely first responders in CPR and AED use, (3) acquiring the necessary emergency equipment, (4) providing a coordinated and practiced response plan, and (5) ensuring access to early defibrillation (see Table for an EAP checklist). The plan should identify the person and/or group responsible for documentation of personnel training, equipment maintenance, actions taken during the emergency, and evaluation of the emergency response.

The EAP should be developed by school or institutional personnel in consultation with local EMS personnel, school public safety officials, on-site first responders, and school administrators.

It is important to designate an EAP coordinator, usually an athletic trainer, team physician, nurse, or sports administrator.

The EAP should be reviewed at least annually with athletic trainers, team and consulting physicians, athletic training students, school and institutional safety personnel, administrators, and coaches.[6] The EAP should be coordinated with the local EMS agency and integrated into the local EMS system.

The local EMS agency is encouraged to conduct a "preincident" survey to identify any problems or poorly accessible areas for EMS personnel.[5]

The National Collegiate Athletic Association recommends that all institution-sponsored collegiate practices or competitions, as well as out-of-season practices and skills sessions, have an EAP. These plans should include the presence of a person qualified to deliver emergency care; planned access to early defibrillation; and planned access, communication, and transport to a medical facility.[56]

Access to Early Defibrillation
Access to early defibrillation is critical in the management of SCA. In developing an EAP, several time-sensitive intervals must be considered to increase the probability of a successful resuscitation for an SCA victim: the time from collapse to EMS activation, the time from collapse to initiation of CPR, the time from collapse to delivery of the first shock, and the time from collapse to arrival of EMS personnel at the victim's side. The EAP should target a collapse-to-EMS call time and CPR initiation of less than 1 minute.[5,19] A second target goal of less than

3 to 5 minutes from time of collapse to first shock is strongly recommended.

The AHA recommends implementation of an AED program in any school that meets one of the following criteria: (1) the frequency of cardiac arrest is such that there is a reasonable probability of AED use within 5 years of rescuer training and AED placement; (2) there are children attending school or adults working at the school who are thought to be at high risk for SCA (eg, children with congenital heart disease); or (3) an EMS call-to-shock interval of less than 5 minutes cannot be reliably achieved with a conventional EMS system, and a collapse-to-shock interval of less than 5 minutes can be reliably achieved (in more than 90% of cases) by training and equipping laypersons to function as first responders by recognizing SCA, activating the EMS system, starting CPR, and using an AED.[5,19]

Schools and institutions sponsoring athletic programs must determine if this target time interval of less than 5 minutes from collapse to defibrillation can be reliably achieved with the conventional EMS system or if an AED program is required to achieve early defibrillation. Studies suggest that, for most EMS systems, the time interval between activating the EMS and arrival of EMS personnel at the victim's side is usually more than 5 minutes (mean 6.1 minutes).[57] In some communities, the time interval from EMS call to EMS arrival may be 7 to 8 minutes or longer.[43,58] Thus, achieving early defibrillation after SCA in athletes is largely dependent on the prompt availability of AEDs for responders. In high school and college athletic programs, coaches, officials, athletic trainers, and other sports medicine professionals are in a unique position to act as first responders to SCA during organized training and competition. Training in CPR and on-site AED programs are likely to be the only means of achieving early defibrillation and improving survival from SCA in athletes.

Emergency Communication

A rapid system for communication must be in place linking all athletic facilities, practice fields, and other parts of the campus to the EMS system. When bystanders recognize an emergency and activate the EMS system, they ensure that basic and advanced life support providers are dispatched to the site of the emergency. The time required for EMS response to each sporting venue should be estimated, and a plan must be in place to efficiently direct EMS personnel to the location.[5]

The communication network can be developed through existing telephones, cellular telephones, walkie-talkies, alarms, or an intercom system that links a rescuer directly to the EMS or to a central location responsible for contacting the EMS and activating on-site responders. Establishing an accessible communication system will prevent critical delays caused by a rescuer running from a distant athletic facility or practice field to activate the EMS system. The communications system should be checked before each practice or competition to ensure proper working order, and a back-up communication plan should be in effect in case the primary communication system fails.

The EAP should be posted at every sporting venue and near appropriate telephones, with the role of the first responder clearly demarcated. A listing of emergency numbers should be available, as well as the street address of the venue and specific directions (eg, cross streets, landmarks) to guide EMS personnel.

When activating the EMS system (calling 911), the caller should alert the EMS to the number and condition of persons injured, if an SCA is suspected, and the first aid treatment rendered. Involving representatives of the EMS system in the initial communications planning before any incidents will improve the onsite transfer of care once EMS personnel arrive on the scene.

Emergency Personnel

The first person to respond to a medical emergency on the field of play will vary widely and may be a coach, official, student, teammate, teacher, school nurse, athletic trainer, physician, or emergency medical technician. All potential rescuers should be familiar and, ideally, trained with the EAP to ensure an effective and coordinated response to an emergency situation.

Each institution or organization with a formal athletic program needs to identify who will be responsible and trained to respond to an SCA. The National Collegiate Athletic Association recommends that all athletics personnel associated with practices, competitions, skills instruction, and strength and conditioning be certified in CPR, first aid, and the

Emergency Action Plan Checklist

The following elements are recommended in the development of a comprehensive emergency action plan (EAP) for sudden cardiac arrest (SCA) in athletics. Actual requirements and implementation may vary depending on the location, school or institution.

I. **Development of an Emergency Action Plan**

☐ Establish a written EAP for each individual athletic venue.

☐ Coordinate the EAP with the local EMS agency, campus public safety officials, on-site first responders, administrators, athletic trainers, school nurses, and team and consulting physicians.

☐ Integrate the EAP into the local EMS response.

☐ Determine the venue-specific access to early defibrillation (<3 to5 minutes from collapse to first shock recommended).

II. **Emergency Communication**

☐ Establish an efficient communication system to activate EMS at each athletic venue.

☐ Establish a communication system to alert on-site responders to the emergency and its location.

☐ Post the EAP at every venue and near telephones, including the role of the first responder, a listing of emergency numbers and street address and directions to guide the personnel.

III. **Emergency Personnel**

☐ Designate an EAP coordinator

☐ Identify who will be responsible and trained to respond to a SCA (likely first responders include athletic trainers, coaches, school nurses and team physicians).

☐ Train targeted responders in CPR and AED use.

☐ Determine who is responsible for personnel training and establish a means of documentation.

☐ Identify the medical coordinator for on-site AED programs.

IV. **Emergency Equipment**

☐ Use on-site or centrally located AED(s) if the collapse-to-shock interval for conventional EMS is estimated to be > 5 minutes.

☐ Notify EMS dispatch centers and agencies of the specific type of AED and the exact location of the AED on school grounds.

☐ Acquire pocket mask or barrier-shield device for rescue breathing.

☐ Acquire AED supplies (scissors, razor and towel) and consider an extra set of AED pads.

☐ Consider bag-valve masks, oxygen delivery systems, oral and nasopharyngeal airways and advanced airways (eg, endotracheal tube, Combitube or laryngeal mask airway).

☐ Consider emergency cardiac medications (eg. aspirin, nitroglycerin).

☐ Determine who is responsible for checking equipment readiness and hos often and establish a means of documentation.

V. **Emergency Transportation**

☐ Determine transportation route for ambulances to enter and exit each venue.

☐ Facilitate access to SCA victim for arriving EMS personnel.

☐ Consider on-site ambulance coverage for high-risk events.

☐ Identify the receiving medical facility equipped in advanced cardiac care.

☐ Ensure that medical coverage is still provided at the athletic event if on-site medical staff accompany the athlete to the hospital.

VI. **Practice and Review of Emergency Action Plan**

☐ Rehearse the EAP at least annually with athletic trainers, athletic training students, team and consulting physicians, school nurses, coaches, campus public safety officials and other targeted responders.

☐ Consider mock SCA scenarios.

☐ Establish an evaluation system for the EAP rehearsal, and modify the EAP if needed.

VII. **Postevent Catastrophic Incident Guidelines**

☐ Establish a contact list of individuals to be notified in case of a catastrophic event.

☐ Determine the procedures for release of information, aftercare services and the postevent evaluation process.

☐ Identify local crisis services and counselors.

☐ Consider pre-established incident report forms to be completed by all responders and the method for system improvement

EMS indicates emergency medical services; CPR, cardiopulmonary resuscitation; and AED, automated external defibrillator.

prevention of disease transmision.[56] For secondary schools, the AHA recommends training of the school nurse and physician, athletic trainer, and several faculty members in the provision of first aid and CPR and that a sufficient number of faculty, staff, and/or students be trained to ensure that a trained rescuer can respond to an SCA within 90 seconds.[5] Because an athletic trainer, physician, or school nurse is not universally present at all extracurricular sporting activities, coaches for every team should receive certified training in CPR and AED use to ensure the presence of a trained rescuer.

Emergency Equipment

All necessary emergency equipment should be at the site or quickly accessible, and personnel must be trained in advance to use it properly. Resuscitation equipment should be placed in a central location that is highly visible and near a telephone or other means of activating the EMS system. All school staff should be instructed on the location of emergency equipment.

For large schools or those with distant or multiple athletic facilities, duplicate equipment may be needed. Emergency equipment should not be placed in a locked box, cabinet, or room, which could delay emergency care. Mounted cabinets with audible alarms that sound when the cabinet door is opened may decrease the theft or vandalism risk.[5]

Basic resuscitation equipment for management of SCA should include a pocket mask or barrier-shield device for rescue breathing, an AED for early defibrillation, and AED application supplies (heavy-duty scissors to remove clothing and expose the chest, a towel to dry the chest, and a razor to shave chest hair). Aluminum chlorhydrate (antiperspirant) spray may help the AED leads stick to sweaty skin, and an extra set of AED pads should be considered in case of misapplication or inadvertent damage.

For high schools and colleges that have physicians and ACLS-certified responders on-site, the acquisition of advanced resuscitation equipment for the management of SCA should be considered based on the skills of the designated responders.

Advanced resuscitation equipment may include bag-valve masks, oxygen delivery systems, oral and nasopharyngeal airways, advanced airways (eg, endotracheal tube, Combitube [Tyco Healthcare Nellcor, Pleasanton, CA], or laryngeal mask airway),

and emergency cardiac medications. The ACLS-certified personnel should have nitroglycerin and aspirin available on-site to use for chest pain without cardiac arrest. The equipment and medications should be assembled in a code bag and stored in an easily accessible central location or at each athletic venue.

If an AED program is implemented, it should be part of the written EAP. The EMS centers should be notified of the specific type of AED and the exact location of the AED on school grounds. If a rescuer is unfamiliar with the school or where an AED is located, he or she can receive instructions from the EMS dispatcher to find and use the AED.[5] All AED programs should include medical or health care provider oversight, appropriate training of anticipated rescuers in CPR and AED use, coordination with the EMS system, appropriate device maintenance, and an ongoing quality improvement program.[5]

If possible, emergency information about the student-athletes, including relevant medical history and contact information, should be accessible to medical personnel at home sporting events and while traveling in case of an emergency.

Emergency Transportation

The EAP should delineate the life support transportation an athlete with SCA will access. In life-threatening emergencies, an athlete should be transported by the EMS personnel to the most appropriate receiving facility that is staffed and equipped to deliver optimal emergency care. Emphasis should be placed on having an ambulance on-site at high-risk events. The EMS response time should be factored in when determining on-site ambulance coverage.

Consideration should be given to the level of transportation service available (eg, basic life support, advanced life support) and the equipment and training level of the personnel who staff the ambulance.[6] If an ambulance is on-site, a location should be designated that allows rapid access to enter and exit the venue. A dedicated staff person should be assigned to each event and be familiar with the directions and access points for arriving EMS personnel to specific athletic facilities on campus. Each site should post written directions to read to the EMS response dispatcher. If air-medical transport may be needed, the global positioning satellite coordinates should also be listed.

Practice and Review of the Emergency Action Plan

The EAP should be reviewed and practiced at least annually with athletic trainers, team and consulting physicians, athletic training students, school and institutional safety personnel, administrators, coaches, and other designated first responders.[6]

More frequent practice sessions will improve the effectiveness, efficiency, and organization of the response team, and any modifications to the EAP based on practice trials should be documented.[59] A mock SCA scenario can be organized using actors or manikins to simulate SCA victims. Evaluation of each emergency response rehearsal should document the time from collapse to EMS activation, the time from collapse to initiation of CPR, the time from collapse to delivery of first shock if an AED is available, and the time from collapse to arrival of EMS personnel at the victim's side.[5]

Post-event Catastrophic Incident Guidelines

The EAP should include a post-event plan outlining the procedures for release of information; aftercare services for responders, teammates, coaches, and families; and the post-event evaluation process. A list of administrative and legal personnel from the school or institution to be contacted after a catastrophic event should be readily accessible in the EAP, and the methods for data collection, reporting, and incident assessment and review should be defined in the plan. Local crisis services and counselors to assist students, teammates, families, and rescuers after a catastrophic event should be defined and available.

The post-event evaluation process is critical both to document the details of the event and to allow system improvement. Pre-established incident report forms to be completed by all responders should be considered to facilitate a summary report with recommendations for site management and modifications to the existing EAP if needed. Feedback, particularly of a positive nature, should also be provided to responders.

Emergency Preparedness: Where Are We Now?

Studies demonstrating that AEDs placed at public locations can substantially improve survival from SCA have accelerated a growing national trend to broadly implement AED programs at public sporting venues and selected athletic facilities. In 2003, 91% of National Collegiate Athletic Association Division

I institutions already had AEDs, with a median of 4 (range 1 to 30) at each of these institutions.[11] The most common location for the AEDs was the athletic training room (82%), followed by the basketball arena (43%), campus police station (40%), football stadium (27%), baseball or softball field (21%), and recreation or fitness facility (21%).[11] A range of 25% to 54% of high schools had at least one AED on school grounds.[44,60,61] Common locations for AEDs in high schools include the school athletic training room, basketball facility or gymnasium, nurse's office, and main lobby.[61,62]

In the university setting, resources to purchase AEDs have largely come from the athletic department budget. In contrast, financial resources at high schools are more limited, and AED acquisition has been primarily funded through donations. In Washington State, 60% of high schools with AEDs acquired them through donated funds, and only 38% were purchased by the school, school district, or athletic department.[61] In the greater Boston area, after a single AED was donated to 35 schools, 25 schools purchased additional AEDs using a combination of donated funds (21), grants (11), and school budget funds (8).[62]

School nurses, athletic trainers, teachers, and coaches may be called on to provide emergency care during school hours and extracurricular sporting activities. However, emergency training for many of these potential first responders varies widely. A survey of school nurses in New Mexico documented that few school nurses and staff had any emergency training.[63]

In 3 midwestern states, one third of teachers surveyed had no first aid training, and 40% had never completed a course in CPR.[64] In Washington State high schools with AEDs, 78% of coaches, 72% of administrators, 70% of school nurses, and 48% of teachers received formal AED training.[61]

Although more schools are placing AEDs on campus grounds, significant deficiencies in emergency planning and coordination still exist. In Washington State, only 25% of high schools coordinated the implementation of AEDs with any outside medical agency, and only 6% of schools coordinated with the local EMS system.[61] In contrast, studies involving AED implementation as part of a more comprehensive emergency plan have demonstrated more success. In the greater Boston area, 35 high schools were given a single donated AED and educated to develop a training protocol for appropriate staff and to assess the need for purchase of additional AEDs.[62] In this study, 90% of schools trained their faculty, 76% trained their staff and custodial workers, 71% trained their athletic trainers, and 48% trained some or all of their student body in AED use.[62] Over a 2-year study period, an AED was successfully used twice for SCA in a football referee and a teacher.

Every school participating in the study considered participation in the AED program to be worthwhile.[62] Similarly, in Wisconsin, Project ADAM has assisted 143 of 400 public high schools in implementing an AED program as part of a comprehensive EAP. The goals of Project ADAM include educating faculty, staff, parents, students, and health care professionals about SCA in children and adolescents and advocating for teaching CPR with AED instruction to all high school students before graduation.[51]

Legislation to require AEDs in schools is also growing but is not uniformly funded. New York and Illinois have already passed legislative mandates for AEDs in public schools, and California, Delaware, Florida, Georgia, Maine, Massachusetts, New Jersey, Nevada, Pennsylvania, Rhode Island, and Virginia have pending legislation.[65] However, unfunded mandates to establish AED programs in schools often lack the necessary emergency planning, coordination, and training that are essential to a successful program.

Obstacles to Implementing Automated External Defibrillators

Although the prevalence of AEDs in schools and at public athletic venues is increasing, budgetary constraints remain an obstacle to initiating public access defibrillation programs.

Policymakers must determine which sites warrant an AED and which must go without. Although uncertainty on where to place the AED (57%) and medical-legal concerns (48%) were also reported as common obstacles, National Collegiate Athletic Association Division I head athletic trainers at institutions without AEDs cited financial resources (70%) as the primary obstacle to acquiring AEDs.[11] In the high school setting, financial resources are the critical barrier to implementing an AED program. In

Washington State, 65% of high schools without AEDs identified monetary resources as the main obstacle to acquiring AEDs.[61] In the greater Boston area, 93% of schools given a single AED reported lack of funding as the reason for not purchasing additional AEDs.[62]

The task force recognizes that budgets for many schools are already challenged, and more research is needed to explore the development of funding programs to assist schools with limited resources. Until the cost of AEDs further declines or government funding is allocated toward emergency preparedness in schools, administrators and those responsible for emergency planning must work within their school districts to elicit financial support from the local community, parenting and fundraising groups, and applicable state and federal grants to fund AED programs. However, the goal is not just to acquire the AED but to do so as part of a comprehensive educational and emergency action plan.

As demonstrated by Project ADAM and the greater Boston area program, donations can fund both the equipment and educational materials for school administrators and lead to the development of a successful program in participating schools.[51,62] The current cost (in 2006) of purchasing a single AED is approximately $1500, and in many communities, local EMS personnel will provide emergency planning consultation at no cost. The additional cost of CPR and AED training for targeted responders must also be considered. However, with the commitment and dedication of school administrators, parents, local businesses, and health care leaders, implementation of an AED program in schools is an obtainable goal.

MANAGEMENT OF SUDDEN CARDIAC ARREST
2005 American Heart Association Guidelines for Cardiopulmonary Resuscitation and Emergency Cardiovascular Care

In December 2005, the AHA released updated guidelines on CPR and ECC.[4] The guidelines are based on the evidence evaluation from the 2005 International Consensus Conference on Cardiopulmonary Resuscitation and Emergency Cardiovascular Care Science With Treatment Recommendations.[66] The AHA adult CPR guidelines apply to any child older than 8 years.[67] Thus, for the purposes of this statement, the protocols discussed are intended for youth and adult athletes greater than 8 years old. The most significant change in these guidelines is a stronger emphasis on chest compressions, increasing the number of chest compressions per minute and reducing the interruptions in chest compressions during CPR. Key changes to the guidelines are listed in the following:

• Elimination of lay rescuer assessment of circulation

• Recommendation of a universal compression-to-ventilation ratio of 30:2 for single rescuers and for all SCA victims in this age group

• Chest compressions ("push hard, push fast") should be at a rate of 100 compressions per minute, allowing complete chest recoil and minimizing interruptions in chest compressions

• CPR should resume immediately after initial shock delivery, beginning with chest compressions

• Rescuers should not check the rhythm or pulse after shock delivery until 5 cycles (or about 2 minutes) of CPR have been performed

• Recommendations that EMS providers consider 5 cycles (or about 2 minutes) of CPR before defibrillation for unwitnessed arrest, particularly if the suspected time from collapse to arrival at the scene is more than 4 to 5 minutes The new recommendations call for only one shock, followed immediately by chest compressions, and represent a major change from traditional treatment protocols involving a sequence of 3 stacked shocks in the treatment of VF and rapid VT. This change is based on the high success rate of a single defibrillation, with first-shock efficacy for VF by current biphasic defibrillators reportedly higher than 90%.[8] In addition, if the first shock fails, CPR may improve oxygen and substrate delivery to the myocardium, making subsequent shocks more likely to be successful. Interruptions in chest compressions for rhythm analysis are associated with lower survival rates and a decreased probability of conversion of VF to another rhythm.[68,69]

Rhythm analysis for a 3-shock sequence in older AEDs results in delays up to 37 seconds between delivery of the first shock and delivery of the first postshock chest compression.[70] The new AHA guidelines necessitate reprogramming of all previously purchased AEDs, as they are programmed with older "stacked shocks" protocols. Institutions that have AEDs with older protocols should contact their vendors to reprogram the AED. If possible,

AED units should also comply with the new AHA recommendations for first shock energy levels, either 360 J for monophasic waveforms or the individual manufacturer's recommendations for biphasic waveforms.[8]

The Collapsed Athlete

Fortunately, most athletes who collapse during or after exercise will not be in SCA. The differential diagnosis of nontraumatic exercise-related syncope includes but is not limited to SCA, exertional heat stroke, heat exhaustion, hyponatremia, hypoglycemia, exercise-associated collapse, neurocardiogenic syncope, seizures, pulmonary embolus, cardiac arrhythmias, valvular disorders, coronary artery disease, cardiomyopathies, ion channel disorders, and other structural cardiac diseases. A collapsed athlete who is also unresponsive should be treated as a potential cardiac arrest until either spontaneous breathing and a pulse are documented or the cardiac rhythm is analyzed.

If SCA is ruled out but the athlete remains unresponsive, further immediate evaluation to determine the cause of collapse is needed, as other emergent medical interventions may still be required.

Exercise-related syncope involves a transient loss of consciousness and postural tone during or immediately after exercise. Exercise-associated collapse describes athletes who are unable to stand or walk unaided as a result of lightheadedness, dizziness, or syncope immediately after exercise.[71] Exertional syncope without SCA in young adults is usually benign but always requires investigation because it can be an indication of a more serious cardiac disorder and the only symptom that precedes SCD.[3,13] Syncope that occurs during exercise tends to be more ominous than syncope occurring after exercise.[72]

Young and otherwise healthy adults who collapse while exercising have a greater probability of an organic cardiac abnormality, such as hypertrophic cardiomyopathy or anomalous coronary artery origin, than do athletes with postexertional or nonexertional syncope.[3,13] The investigation of exercise-related syncope should specifically exclude known pathologic diagnoses before a complete return to activity is permitted.

Recognition of Sudden Cardiac Arrest

Prompt identification of SCA is critical in the

management of this life-threatening emergency. Any collapsed athlete who is unresponsive requires an immediate assessment for SCA. Although SCA is relatively uncommon in the athletic setting, on-site responders must maintain a high index of suspicion, as unrecognized SCA in a collapsed athlete causes critical delays in CPR and defibrillation. Resuscitation is often delayed because the victim is reported to have signs of life.[73] Sudden cardiac arrest can be misdiagnosed as a seizure in the form of involuntary myoclonic jerks; seizure-like activity is present in approximately 20% of patients with cardiogenic collapse.[74]

Seizure-like activity has also been reported in 3 of 10 athletes with SCA.[75] To avoid life-threatening delays in resuscitation, brief seizure-like activity should be assumed to be due to SCA and initial management steps for SCA taken immediately until a noncardiac cause of the collapse is clearly determined.

Other barriers to recognizing SCA in athletes include inaccurate rescuer assessment of pulse or respirations. Occasional or agonal gasping can occur in the first minutes after SCA and is often misinterpreted as normal breathing, especially by lay responders.[76] Occasional gasping does not represent adequate breathing and, if present, should not prevent rescuers from initiating CPR. Assessment of signs of circulation and the presence of a pulse by lay rescuers and health care professionals can also be inaccurate. Lay rescuers fail to recognize the absence of a pulse in 10% of pulseless victims and fail to detect a pulse in 40% of victims with a pulse.[7,77]

The updated AHA CPR guidelines eliminate lay rescuer assessment of pulse and recommend that cardiac arrest be assumed if the unresponsive victim does not demonstrate normal breathing.[4] Health care providers may also have difficulty accurately determining if a pulse is present or take too long in their assessment. Health care providers should take no longer than 10 seconds to check for a pulse and should proceed with chest compressions if a pulse is not definitively detected.[7]

Sports medicine professionals and other potential first responders to an SCA in athletes must understand these potential obstacles to recognizing SCA, as inaccurate initial assessment of SCA results in critical delays or even failure to activate the EMS system, initiate CPR, and provide early defibrillation.

Management of Sudden Cardiac Arrest: Witnessed Collapse

Sudden cardiac arrest in the athletic setting is likely to be witnessed by a bystander, coach, official, teammate, or athletic trainer. When more than one person is present at the scene, several management steps can be taken simultaneously.

Management of a collapsed athlete begins with an initial assessment of responsiveness. The rescuer should check the victim for a response by tapping the victim on the shoulder and asking, "Are you all right?"[7] If the athlete is unresponsive, one or more trained rescuers should begin CPR while another bystander activates the EMS system by calling 911 or the local emergency number and retrieves the AED if available.

When contacting the EMS system, the rescuer should be prepared to provide the exact location of the emergency and a brief account of what happened and the initial care given.

In the case of a lone rescuer and a witnessed arrest, the rescuer should first activate the EMS system by calling 911 or the local emergency number, obtain an AED if readily available, and return to the victim to initiate CPR and AED use. If an on-site response system is activated, the central communication center is responsible for contacting the EMS and activating on-site responders to facilitate transport of an AED to the victim.

An AED should be applied to the victim as soon as possible and turned on for rhythm analysis and defibrillation if indicated. If an AED is not immediately available, the rescuer should open the airway by using the head tilt–chin lift maneuver and then "look, listen, and feel" for breathing. If a cervical spine injury is suspected, the modified jaw thrust maneuver is recommended to open the airway. The presence of normal breathing should distinguish the victim who has collapsed but does not require CPR. Agonal or occasional gasping should not be mistaken for normal breathing and should be recognized as a sign of SCA.[67] If a collapsed athlete is determined not to be in SCA and does not become normally responsive, the athlete should be continually reassessed for signs of, or progression to, SCA. The athlete may require other medical interventions depending on the specific cause of collapse.

If normal breathing is not detected within 10 seconds, 2 rescue breaths should be given, followed by chest compressions.[7] Lay rescuers (coaches, officials, and other bystanders) should not assess the athlete for a pulse or signs of circulation. Health care providers (athletic trainers, school nurses, emergency medical technicians, and physicians) should deliver 2 rescue breaths and may consider checking for a pulse. If the health care provider does not definitively feel a pulse within 10 seconds, CPR should be initiated. Rescue breaths are provided by pinching the victim's nose, creating an airtight mouth-to-mouth seal, and giving one breath over 1 second that produces a visible chest rise. If the victim's chest does not rise with the first rescue breath, the head tilt–chin lift maneuver should be repeated before the second breath in an attempt to open the airway. If the rescuer is unable or unwilling to give rescue breaths, then chest compressions should be initiated.

Effective chest compressions in adults are performed by compressing the lower half of the sternum, using the heels of the hands, and should depress the chest a depth of 3.8 to 5.1 cm; complete chest recoil permits venous return between compressions. Rescuers should "push hard and push fast."[67] The CPR should be performed using the universal compression-to-ventilation ratio of 30:2 at a rate of 100 compressions per minute. When multiple rescuers are present, they should rotate the compressor role about every 2 minutes or earlier if fatigue develops.

An AED or a manual defibrillator should be applied for rhythm analysis as soon as it arrives. All interruptions in chest compressions for analyzing the rhythm or delivering a shock should be minimized. With 2 or more rescuers, CPR can be continued while attaching the AED leads. Defibrillation is more likely to be successful with a shorter time between chest compressions and delivery of a shock.[78,79] If VF or rapid VT is detected, the AED will instruct the rescuer to deploy a shock. The rescuer should deliver 1 shock and then immediately resume CPR, beginning with chest compressions. When 2 rescuers are present, the rescuer operating the AED should be prepared to deliver a shock as soon as the compressor removes his or her hands from the chest and all rescuers are clear of contact with the victim. The rescuer should not delay resuming chest compressions to allow for repeat rhythm analysis, and CPR should be continued for 5 cycles or about 2 minutes before rechecking the rhythm or until the

victim becomes responsive. If no shock is advised after rhythm analysis, CPR should be immediately resumed and continued for 5 cycles before rechecking the rhythm or until advanced life support measures are available.

Some advanced airway devices such as an endotracheal tube, esophageal-tracheal Combitube, or laryngeal mask airway can be used by health care professionals with sufficient training and experience. Once an advanced airway is in place, pauses or interruptions in chest compressions for ventilation are no longer necessary. Rescuers should deliver 100 compressions per minute and 8 to 10 breaths per minute continuously.[67] If available, bag-mask ventilation can also be performed by health care providers with the use of supplementary oxygen at a minimum flow rate of 10 to 12 L/min.[7]

Management of Sudden Cardiac Arrest: Unwitnessed Collapse

If an athlete is found collapsed and unresponsive and the time lapse from onset of SCA is unknown, rescuers may consider 5 cycles or 2 minutes of CPR before checking the rhythm and attempting defibrillation.[7,8] After a prolonged cardiac arrest, a brief period of CPR can deliver oxygen and energy substrates, perhaps increasing the likelihood that a perfusing rhythm will return if defibrillation is possible.

SPECIAL CIRCUMSTANCES
Cervical Spine Injury

Any athlete suspected of having a cervical spine injury should not be moved, and the cervical spine should be immobilized. Unconscious athletes in collision sports are presumed to have unstable spine injuries until proved otherwise.

High cervical spine injuries can cause apnea, ineffective breathing patterns, and paralysis of the phrenic nerve. Although rare, prolonged hypoxemia can lead to cardiac arrest.

Protective equipment used in collision sports such as football and hockey makes the management of SCA in a spine-injured athlete difficult. The facemask should be removed (leaving the helmet in place) as soon as possible before transportation, regardless of respiratory status and even if the athlete is conscious.[80] Shoulder pads should also be opened (but not removed) before transportation to provide access to the chest if CPR or defibrillation is required. A designated rescuer must be responsible for manually stabilizing the head and neck during CPR and any transfer of the victim. The rescuer responsible for neck stabilization should disengage if defibrillation is necessary.

Commotio Cordis
Commotio cordis, also called cardiac concussion, involves a blunt, nonpenetrating blow to the chest during a vulnerable phase of ventricular repolarization, leading to a ventricular arrhythmia with no structural damage or cardiac contusion present. Commotio cordis occurs most commonly in young male adolescents (mean age = 13.6 years) with compliant chest walls.[47] Approximately 80% of cases involve blunt chest impact by a firm projectile, such as a baseball, softball, hockey puck, or lacrosse ball, and 20% of cases are due to chest contact with another person.[47]

To date, commercially available chest protectors have not been shown to prevent commotio cordis.[82] Survival after commotio cordis closely depends on the time to defibrillation.[54] Overall survival as reported from the United States Commotio Cordis Registry was only 16%, but for those victims still in VF who were reached in time to receive defibrillation, the survival rate was 46%.[47]

Young athletes who collapse shortly after being struck in the chest should be suspected of having commotio cordis until the athlete is clearly responsive. Rescuers can improve survival by promptly recognizing SCA due to commotio cordis, activating the EMS system, immediately initiating CPR, and using an AED as soon as possible.

Exertional Heat Stroke
Heat stroke is a life-threatening emergency, and treatment of concurrent cardiac arrest requires simultaneously cooling the athlete and performing CPR. The presence of exertional heat stroke in a collapsed athlete must be suspected in hot, humid environments, especially if the athlete is wearing athletic clothing and equipment that limits heat loss, and the EMS system must be activated.

Both heat exhaustion and heat stroke can cause syncope in the athlete. Heat stroke is differentiated by the presence of mental status changes and a core temperature of greater than 40 degrees C (104 degrees F). Untreated exertional heat stroke can progress to end-organ damage, adult respiratory distress syndrome, disseminated intravascular coagulation, neurologic injury, cardiac arrest, and death. The diagnosis of heat stroke can be confirmed on-site with a rectal temperature measurement.

If the athlete is unresponsive but has normal breathing and circulation, rapid cooling by ice water bath immersion is recommended.[83] If an ice water tub is not available or if concurrent SCA is suspected, rotating ice water towels applied to the head, trunk, and extremities and ice packs applied to the neck, axilla, and groin represent an alternative method for cooling while performing CPR and using an AED. Because prompt temperature reduction is critical, transport to the emergency department for heat stroke victims without SCA should be delayed if sideline cooling measures, such as ice water bath immersion, are available.[83] Cooling should also be continued during transport if needed.

Lightning
Lightning presents an environmental hazard with the potential for multiple victims. If the lightning storm is ongoing, rescuers must ensure their personal safety by moving an SCA victim indoors if possible. Spine immobilization should be considered. Cardiac arrest from lightning strike is associated with significant mortality and requires modification of standard ACLS measures to achieve successful resuscitation. Most lightning strike victims have associated multisystem involvement, including neurologic complications, cutaneous burns, soft tissue injury such as rhabdomyolysis, and associated blunt trauma.[84]

When managing several lightning strike victims, the normal multiple casualty triage priorities are reversed. Casualties who appear unresponsive require prompt, aggressive resuscitation using standard CPR and ACLS protocols, including defibrillation and cardiac pharmacotherapy.[84] The chance for a successful outcome is greater for lightning-related cardiac arrest, even with initial rhythms that are traditionally unresponsive to therapy.

Mass Events
Emergency preparation and management of SCA at mass athletic events require additional planning. Schools and institutions may have their own athletic staffs with them, and advanced communication with

the host organization is helpful to ensure that visiting athletic staffs are familiar with the EAP and central medical area or equipment. Distance events such as cross-country meets, triathlons, and marathons present an additional challenge because running or biking courses are often spread out over long distances, sometimes in remote areas.

Among marathoners, SCA occurs in approximately 1 in 40,000 runners across the age spectrum.[85] Distributing medical staff and AEDs along the course or field of play and using bicycle or "golf-cart" rescue teams will improve response times should an emergency arise.

Rainy, Wet, Ice, and Metal Surfaces

Defibrillators used in a wet environment or on an ice playing surface are considered safe and do not pose a shock hazard for rescuers or bystanders. If a collapsed victim with suspected SCA is lying on a wet surface or in a puddle, the patient should not be moved to avoid delays in initiating CPR. Simulation of a patient and a rescuer in a wet environment does not show a significant risk of electric shock.[86]

Responders to an SCA on an ice playing surface should consider foot traction devices and helmets for their own safety.[87,88] In contrast, SCA victims found immersed in a pool or contained body of water should be removed from the water before defibrillation. Any SCA victims lying on metal conducting surfaces (eg, bleachers) should be moved to a nonmetal surfaces or placed onto spine boards before defibrillation if that can be done quickly and without significant delays.

CONCLUSIONS

The most important factor in SCA survival is the presence of a trained rescuer who can initiate CPR and has access to early defibrillation. The athletic community is in a unique position to have trained coaches, officials, and other targeted responders, and, in some circumstances, on-site athletic trainers, school nurses, and team physicians respond immediately to SCA at organized athletic events and practices.

Comprehensive emergency planning is needed for high school and college athletic programs to ensure an efficient and structured response to SCA. Essential elements to an EAP include establishing an effective communication system, training of anticipated responders in CPR and AED use, access to an AED for early defibrillation, acquisition of necessary emergency equipment, coordination and integration of on-site responder and AED programs with the local EMS system, and practice and review of the response plan. High suspicion of SCA should be maintained in any collapsed and unresponsive athlete, with application of an AED as soon as possible for rhythm analysis and defibrillation if indicated. Interruptions in chest compressions for rhythm analysis and shock delivery should be minimized, and rescuers should be prepared to resume CPR, beginning with chest compressions, as soon as a shock is delivered. Improved education in the recognition of SCA, enhanced emergency preparedness, training in current CPR protocols, and increased access to AEDs for early defibrillation are needed to improve survival from SCA in athletics.

DISCLAIMER

The National Athletic Trainers' Association and the Inter-Association Task Force advise individuals, schools, and institutions to carefully and independently consider each of the recommendations. The information contained in the statement is neither exhaustive nor exclusive to all circumstances or individuals.

Variables such as institutional human resource guidelines, state or federal statutes, rules, or regulations, as well as regional environmental conditions, may impact the relevance and implementation of these recommendations. The NATA and the Inter-Association Task Force advise their members and others to carefully and independently consider each of the recommendations (including the applicability of same to any particular circumstance or individual). The foregoing statement should not be relied on as an independent basis for care but rather as a resource available to NATA members or others. Moreover, no opinion is expressed herein regarding the quality of care that adheres to or differs from any of NATA's position statements. The NATA and the Inter-Association Task Force reserve the right to rescind or modify their statements at any time.

REFERENCES
1. Maron BJ. Sudden death in young athletes. *N Engl J Med*. 2003;349: 1064–1075.
2. Van Camp SP, Bloor CM, Mueller FO, Cantu RC, Olson HG. Nontraumatic sports death in high school and college athletes. *Med Sci Sports Exerc*. 1995;27:641–647.
3. Maron BJ, Shirani J, Poliac LC, Mathenge R, Roberts WC, Mueller FO. Sudden death in young competitive athletes: clinical, demographic, and pathological profiles. *JAMA*. 1996;276:199–204.
4. ECC Committee, Subcommittees and Task Forces of the American Heart Association. 2005 American Heart Association guidelines for cardiopulmonary resuscitation and emergency cardiovascular care. *Circulation*. 2005;112(suppl 24):IV1–203.
5. Hazinski MF, Markenson D, Neish S, et al. Response to cardiac arrest and selected life-threatening medical emergencies: the medical emergency response plan for schools. A statement for healthcare providers, policymakers, school administrators, and community leaders. *Circulation*. 2004; 109:278–291.

6. Andersen J, Courson RW, Kleiner DM, McLoda TA. National Athletic Trainers' Association position statement: emergency planning in athletics. *J Athl Train*. 2002;37:99–104.

7. ECC Committee, Subcommittees and Task Forces of the American Heart Association. 2005 American Heart Association guidelines for cardiopulmonary resuscitation and emergency cardiovascular care, part 4: adult basic life support. *Circulation*. 2005;112(suppl 24):IV19–34.

8. ECC Committee, Subcommittees and Task Forces of the American Heart Association. 2005 American Heart Association guidelines for cardiopulmonary resuscitation and emergency cardiovascular care, part 5: electrical therapies. Automated external defibrillators, defibrillation, cardioversion, and pacing. *Circulation*. 2005;112(suppl 24):IV35–46.

9. Ellsworth EG, Ackerman MJ. The changing face of sudden cardiac death in the young. *Heart Rhythm*. 2005;2:1283–1285.

10. Sen-Chowdhry S, McKenna WJ. Sudden cardiac death in the young: a strategy for prevention by targeted evaluation. *Cardiology*. 2006;105:196–206.

11. Drezner JA, Rogers KJ, Zimmer RR, Sennett BJ. Use of automated external defibrillators at NCAA Division I universities. *Med Sci Sports Exerc*. 2005;37:1487–1492.

12. Maron BJ, Doerer JJ, Haas TS, Tierney DM, Mueller FO. Profile and frequency of sudden death in 1463 young competitive athletes: from a 25 year U.S. national registry, 1980–2005. American Heart Association Scientific Sessions; November 12-15, 2006; Chicago, IL.

13. Basso C, Maron BJ, Corrado D, Thiene G. Clinical profile of congenital coronary artery anomalies with origin from the wrong aortic sinus leading to sudden death in young competitive athletes. *J Am Coll Cardiol*. 2000;35:1493–1501.

14. Maron BJ, Thompson PD, Puffer JC, et al. Cardiovascular preparticipation screening of competitive athletes: a statement for health professionals from the Sudden Death Committee (clinical cardiology) and Congenital Cardiac Defects Committee (cardiovascular disease in the young), American Heart Association. *Circulation*. 1996;94:850–856.

15. American Academy of Family Physicians, American Academy of Pediatrics, American College of Sports Medicine, American Medical Society for Sports Medicine, American Orthopaedic Society for Sports Medicine, American Osteopathic Academy of Sports Medicine. *Preparticipation Physical Evaluation*. 3rd ed. New York, NY: McGraw-Hill; 2005.

16. Maron BJ, Douglas PS, Graham TP, Nishimura RA, Thompson PD. Task Force 1: preparticipation screening and diagnosis of cardiovascular disease in athletes. *J Am Coll Cardiol*. 2005;45:1322–1326.

17. Rea TD, Eisenberg MS, Sinibaldi G, White RD. Incidence of EMS-treated out-of-hospital cardiac arrest in the United States. *Resuscitation*. 2004;63:17–24.

18. Larsen MP, Eisenberg MS, Cummins RO, Hallstrom AP. Predicting survival from out-of-hospital cardiac arrest: a graphic model. *Ann Emerg Med*. 1993;22:1652–1658.

19. The American Heart Association in collaboration with the International Liaison Committee on Resuscitation. Guidelines 2000 for cardiopulmonary resuscitation and emergency cardiovascular care, part 4: the automated external defibrillator. Key link in the chain of survival. *Circulation*. 2000;102(suppl 8):I60–76.

20. Valenzuela TD, Roe DJ, Cretin S, Spaite DW, Larsen MP. Estimating effectiveness of cardiac arrest interventions: a logistic regression survival model. *Circulation*. 1997;96:3308–3313.

21. White RD, Russell JK. Refibrillation, resuscitation and survival in out-of-hospital sudden cardiac arrest victims treated with biphasic automated external defibrillators. *Resuscitation*. 2002;55:17–23.

22. Berg MD, Clark LL, Valenzuela TD, Kern KB, Berg RA. Post-shock chest compression delays with automated external defibrillator use. *Resuscitation*. 2005;64:287–291.

23. Carpenter J, Rea TD, Murray JA, Kudenchuk PJ, Eisenberg MS. Defibrillation waveform and post-shock rhythm in out-of-hospital ventricular fibrillation cardiac arrest. *Resuscitation*. 2003;59:189–196.

24. Herlitz J, Ekstrom L, Wennerblom B, Axelsson A, Bang A, Holmberg S. Effect of bystander initiated cardiopulmonary resuscitation on ventricular fibrillation and survival after witnessed cardiac arrest outside hospital. *Br Heart J*. 1994;72:408–412.

25. Stiell I, Nichol G, Wells G, et al. Health-related quality of life is better for cardiac arrest survivors who received citizen cardiopulmonary resuscitation. *Circulation*. 2003;108:1939–1944.

26. Wik L, Kramer-Johansen J, Myklebust H, et al. Quality of cardiopulmonary resuscitation during out-of-hospital cardiac arrest. *JAMA*. 2005;293:299–304.

27. Kerber RE, Becker LB, Bourland JD, et al. Automatic external defibrillators for public access defibrillation: recommendations for specifying and reporting arrhythmia analysis algorithm performance, incorporating new waveforms, and enhancing safety. A statement for health professionals from the American Heart Association Task Force on Automatic External Defibrillation, Subcommittee on AED Safety and Efficacy. *Circulation*. 1997;95:1677–1682.

28. Gundry JW, Comess KA, DeRook FA, Jorgenson D, Bardy GH. Comparison of naive sixth-grade children with trained professionals in the use of an automated external defibrillator. *Circulation*. 1999;100:1703–1707.

29. Weisfeldt ML, Becker LB. Resuscitation after cardiac arrest: a 3-phase time-sensitive model. *JAMA*. 2002;288:3035–3038.

30. Yakaitis RW, Ewy GA, Otto CW, Taren DL, Moon TE. Influence of time and therapy on ventricular defibrillation in dogs. *Crit Care Med*. 1980;8:157–163.

31. Niemann JT, Cairns CB, Sharma J, Lewis RJ. Treatment of prolonged ventricular fibrillation. Immediate countershock versus high-dose epinephrine and CPR preceding countershock. *Circulation*. 1992;85:281–287.

32. Cobb LA, Fahrenbruch CE, Walsh TR, et al. Influence of cardiopulmonary resuscitation prior to defibrillation in patients with out-of-hospital ventricular fibrillation. *JAMA*. 1999;281:1182–1188.

33. Wik L, Hansen TB, Fylling F, et al. Delaying defibrillation to give basic cardiopulmonary resuscitation to patients with out-of-hospital ventricular fibrillation: a randomized trial. *JAMA*. 2003;289:1389–1395.

34. Vanden Hoek TL, Shao Z, Li C, Zak R, Schumacker PT, Becker LB. Reperfusion injury on cardiac myocytes after simulated ischemia. *Am J Physiol*. 1996;270(4 Pt 2):H1334–H1341.

35. Caffrey SL, Willoughby PJ, Pepe PE, Becker LB. Public use of automated external defibrillators. *N Engl J Med*. 2002;347:1242–1247.

36. Hallstrom AP, Ornato JP, Weisfeldt M, et al. Public-access defibrillation and survival after out-of-hospital cardiac arrest. *N Engl J Med*. 2004;351:637–646.

37. Page RL, Joglar JA, Kowal RC, et al. Use of automated external defibrillators by a U.S. airline. *N Engl J Med*. 2000;343:1210–1216.

38. Valenzuela TD, Roe DJ, Nichol G, Clark LL, Spaite DW, Hardman RG. Outcomes of rapid defibrillation by security officers after cardiac arrest in casinos. *N Engl J Med*. 2000;343:1206–1209.

39. Weaver WD, Hill D, Fahrenbruch CE, et al. Use of the automatic external defibrillator in the management of out-of-hospital cardiac arrest. *N Engl J Med*. 1988;319:661–666.

40. White RD, Asplin BR, Bugliosi TF, Hankins DG. High discharge survival rate after out-of-hospital ventricular fibrillation with rapid defibrillation by police and paramedics. *Ann Emerg Med*. 1996;28:480–485.

41. Myerburg RJ, Fenster J, Velez M, et al. Impact of community-wide police car deployment of automated external defibrillators on survival from out-of-hospital cardiac arrest. *Circulation*. 2002;106:1058–1064.

42. White RD, Bunch TJ, Hankins DG. Evolution of a community-wide early defibrillation programme experience over 13 years using police/fire personnel and paramedics as responders. *Resuscitation*. 2005;65:279–283.

43. Mosesso VN Jr, Davis EA, Auble TE, Paris PM, Yealy DM. Use of automated external defibrillators by police officers for treatment of out-of-hospital cardiac arrest. *Ann Emerg Med*. 1998;32:200–207.

44. Jones E, Vijan S, Fendrick AM, Deshpande S, Cram P. Automated external defibrillator deployment in high schools and senior centers. *Prehosp Emerg Care*. 2005;9:382–385.

45. Coris EE, Miller E, Sahebzamani F. Sudden cardiac death in Division I collegiate athletics: analysis of automated external defibrillator utilization in National Collegiate Athletic Association Division I athletic programs. *Clin J Sport Med*. 2005;15:87–91.

46. Drezner JA, Rogers KJ. Sudden cardiac arrest in intercollegiate athletes: detailed analysis and outcomes of resuscitation in nine cases. *Heart Rhythm*. 2006;3:755–759.

47. Maron BJ, Gohman TE, Kyle SB, Estes NA 3rd, Link MS. Clinical profile and spectrum of commotio cordis. *JAMA*. 2002;287:1142–1146.

48. Maron BJ, Wentzel DC, Zenovich AG, Estes NA 3rd, Link MS. Death in a young athlete due to commotio cordis despite prompt external defibrillation. *Heart Rhythm*. 2005;2:991–993.

49. Salib EA, Cyran SE, Cilley RE, Maron BJ, Thomas NJ. Efficacy of bystander cardiopulmonary resuscitation and out-of-hospital automated external defibrillation as life-saving therapy in commotio cordis. *J Pediatr*.

2005;147:863–866.

50. Strasburger JF, Maron BJ. Images in clinical medicine: commotio cordis. *N Engl J Med*. 2002;347:1248.

51. Berger S, Utech L, Hazinski MF. Lay rescuer automated external defibrillator programs for children and adolescents. *Pediatr Clin North Am*. 2004;51:1463–1478.

52. Maron BJ, Shen WK, Link MS, et al. Efficacy of implantable cardioverter-defibrillators for the prevention of sudden death in patients with hypertrophic cardiomyopathy. *N Engl J Med*. 2000;342:365–373.

53. Begley DA, Mohiddin SA, Tripodi D, Winkler JB, Fananapazir L. Efficacy of implantable cardioverter defibrillator therapy for primary and secondary prevention of sudden cardiac death in hypertrophic cardiomyopathy. *Pacing Clin Electrophysiol*. 2003;26:1887–1896.

54. Link MS, Maron BJ, Stickney RE, et al. Automated external defibrillator arrhythmia detection in a model of cardiac arrest due to commotio cordis. *J Cardiovasc Electrophysiol*. 2003;14:83–87.

55. Holmberg M, Holmberg S, Herlitz J. Effect of bystander cardiopulmonary resuscitation in out-of-hospital cardiac arrest patients in Sweden. *Resuscitation*. 2000;47:59–70.

56. Guideline 1c: Emergency Care and Coverage. NCAA Sports Medicine Handbook 2006-07. Available at: http://www.ncaa.org/library/sports_sciences/sports_med_handbook/2006-07/2006-07_sports_medicine_handbook.pdf. Accessed September 4, 2006.

57. Nichol G, Stiell IG, Laupacis A, Pham B, De Maio VJ, Wells GA. A cumulative meta-analysis of the effectiveness of defibrillator-capable emergency medical services for victims of out-of-hospital cardiac arrest. *Ann Emerg Med*. 1999;34(4 Pt 1):517–525.

58. Eisenberg MS, Horwood BT, Cummins RO, Reynolds-Haertle R, Hearne TR. Cardiac arrest and resuscitation: a tale of 29 cities. *Ann Emerg Med*. 1990;19:179–186.

59. Sideline preparedness for the team physician: consensus statement. *Med Sci Sports Exerc*. 2001;33:846–849.

60. Berger S, Whitstone BN, Frisbee SJ, et al. Cost-effectiveness of Project ADAM: a project to prevent sudden cardiac death in high school students. *Pediatr Cardiol*. 2004;25:660–667.

61. Rothmier JR, Drezner JA, Harmon KG. Automated external defibrillators in Washington State high schools: an assessment of emergency preparedness. *Clin J Sport Med*. 2006;16:434.

62. England H, Hoffman C, Hodgman T, et al. Effectiveness of automated external defibrillators in high schools in greater Boston. *Am J Cardiol*. 2005;95:1484–1486.

63. Sapien RE, Allen A. Emergency preparation in schools: a snapshot of a rural state. *Pediatr Emerg Care*. 2001;17:329–333.

64. Gagliardi M, Neighbors M, Spears C, Byrd S, Snarr J. Emergencies in the school setting: are public school teachers adequately trained to respond? *Prehospital Disaster Med*. 1994;9:222–225.

65. England H, Weinberg PS, Estes NA 3rd. The automated external defibrillator: clinical benefits and legal liability. *JAMA*. 2006;295:687–690.

66. International Liaison Committee on Resuscitation. 2005 International Consensus on Cardiopulmonary Resuscitation and Emergency Cardiovascular Care Science with Treatment Recommendations, part 1: introduction. *Resuscitation*. 2005;67:181–186.

67. ECC Committee, Subcommittees and Task Forces of the American Heart Association. 2005 American Heart Association guidelines for cardiopulmonary resuscitation and emergency cardiovascular care, part 3: overview of CPR. *Circulation*. 2005;112(suppl 24):IV12–18.

68. Eftestol T, Sunde K, Steen PA. Effects of interrupting precordial compressions on the calculated probability of defibrillation success during out-of-hospital cardiac arrest. *Circulation*. 2002;105:2270–2273.

69. Kern KB, Hilwig RW, Berg RA, Sanders AB, Ewy GA. Importance of continuous chest compressions during cardiopulmonary resuscitation: improved outcome during a simulated single lay-rescuer scenario. *Circulation*. 2002;105:645–649.

70. Yu T, Weil MH, Tang W, et al. Adverse outcomes of interrupted precordial compression during automated defibrillation. *Circulation*. 2002;106:368–372.

71. Roberts WO. Exercise-associated collapse in endurance events: a classification system. *Physician Sportsmed*. 1989;15(5):49–59.

72. O'Connor FG, Oriscello RG, Levine BD. Exercise-related syncope in the young athlete: reassurance, restriction or referral? *Am Fam Physician*.

1999;60:2001–2008.

73. Hauff SR, Rea TD, Culley LL, Kerry F, Becker L, Eisenberg MS. Factors impeding dispatcher-assisted telephone cardiopulmonary resuscitation. *Ann Emerg Med*. 2003;42:731–737.

74. Bergfeldt L. Differential diagnosis of cardiogenic syncope and seizure disorders. *Heart*. 2003;89:353–358.

75. Terry GC, Kyle JM, Ellis JM Jr, Cantwell J, Courson R, Medlin R. Sudden cardiac arrest in athletic medicine. *J Athl Train*. 2001;36:205–209.

76. Ruppert M, Reith MW, Widmann JH, et al. Checking for breathing: evaluation of the diagnostic capability of emergency medical services personnel, physicians, medical students, and medical laypersons. *Ann Emerg Med*. 1999;34:720–729.

77. Eberle B, Dick WF, Schneider T, Wisser G, Doetsch S, Tzanova I. Checking the carotid pulse check: diagnostic accuracy of first responders in patients with and without a pulse. *Resuscitation*. 1996;33:107–116.

78. Eftestol T, Sunde K, Ole Aase S, Husoy JH, Steen PA. Predicting outcome of defibrillation by spectral characterization and nonparametric classification of ventricular fibrillation in patients with out-of-hospital cardiac arrest. *Circulation*. 2000;102:1523–1529.

79. Eftestol T, Wik L, Sunde K, Steen PA. Effects of cardiopulmonary resuscitation on predictors of ventricular fibrillation defibrillation success during out-of-hospital cardiac arrest. *Circulation*. 2004;110:10–15.

80. Kleiner DM. Inter-Association Task Force for Appropriate Care of the Spine-Injured Athlete. Prehospital care of the spine-injured athlete: monograph summary. *Clin J Sport Med*. 2003;13:59–61.

81. Prehospital Care of the Spine-Injured Athlete: A Document from the Inter-Association Task Force for Appropriate Care of the Spine-Injured Athlete. National Athletic Trainers' Association. Available at: http://www.nata.org/statements/consensus/NATAPreHospital.pdf. Accessed September 4, 2006.

82. Weinstock J, Maron BJ, Song C, Mane PP, Estes NA 3rd, Link MS. Failure of commercially available chest wall protectors to prevent sudden cardiac death induced by chest wall blows in an experimental model of commotio cordis. *Pediatrics*. 2006;117:e656–e662.

83. Smith JE. Cooling methods used in the treatment of exertional heat illness. *Br J Sports Med*. 2005;39:503–507.

84. Fontanarosa PB. Electrical shock and lightning strike. *Ann Emerg Med*. 1993;22:378–387.

85. Roberts WO, Maron BJ. Evidence for decreasing occurrence of sudden cardiac death associated with the marathon. *J Am Coll Cardiol*. 2005;46:1373–1374.

86. Lyster T, Jorgenson D, Morgan C. The safe use of automated external defibrillators in a wet environment. *Prehosp Emerg Care*. 2003;7:307–311.

87. Gao C, Abeysekera J. A systems perspective of slip and fall accidents on icy and snowy surfaces. *Ergonomics*. 2004;47:573–598.

88. McKiernan FE. A simple gait-stabilizing device reduces outdoor falls and nonserious injurious falls in fall-prone older people during the winter. *J Am Geriatr Soc*. 2005;53:943–947.

Jonathan A. Drezner, MD, and Ron W. Courson, ATC, PT, NREMT-I, contributed to conception and design; acquisition and analysis and interpretation of the data; and drafting, critical revision, and final approval of the article. William O. Roberts, MD, FACSM; Vincent N. Mosesso, Jr, MD; Mark S. Link, MD, FACC; and Barry J. Maron, MD, FACC, contributed to acquisition and analysis and interpretation of the data; and drafting, critical revision, and final approval of the article.

Address correspondence to Jonathan A. Drezner, MD, University of Washington, 4245 Roosevelt Way NE, Box 354775, Seattle, WA 98105. Address e-mail to jdrezner@fammed.washington.edu.

Appendix. Task Force Members and Participating National Organizations

Inter-Association Task Force Members

Co-Chairs

Ron W. Courson, ATC, PT, NREMT-I
Director of Sports Medicine, University of Georgia
Jonathan A. Drezner, MD
Associate Professor and Team Physician
Department of Family Medicine, University of Washington

Invited speakers

Randy Cohen, ATC, PT
Director of C.A.T.S.
Athletic Treatment Center, University of Arizona

Bernie DePalma, ATC, PT
Assistant Director of Athletics for Sports Medicine,
Cornell University

Chuck Kimmel, ATC
President, National Athletic Trainers' Association
Austin Peay State University

David Klossner, PhD, ATC
Associate Director of Education Outreach
National Collegiate Athletic Association

Mark S. Link, MD, FACC
Director, Center for the Evaluation of Athletes
Tufts-New England Medical Center

Michael Meyer, MS, ATC
Assistant Athletic Trainer, Vanderbilt University

Tim Neal, MS, ATC
Assistant Athletic Director for Sports Medicine
Syracuse University

Robert Schriever
President, Sudden Cardiac Arrest Association

Andrew Smith, MS, ATC
Head Athletic Trainer, Canisius College

Invited participants

Glenn Henry, NREMT-P
Medical Director, Ware County Emergency Medical Services,
Waycross, GA

James Kyle, MD, FACSM
Family, Athletic, and Recreational Medicine, Ponte Vedra, FL

Barry J. Maron, MD, FACC
Director, Hypertrophic Cardiomyopathy Center
Minneapolis Heart Institute Foundation

John Payne, MD
Director, Cardiac Electrophysiology
University of Mississippi Medical Center

Fred Reifsteck, MD
Team Physician, University of Georgia

Representatives from national organizations

Jon Almquist, ATC
National Athletic Trainers' Association Secondary School Athletic Training Committee

Jeffrey Anderson, MD, *American Medical Society for Sports Medicine*

Jeffrey Bytomski, DO, *American Osteopathic Academy of Sports Medicine*

Steven Chudik, MD, *American Orthopaedic Society for Sports Medicine*

Ian Greenwald, MD, *American College of Emergency Physicians*

Michael Krauss, MD, *National Collegiate Athletic Association Competitive Safeguards Committee*

Shahram Lotfipour, MD, MPH,
American Academy of Emergency Medicine

Eugene Luckstead, Sr, MD, *American Academy of Pediatrics*

Raina Merchant, MD, *American Heart Association*

Connie Meyer, MICT
National Association of Emergency Medical Technicians

Vincent N. Mosesso, Jr, MD
National Association of Emergency Medical Service Physicians

William O. Roberts, MD, FACSM, *American College of Sports Medicine*

Johnny Scott, PhD, MD
National Federation of State High School Associations

Michele Weinstein, PT, MS, SCS, ATC
American Physical Therapy Association Sports Physical Therapy Section

Staff

Rachael Oats
Special Projects Manager, National Athletic Trainers' Association

Teresa Foster Welch, CAE
Assistant Executive Director, National Athletic Trainers' Association

Participating national organizations

American Academy of Emergency Medicine

American Academy of Pediatrics

American College of Emergency Physicians

American College of Sports Medicine

American Heart Association

American Medical Society for Sports Medicine

American Orthopedic Society for Sports Medicine

American Osteopathic Academy of Sports Medicine

American Physical Therapy Association Sports Physical Therapy Section

National Association of Emergency Medical Service Physicians

National Association of Emergency Medical Technicians

National Athletic Trainers' Association

National Collegiate Athletic Association

National Federation of State High School Associations

Sudden Cardiac Arrest Association

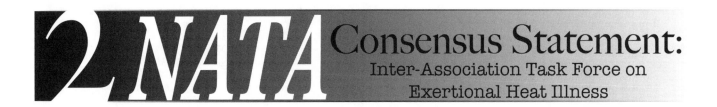

2 NATA Consensus Statement:
Inter-Association Task Force on Exertional Heat Illness

In This Section: The following statement provides suggestions for handling exertional heat illnesses. Included are tips on prevention and treatment as well as guidelines on how to handle dehydration, heat exhaustion, heat cramps and external hyponatremia.

Overall Strategies for the Prevention of Exertional Heat Illnesses

Every athletic organization should have a policy, procedure or emergency plan established to address exertional heat illnesses. A thorough plan includes the key factors to prevent, identify and treat exertional heat illnesses.

Scientific evidence indicates the following factors may increase the risk associated with exercise in the heat. Although some factors can be optimized (e.g., heat acclimatization), others cannot (e.g., health problems). Regardless, these factors may help in developing a proactive approach to preventing exertional heat illnesses.

Intrinsic factors include:
- History of exertional heat illnesses
- Inadequate heat acclimatization
- Lower level of fitness status
- Higher percent body fat
- Dehydration or overhydration
- Presence of a fever
- Presence of gastrointestinal illness
- Salt deficiency
- Skin condition (e.g., sunburn, skin rash, etc.)
- Ingestion of certain medications (e.g., antihistamines, diuretics, etc.) or dietary supplements (e.g., ephedra, etc.)
- Motivation to push oneself/warrior mentality
- Reluctance to report problems, issues, illness,
- Pre-pubescence

Extrinsic factors include:
- Intense or prolonged exercise with minimal breaks
- High temperature/humidity/sun exposure (Table 1 and Figure 1), as well as exposure to heat/humidity in preceding days
- Inappropriate work/rest ratios based on intensity, wet bulb globe temperature (WBGT), clothing, equipment, fitness and athlete's medical condition
- Lack of education and awareness of heat illnesses among coaches, athletes and medical staff
- No emergency plan to identify and treat exertional heat illnesses
- No access to shade during exercise or during rest breaks
- Duration and number of rest breaks is limited
- Minimal access to fluids before and during practice and rest breaks
- Delay in recognition of early warning signs

General Considerations for Risk Reduction
- Encourage proper education regarding heat illnesses (for athletes, coaches, parents, medical staff, etc.). Education about risk factors should focus on hydration needs, acclimatization, work/rest ratio, signs and symptoms of exertional heat illnesses, treatment, dietary supplements, nutritional issues and fitness status.
- Provide medical services onsite (e.g., certified athletic trainer [ATC], emergency medical technician [EMT], physician).
- Ensure pre-participation physical examination that includes specific questions regarding fluid intake, weight changes during activity, medication and supplement use and history of cramping/heat illnesses has been completed.
- Assure that onsite medical staff has authority to alter work/rest ratios, practice schedules, amount of equipment and withdrawal of individuals from participation based on environment and/or athlete's medical condition.

DEHYDRATION

Factors Contributing to Onset of Condition

When athletes do not replenish lost fluids, they become dehydrated. Mild dehydration (<2% body weight loss [BWL]) is often unavoidable because athletes cannot always replenish fluids at a rate equal to that being lost. Dehydration as minimal as 2% BWL can begin to hinder performance and thermoregulatory function.

Optimal hydration is the replacement of fluids and electrolytes in accordance with individual needs. Fluid intake should nearly approximate fluid losses. Athletes must personally establish and monitor fluid requirements and modify behavior to ensure optimal hydration status. Fluid intake beyond fluid needs for many hours also can be quite harmful (see Exertional Hyponatremia).

Recognition

Indicators include dry mouth, thirst, irritability, general discomfort, headache, apathy, weakness, dizziness, cramps, chills, vomiting, nausea, head or neck heat sensations, excessive fatigue and/or decreased performance.

Treatment

The following procedures are recommended if dehydration is suspected:

- Dehydrated athletes should move to a cool environment and rehydrate.
- Maintaining normal hydration (as indicated by baseline body weight) is critical to avoiding heat illnesses. If an athlete's BWL is greater than 1% to 2% within a given day or on consecutive days, that athlete should return to normal hydration status before being allowed to practice. (Remember that pre-exercise/event/participation examination body weight baseline measures may not accurately assess hydration status if post-practice body weight is being compared to a baseline that is measured in a dehydrated state. Urine specific gravity or urine color can help with this assessment if an athlete is suspected to be dehydrated at the time baseline measurements are taken.)

- Athletes should begin exercise sessions properly hydrated. Any fluid deficits should be replaced within 1 to 2 hours after exercise is complete.
- Given the nature of sweat and variability and timing of nutritional intake, hydrating with a sports drink containing carbohydrates and electrolytes (i.e., sodium and potassium) before and during exercise is optimal to replace losses and provide energy. Because athletes replace only about half of the fluid lost when drinking water, a flavored sports drink may promote an increase in the quantity of fluids consumed.
- Replacing lost sodium after exercise is best achieved by consuming food in combination with a rehydration beverage.
- Athletes should have convenient access to fluids throughout practice and be allowed to hydrate in addition to prescribed breaks. These factors can minimize dehydration and may maximize performance.
- A nauseated or vomiting athlete should seek medical attention to replace fluids via an intravenous line.

Return-to-Play Considerations

If the degree of dehydration is minor and the athlete is symptom free, continued participation is acceptable. The athlete must maintain hydration status and should receive periodic checks from onsite medical personnel.

Table 1
Wet Bulb Globe Temperature Risk Chart

WBGT	Flag Color	Level of Risk	Comments
<65°F (<18°C)	Green	Low	Risk low but still exists on the basis of risk factors
65°-73°F (18°-23°C)	Yellow	Moderate	Risk level increases as event progresses through the day
73°-82°F (23°-28°C)	Red	High	Everyone should be aware of injury potential; individuals at risk should not compete
>82°F (>28°C)	Black	Extreme or hazardous	Consider rescheduling or delaying the event until safer conditions prevail; if the event must take place, be on high alert. Take steps to reduce risk factors (e.g., more and longer rest breaks, reduced practice time, reduced exercise intensity, access to shade, minimal clothing and equipment, cold tubs at practice site, etc.).

The WBGT can be measured with a WBGT meter. The calculation for the determination of WBGT is: WBGT = .7 (Wet Bulb Temperature) + .2 (Black Globe Temperature) + .1 (Dry Bulb Temperature).

This table was originally printed in Roberts WO. Medical management and administration manual for long distance road racing. In: Brown CH, Gudjonsson B, *IAAF Medical Manual for Athletics and Road Racing Competitions: a Practical Guide.* Monaco: International Association of Athletics Federations;1998:39-75.

EXERTIONAL HEAT STROKE

Factors Contributing to Onset of Condition

Exertional heat stroke is a severe illness characterized by central nervous system (CNS) abnormalities and potentially tissue damage resulting from elevated body temperatures induced by strenuous physical exercise and increased environmental heat stress.

Recognition

The ability to rapidly and accurately assess core body temperature and CNS functioning is critical to the proper evaluation of EHS; axillary, oral and tympanic temperatures are not valid measures in individuals exercising in hot environments. Medical staff should be properly trained and equipped to assess core temperature via rectal thermometer when feasible.

Most critical criteria for determination are (1) CNS dysfunction (altered consciousness, coma, convulsions, disorientation, irrational behavior, decreased mental acuity, irritability, emotional instability, confusion, hysteria, apathy) and (2) hyperthermic (rectal temperature usually >104°F/40°C) immediately post-incident.

Other possible salient findings include (1) nausea, vomiting, diarrhea, (2) headache, dizziness, weakness, (3) hot and wet or dry skin (important to note that skin may be wet or dry at time of incident), (4) increased heart rate, decreased blood pressure, increased respiratory rate, (5) dehydration and (6) combativeness.

Treatment

Aggressive and immediate whole-body cooling is the key to optimizing treatment. The duration and degree of hyperthermia may determine adverse outcomes. If untreated, hyperthermia-induced physiological changes resulting in fatal consequences may occur within vital organ systems (e.g., muscle, heart, brain, liver, kidneys, etc.). Due to superior cooling rates, immediate whole-body cooling via cold water immersion is the best treatment for EHS and should be initiated within minutes post-incident.

Provided that adequate emergency medical care is available onsite (i.e., ATC, EMT or physician), it is recommended to cool first via cold water immersion, then transport second.

Cooling can be successfully verified by measuring rectal temperature. If onsite rapid cooling via cold water immersion is not an option or if other complications develop that would be considered life threatening (i.e., airway, breathing, circulation), immediate transport to the nearest medical facility is essential.

The following procedures are recommended if EHS is suspected:

- Immediately immerse athlete in tub of cold water (approximately 35°-58°F/1.67°-14.5°C), onsite if possible. Remove clothing/equipment. (Immersion therapy should include constant monitoring of core temperature by rectal thermistor [or thermometer].)
- If immersion is not possible, transport

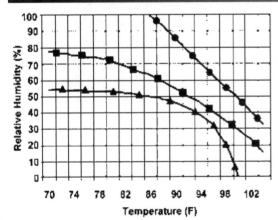

Adapted with permission from Kulka J, Kenney WL. Heat balance limits in football uniforms: how different uniform ensembles alter the equation. *Physician Sportsmed.* 2002;30(7):29-39.

Figure 1. Heat stress risk temperature and humidity graph. Heat stroke risk rises with increasing heat and relative humidity. Fluid breaks should be scheduled for all practices and scheduled more frequently as the heat stress rises. Add 5° to temperature between 10 a.m. and 4 p.m. from mid-May to mid-September on bright, sunny days. Practices should be modified for the safety of the athletes to reflect the heat stress conditions. Regular practices with full practice gear can be conducted for conditions that plot to the left of the triangles. Cancel all practices when the temperature and relative humidity plot is to the right of the circles; practices may be moved into air-conditioned spaces or held as walk through sessions with no conditioning activities.

Conditions that plot between squares and circles: use work/rest ratio with 15 to 20 minutes of activity followed by 5- to 10-minute rest and fluid breaks, practice should be in shorts only (with all protective equipment removed, if worn for activity).

Conditions that plot between triangles and squares: use work/rest ratio with 20 to 25 minutes of activity followed by 5- to 10-minute rest and fluid breaks; practice should be in shorts (with helmets and shoulder pads only, not full equipment, if worn for activity).

Conditions that plot beneath triangles (through remaining range of chart): use work/rest ratio with 25 to 30 minutes of activity followed by 5- to 10-minute rest and fluid breaks.

immediately. Alternative cooling strategies should be implemented while waiting for and during transport. These strategies could include: spraying the body with cold water, fans, ice bags or ice over as much of the body as possible and/or cold towels (replace towels frequently).

- Monitor airway, breathing, circulation, core temperature, and CNS status (cognitive, convulsions, orientation, consciousness, etc.) at all times.
- Place an intravenous line using normal saline (if appropriate medical staff is available).
- Cease aggressive cooling when core temperature reaches approximately 101°-102°F (38.3°-38.9°C); continue to monitor.
- If rapid onsite cooling was administered and rectal temperature has reached approximately 101°-102°F (38.3°-38.9°C), transport athlete to medical facility for monitoring of possible organ system damage.

Return-to-Play Considerations

Physiological changes may occur after an episode of EHS. For example, the athlete's heat tolerance may be temporarily or permanently compromised. To ensure a safe return to full participation, a careful return-to-play strategy should be decided by the athlete's physician and implemented with the assistance of the ATC or other qualified health care professional.

The following guidelines are recommended for return-to-play after EHS:

- Physician clearance is necessary before returning to exercise. The athlete should avoid all exercise until completely asymptomatic and all laboratory tests are normal.
- Severity of the incident should dictate the length of recovery time.
- The athlete should avoid exercise for the minimum of one week after release from medical care.
- The athlete should cautiously begin a gradual return to physical activity to regain peak fitness and acclimatization under the supervision of an ATC or other qualified health care professional. Type and length of exercise should be determined by the athlete's physician and might follow this pattern:

1. Easy-to-moderate exercise in a climate controlled environment for several days, followed by strenuous exercise in a climate-controlled environment for several days.

2. Easy-to-moderate exercise in heat for several days, followed by strenuous exercise in heat for several days.

3. (If applicable) Easy-to-moderate exercise in heat with equipment for several days, followed by strenuous exercise in heat with equipment for several days.

HEAT EXHAUSTION

Factors Contributing to Onset of Condition

Heat exhaustion is a moderate illness characterized by the inability to sustain adequate cardiac output, resulting from strenuous physical exercise and environmental heat stress.

Inherent needs to maintain blood pressure and essential organ function, combined with a loss of fluid due to acute dehydration, create a challenge the body cannot meet, especially if intense exercise were to continue unabated.

Recognition

Most critical criteria for determination are (1) athlete has obvious difficulty continuing intense exercise in heat, (2) lack of severe hyperthermia (usually <104°F/40°C), although it would be expected to find mild hyperthermia at the time of the incident (more commonly, 100°-103°F/37.7°-39.4°C) and (3) lack of severe CNS dysfunction. If any CNS dysfunction (see symptoms listed under EHS) is present, it will be mild and symptoms will subside quickly with treatment and as activity is discontinued.

Other possible salient findings include (1) physical fatigue, (2) dehydration and/or electrolyte depletion, (3) ataxia and coordination problems, syncope, dizziness, (4) profuse sweating, pallor, (5) headache, nausea, vomiting, diarrhea, (6) stomach/intestinal cramps, persistent muscle cramps and (7) rapid recovery with treatment.

Treatment

The following procedures are recommended if heat exhaustion is suspected:

- Remove athlete from play and immediately move to a shaded or air-conditioned area.
- Remove excess clothing and equipment.
- Cool athlete until rectal temperature is approximately 101°F (38.3°C).

- Have athlete lie comfortably with legs propped above heart level.
- If athlete is not nauseated, vomiting or experiencing any CNS dysfunction, rehydrate orally with chilled water or sports drink. If athlete is unable to take oral fluids, implement intravenous infusion of normal saline.
- Monitor heart rate, blood pressure, respiratory rate, rectal temperature and CNS status.
- Transport to an emergency facility if rapid improvement is not noted with prescribed treatment.

Return-to-Play Considerations

The following guidelines are recommended for return-to-play after heat exhaustion:
- Athlete should be symptom free and fully hydrated.
- Recommend physician clearance or, at minimum, a discussion with supervising physician before return.
- Rule out underlying condition or illness that predisposed athlete for continued problems.
- Avoid intense practice in heat until at least the next day to ensure recovery from fatigue and dehydration. (In severe cases, intense practice in heat should be delayed for more than 1 day.)
- If underlying cause was lack of acclimatization and/or fitness level, correct this problem before athlete returns to full-intensity training in heat (especially in sports with equipment).

HEAT CRAMPS

Factors Contributing to Onset of Condition

The etiology of muscle cramps is not well understood and there may be a number of causes. Heat cramps are often present in athletes who perform strenuous exercise in the heat. Conversely, cramps also occur in the absence of warm or hot conditions (e.g., common in ice hockey players).

Whether or not heat related, cramps tend to occur later in an activity, in conjunction with muscle fatigue and after fluid and electrolyte imbalances have reached a critical level.

Dehydration, diet poor in minerals, and large losses of sodium and other electrolytes in sweat appear to increase the risk of severe, often whole-body, muscle cramps. Muscle cramps can largely be avoided with adequate conditioning, acclimatization, rehydration, electrolyte replacement and appropriate dietary practices.

Table 2

Sample Sweat Rate Calculation*

A	B	C	D	E	F	G	H	I	J
		Before Exercise	After Exercise	Change in BW (C-D)			Sweat Loss (E+F-G)	Exercise Time	Sweat Rate (H/I)
Name	Date	kg	kg	g	Drink Volume mL	Urine Volume † mL	mL	min	mL/min
		(lb/2.2)	(lb/2.2)	(kg x 1000)	(oz x 30)	(oz x 30)	(oz x 30)	h	mL/h
		kg	kg	g	mL	mL	mL	min	mL/min
		(lb/2.2)	(lb/2.2)	(kg x 1000)	(oz x 30)	(oz x 30)	(oz x 30)	h	mL/h
		kg	kg	g	mL	mL	mL	min	mL/min
		(lb/2.2)	(lb/2.2)	(kg x 1000)	(oz x 30)	(oz x 30)	(oz x 30)	h	mL/h
		kg	kg	g	mL	mL	mL	min	mL/min
		(lb/2.2)	(lb/2.2)	(kg x 1000)	(oz x 30)	(oz x 30)	(oz x 30)	h	mL/h
Kelly K. ‡	9/15	61.7 kg	60.3 kg	1400 g	420 mL	90 mL	1730 mL	90 min	19 mL/min
		(lb/2.2)	(lb/2.2)	(kg x 1000)	(oz x 30)	(oz x 30)	(oz x 30)	1.5 h	1153 mL/h

* Reprinted with permission from Murray R. Determining sweat rate. *Sports Sci Exch.* 1996; 9 (Suppl 63).
† Weight of urine should be subtracted *if urine was excreted prior to post-exercise body weight.*
‡ In the example, Kelly K. should drink about 1 L (32 oz.) of fluid during each hour of activity to remain well hydrated.

Formula for Calculating Sweat Rate

When calculating an athlete's sweat rate (sweat rate = pre-exercise body weight - post-exercise body weight + fluid intake - urine volume/exercise time in hours), do so for a representative range of environmental conditions, practices and competitions.

The simplest way to get athletes to focus on their hydration needs is to teach them to compare pre-exercise and post-exercise body weights. If the athletes lost weight, they need to drink more at the next practice; if they gained weight, they should drink less. This gives the athletes immediate feedback about their drinking habits.

Recognition

Most critical criteria for determination are (1) intense pain (not associated with acute muscle strain) and (2) persistent muscle contractions in working muscles during and after prolonged exercise and most often associated with exercise in heat.

Other possible salient findings include (1) "salty sweaters" (those with high salt concentration in sweat), (2) high sweat rate, heavy sweating, (3) lack of heat acclimatization, (4) insufficient sodium intake (during meals and practice), (5) dehydration, thirsty, (6) irregular meals, (7) increased fatigue and (8) previous cramping history.

Treatment

The following procedures are recommended if heat cramps are suspected:

* Re-establish normal hydration status and replace some sodium losses with a sports drink or other sodium source.
* Some additional sodium may be needed (especially in those with a history of heat cramps) earlier in the activity (pre-cramps) and is best administered by dilution into sports drink. For example, 1/2 g of sodium (equal to the amount of sodium found in 1/4 tsp of table salt) dissolved in about 1 L (approximately 32 oz) of a sports drink early in the exercise session provides ample fluids and sodium, and the flavor (while certainly saltier) is still very palatable.
* Light stretching, relaxation and massage of the involved muscle may help acute pain of a muscle cramp.

Return-to-Play Considerations

Athletes should be assessed to determine if they can perform at the level needed for successful participation. After an acute episode, diet, rehydration practices, electrolyte consumption, fitness status, level of acclimatization and use of dietary supplements should be reviewed and possibly modified to decrease risk of recurring heat cramps.

EXERTIONAL HYPONATREMIA

Factors Contributing to Onset of Condition
When an athlete consumes more fluids (especially water) than necessary, and/or sodium lost in sweat is not adequately replaced, sodium in the bloodstream can become diluted and cause cerebral and/or pulmonary edema. This is called hyponatremia (low blood-sodium levels) and tends to occur during warm/hot weather activities.

The risk of acquiring hyponatremia can be substantially reduced if fluid consumption during activity does not exceed fluid losses and sodium is adequately replaced.

Because progressive dehydration may also compromise thermoregulatory function, it is of great value for an athlete to be aware of individual fluid needs to protect against both dehydration and overhydration.

Fluid needs can be determined by establishing an athlete's "sweat rate" (liters per hour) or the amount of fluid lost in a given length of time (usually discussed in an amount per hour) during a given intensity of activity, while wearing a given amount of clothing/equipment, for a given set of environmental conditions (Table 2). Variations can exist in sweat rates, so individual assessments can be quite helpful (especially in at-risk individuals). When establishing fluid needs, it is best to mimic the same conditions of the athletic event to establish an accurate sweat rate.

Recognition

Most critical criteria for determination are (1) low bloodsodium levels (<130 mmol/L). Severity of condition increases as sodium levels decrease, (2) likelihood of excessive fluid consumption before, during and after exercise (weight gain during activity), (3) low sodium intake, (4) likelihood of sodium deficits before, during and after exercise and (5) if condition progresses, CNS changes (e.g., altered consciousness, confusion, coma, convulsions, altered cognitive functioning) and respiratory changes resulting from cerebral and/or pulmonary edema, respectively.

Other possible salient findings include (1) increasing headache, (2) nausea, vomiting (often repetitive), (3) swelling of extremities (hands and feet), (4) irregular diet (e.g., inadequate sodium intake), (5) during prolonged activity (often lasting >4 hours), (6) copious urine with low specific gravity following exercise, (7) lethargy/apathy, (8) agitation and (9) absence of severe hyperthermia (most commonly <104°F/40°C).

Treatment

The following procedures are recommended if exertional hyponatremia is suspected:

- If blood sodium levels cannot be determined onsite, hold off on rehydrating athlete (may worsen condition) and transport immediately to a medical facility.
- The delivery of sodium, certain diuretics or intravenous solutions may be necessary. All will be monitored in the emergency department to ensure no complications develop.

Return-to-Play Considerations

The following guidelines are recommended for return-to-play after exertional hyponatremia:

- Physician clearance is strongly recommended in all cases.
- In mild cases, activity can resume a few days after completing an educational session on establishing an individual-specific hydration protocol. This will ensure the proper amount and type of beverages and meals are consumed before, during and after physical activity (see Table 2).

EXPERT PANEL

Oded Bar-Or, MD, FACEP
American Academy of Pediatrics

Stephen Cantrill, MD, FACEP
American College of Emergency Physicians

W. Larry Kenney, PhD, FACSM
American College of Sports Medicine

Suzanne Nelson Steen, DSc, RD
American Dietetic Association

Kim Fagan, MD
American Medical Society for Sports Medicine

Rick Wilkerson, DO, FAAOS
American Orthopaedic Society for Sports Medicine

Phillip Zinni III, DO, FAOASM, ATC
American Osteopathic Academy of Sports Medicine

Michael N. Sawka, PhD, FACSM
American Physiological Society

C. Dexter (Bo) Kimsey, Jr, PhD, MSEH
CDC- Nutrition and Physical Activity

John W. Gardner, MD, DrPH;COL,MC,FS,USA
Department of Defense Health Affairs

Bob Murray, PhD
Gatorade Sports Science Institute

Bareket Falk, PhD
North American Society for Pediatric Exercise Medicine

Christine Bolger
National Association of Sport and Physical Education/AAHPERD

Douglas J. Casa, PhD, ATC, FACSM, Chair
Jon Almquist, ATC
Scott Anderson, ATC
Michelle A. Cleary, PhD, ATC
Ron Courson, ATC, PT, NREMT-1, CSCS
Robert L. Howard, MA, ATC
Michelle Ryan, ATC, PT
Chris Troyanos, ATC
Katie Walsh, EdD, ATC
National Athletic Trainers' Association

Maria Dastur, MBA, ATC
National SAFE KIDS Campaign

Michael Barnes, MEd, CSCS*D, NSCA-CPT
National Strength and Conditioning Association

Terrence Lee, MPH
U.S. Army Center for Health Promotion and Preventative Medicine

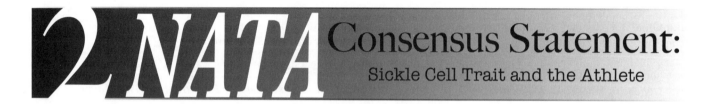

2 NATA Consensus Statement:
Sickle Cell Trait and the Athlete

In This Section: **The following statement describes how sickle cell trait impacts athletes. It explains necessary precautions and the treatment that should be taken in the event of a sickling collapse.**

Consensus Statement *NATA*

Sickle Cell Trait and the Athlete

Introduction

Sickle cell trait is the inheritance of one gene for sickle hemoglobin and one for normal hemoglobin. During intense or extensive exertion, the sickle hemoglobin can change the shape of red cells from round to quarter-moon, or "sickle." This change, exertional sickling, can pose a grave risk for some athletes. In the past seven years, exertional sickling has killed nine athletes, ages 12 through 19.

Research shows how and why sickle red cells can accumulate in the bloodstream during intense exercise. Sickle cells can "logjam" blood vessels and lead to collapse from ischemic rhabdomyolysis, the rapid breakdown of muscles starved of blood. Major metabolic problems from explosive rhabdomyolysis can threaten life. Sickling can begin in 2-3 minutes of any all-out exertion – and can reach grave levels soon thereafter if the athlete continues to struggle. Heat, dehydration, altitude, and asthma can increase the risk for and worsen sickling, even when exercise is not all-out. Despite telltale features, collapse from exertional sickling in athletes is under-recognized and often misdiagnosed. Sickling collapse is a medical emergency.

We recommend confirming sickle cell trait status in all athletes' pre-participation physical examinations. As all 50 states screen at birth, this marker is a base element of personal health information that should be made readily available to the athlete, the athlete's parents, and the athlete's healthcare provider, including those providers responsible for determination of medical eligibility for participation in sports.

Knowledge of sickle cell trait status can be a gateway to education and simple precautions that may prevent sickling collapse and enable athletes with sickle cell trait to thrive in sport. Nearly all of the 13 deaths in college football have been at institutions that did not screen for sickle cell trait or had a lapse in precautions for it. Small numbers preclude cogent evidence to support screening. All considered, however, we believe that each institution should carefully weigh the decision to screen based on the potential to provide key clinical information and targeted education that can save lives. Irrespective of screening, the institution should educate staff, coaches, and athletes on the potentially lethal nature of this condition.

Background

A condition of inheritance versus race, the sickle gene is common in people whose origin is from areas where malaria is widespread. Over the millennia, carrying one sickle gene fended off death from malaria, leaving one in 12 African-Americans (versus one in 2,000 to one in 10,000 white Americans) with sickle cell trait. The sickle gene is also present in those of Mediterranean, Middle Eastern, Indian, Caribbean and South and Central American ancestry; hence, the required screening of all newborns in the United States.

In the past four decades, exertional sickling has killed at least 15 football players. In the past seven years alone, sickling has killed nine athletes: five college football players in training, two high school athletes (one a 14-year-old female basketball player), and two 12-year-old boys training for football. Of 136 sudden, non-traumatic sports deaths in high school and college athletes over a decade, seven (5%) were from exertional sickling[1].

The U. S. military tied sickle cell trait to sudden death during recruit basic training. The relative risk of exercise-related death in sickle cell trait was about 30[2]. In other words, recruits with sickle cell trait were 30 times more likely to die during basic training. The main cause of death was rhabdomyolysis – and the risk of exertional rhabdomyolysis was about 200 times greater for those with sickle cell trait[3].

In sickle cell trait, strenuous exercise evokes four forces that in concert foster sickling, 1) severe hypoxemia, 2) metabolic acidosis 3) hyperthermia in muscles, and 4) red-cell dehydration. Evidence supports this syndrome. Military research shows that, during intense exertion and hypoxemia, sickle cells can accumulate in the blood[4]. Recent research also shows that systemic dehydration worsens exertional sickling[5]. Field studies in Africa suggest that sickle-trait runners are limited not in single sprints but in middle distance or altitude running[6]. The pattern in American athletes is similar.

Sickling Collapse: Football and Other Sports

The first known sickling death in college football was in 1974. A defensive back from Florida ran a conditioning test on the first day of practice at altitude in Colorado. He had collapsed on the first day of practice the year before.

This time, near the end of the first long sprint, at about 700 meters, he collapsed again – and died the next day. The most recent sickling death, a freshman defensive back at Rice University in the fall of 2006, is similar. He collapsed after running 16 sprints of 100 yards each – and died the next morning. The cause of death for both athletes was acute exertional rhabdomyolysis associated with sickle cell trait.

Up to 13 college football players have died after a sickling collapse. The setting and syndrome in most are similar:

- Sickling players may be on-field only briefly, sprinting only 800-1,600 meters, often early in the season.

- Sickling can also occur during repetitive running of hills or stadium steps, during intense sustained strength training, if the tempo increases late in intense one-hour drills, or at the end of practice when players run "gassers."

- Sickling can even occur rarely in the game, as when a running back is in constant action during a long, frantic drive downfield[7].

Sickling collapse is not limited to football. It has occurred in distance racing and has killed or nearly killed several college or high school basketball players (two were females) in training, typically during "suicide sprints" on the court, laps on a track, or a long training run.

The harder and faster athletes go, the earlier and greater the sickling, which likely explains why exertional collapse occurs "sooner" in college football players sprinting than in military recruits running longer distances. Sickling can begin in only 2-3 minutes of sprinting – or in any other all-out exertion – and sickling can quickly increase to grave levels if the stricken athlete struggles on or is urged on by the coach.

Sickling Collapse: Telltale Features

Sickling collapse has been mistaken for cardiac collapse or heat collapse. But unlike sickling collapse, cardiac collapse tends to be "instantaneous," has no "cramping" with it, and the athlete (with ventricular fibrillation) who hits the ground no longer talks. Unlike heat collapse, sickling collapse often occurs within the first half hour onfield, as during initial windsprints. Core temperature is not greatly elevated.

Sickling is often confused with heat cramping; but, athletes who have had both syndromes know the difference, as indicated by the following distinctions:**1)** Heat cramping often has a prodrome of muscle twinges; whereas, sickling has none;
2) The pain is different – heat-cramping pain is more excruciating;
3) What stops the athlete is different – heat crampers hobble to a halt with "locked-up" muscles, while sickling players slump to the ground with weak muscles;
4) Physical findings are different – heat crampers writhe and yell in pain, with muscles visibly contracted and rock-hard; whereas, sicklers lie fairly still, not yelling in pain, with muscles that look and feel normal;
5) The response is different – sickling players caught early and treated right recover faster than players with major heat cramping[7].

This is not to say that all athletes who sickle present exactly the same way. How they react differs, including some stoic players who just stop, saying "I can't go on." As the player rests, sickle red cells regain oxygen in the lungs and most then revert to normal shape, and the athlete soon feels good again and ready to continue. This self-limiting feature surely saves lives.

Precautions and Treatment

No sickle-trait athlete is ever disqualified, because simple precautions seem to suffice. For the athlete with sickle cell trait, the following guidelines should be adhered to:
1) Build up slowly in training with paced progressions, allowing longer periods of rest and recovery between repetitions.
2) Encourage participation in preseason strength and conditioning programs to enhance the preparedness of athletes for performance testing which should be

sports-specific. Athletes with sickle cell trait should be excluded from participation in performance tests such as mile runs, serial sprints, etc., as several deaths have occurred from participation in this setting.

3) Cessation of activity with onset of symptoms [muscle 'cramping', pain, swelling, weakness, tenderness; inability to "catch breath", fatigue].

4) If sickle-trait athletes can set their own pace, they seem to do fine.

5) All athletes should participate in a year-round, periodized strength and conditioning program that is consistent with individual needs, goals, abilities and sport-specific demands. Athletes with sickle cell trait who perform repetitive high speed sprints and/or interval training that induces high levels of lactic acid should be allowed extended recovery between repetitions since this type of conditioning poses special risk to these athletes.

6) Ambient heat stress, dehydration, asthma, illness, and altitude predispose the athlete with sickle trait to an onset of crisis in physical exertion.

    a. Adjust work/rest cycles for environmental heat stress

    b. Emphasize hydration

    c. Control asthma

    d. No workout if an athlete with sickle trait is ill

    e. Watch closely the athlete with sickle cell trait who is new to altitude. Modify training and have supplemental oxygen available for competitions

7) Educate to create an environment that encourages athletes with sickle cell trait to report any symptoms immediately; any signs or symptoms such as fatigue, difficulty breathing, leg or low back pain, or leg or low back cramping in an athlete with sickle cell trait should be assumed to be sickling[7].

    In the event of a sickling collapse, treat it as a medical emergency by doing the following:

    1) Check vital signs.

    2) Administer high-flow oxygen, 15l pm (if available), with a non-rebreather face mask.

    3) Cool the athlete, if necessary.

    4) If the athlete is obtunded or as vital signs decline, call 911, attach an AED, start an IV, and get the athlete to the hospital fast.

    5) Tell the doctors to expect explosive rhabdomyolysis and grave metabolic complications.

    6) Proactively prepare by having an Emergency Action Plan and appropriate emergency equipment for all practices and competitions.

Immediate action can save lives.

What We Can Do

Though screening is done at birth; many athletes do not know their sickle-trait status, rendering self-report in a questionnaire unreliable. Many institutions have employed screening strategies to rectify this. A recent survey of NCAA Division I-A schools found that 64% (of respondents) screen[8]. The NFL Scouting Combine screens for sickle cell trait. All considered, despite no evidence-based proof yet that screening saves lives, each institution should carefully weigh the decision to screen in the absence of documented newborn screen results.

The Consensus of this Task Force is:

1) There is no contraindication to participation in sport for the athlete with sickle cell trait.

2) Red blood cells can sickle during intense exertion, blocking blood vessels and posing a grave risk for athletes with sickle cell trait.

3) Screening and simple precautions may prevent deaths and help athletes with sickle cell trait thrive in their sport.

4) Efforts to document newborn screening results should be made during the PPE.

5) In the absence of newborn screening results, institutions should carefully weigh the decision to screen based on the potential to provide key clinical information and targeted education that may save lives.

6) Irrespective of screening, institutions should educate staff, coaches, and athletes on the potentially lethal nature of this condition.

7) Education and precautions work best when targeted at those athletes who need it most; therefore, institutions should carefully weigh this factor in deciding whether to screen. All told, the case for screening is strong.

GLOSSARY

Acute Ischemic rhabdomyolysis: the rapid breakdown of muscle tissue starved of blood

Acute Rhabdomyolysis: a serious and potentially fatal condition involving the breakdown of skeletal muscle fibers resulting in the release of muscle fiber contents into the circulation

Contraindication: circumstance or condition that

makes participation unsafe or inappropriate

Exertional rhabdomyolysis: muscle breakdown triggered by physical activity

Exertional sickling: hemoglobin [red blood cell] sickling due to intense or sustained physical exertion

Hyperthermia: body temperature elevated above the normal range

Hypoxemia: decreased oxygen content of arterial blood

Ischemia: a deficiency of blood flow to tissue

Metabolic acidosis: a condition in which the pH of the blood is too acidic because of the production of certain types of acids

Nontraumatic: not related to a physical injury caused by an external force

Obtunded: having diminished arousal and awareness; mentally dull

Sickling collapse: the collapse of an athlete who shows features consistent with exertional sickling

Ventricular Fibrillation: a condition in which there is uncoordinated contraction of the cardiac muscle of the ventricles in the heart

REFERENCES

1. Van Camp SP, Bloor CM, Mueller FO, Cantu RC, Olson HG. Nontraumatic sports death in high school and college athletes. *Med Sci Sports Exerc*. 1995;27:641-647.

2. Kark JA, Ward FT. Exercise and hemoglobin S. *Semin in Hematol*. 1994;31:181-225.

3. Gardner JW, Kark JA. Fatal rhabdomyolysis presenting as mild heat illness in military training. *Milit. Med*. 1994;159:160-163.

4. Martin TW, Weisman IM, Zeballos RJ, Stephenson RS. Exercise and hypoxia increase sickling in venous blood from an exercising limb in individuals with sickle cell trait. *Am J Med*. 1989;87:48-56.

5. Bergeron MF, Cannon JG, Hall EL, Kutlar A. Erythrocyte sickling during exercise and thermal stress. *Clin J Sport Med*. 2004;14:354-356.

6. Marlin L, Etienne-Julan M, Le Gallais D, Hue O. Sickle cell trait in French West Indian elite sprint athletes. *Int J Sports Med*. 2005;26:622-625.

7. Eichner ER. Sickle cell trait. *J Sport Rehab*, 2007 (May), in press.

8. Clarke CE, Paul S, Stilson M, Senf J. Sickle cell trait preparticipation screening practices of collegiate physicians. *Clin J Sport Med* 2006;16:440a.

TASK FORCE PARTICIPANTS

The following individuals and associations were members of the Inter-Association Task Force on Sickle Cell Trait and the Athlete. Their participation is not an endorsement of this document.

Co-Chairs
Scott Anderson, ATC
E. Randy Eichner, MD

At-Large Members:
Mary L. Anzalone, MD
James C. Puffer MD
Brock Schnebel, MD

American Academy of Pediatrics
Jorge Gomez, MD

American College of Sports Medicine
Michael F. Bergeron, PhD, FACSM
Don Porter, MD

American Medical Society for Sports Medicine
James Moriarity, MD

American Orthopaedic Society for Sports Medicine
James C. Walter, II, MD

American Osteopathic Academy of Sports Medicine
Jeffrey Bytomski, DO
Angela Cavanna, DO, FAOASM

Association of Black Cardiologists
B. Waine Kong, PhD, JD

College of American Pathologists
Michael J. Dobersen, MD, PhD

Gatorade Sports Science Institute
Jeff Kearney
Craig Horswill, PhD
Magie Lacambra, MEd, ATC

Military Medicine
Fred Brennan, Jr., DO

National Association of Basketball Coaches
Reggie Minton

National Association of EMTs
Connie Meyer, MICT

National Association of Medical Examiners
Jeffery Barnard, MD

National Athletic Trainers' Association
Veronica Ampey, MS, ATC
Douglas Casa, PhD, ATC, FACSM
Terry Dewitt, PhD, ATC
Scott Galloway, ATC, LAT
Chris A. Gillespie, MEd, ATC, LAT
Eric Howard, EdD, MS, ATC
Bob Toth, MS, ATC
Torrance Williams, ATC, LAT

National Basketball Athletic Trainers' Association
Dionne Calhoun, ATC
National Collegiate Athletics Association
David Klossner, PhD, ATC
John W. Scott, PhD, MD
Tracy Ray, MD

National Federation of State High School Associations
Bob Colgate

National Football League
Gary W. Dorshimer, MD, FACP

National Strength and Conditioning Association
Avery Faigenbaum, EdD, CSCS

Professional Football Athletic Trainers' Society
Corey Oshikoya, ATC

The Sickle Cell Disease Association of America, Inc.
National Medical Association
Betty S. Pace, MD

The Sickle Cell Foundation of Georgia, Inc.
Rudolph Jackson, MD

Women's Basketball Coaches Association
Marsha Sharp

3 NATA Official Statements:

1. Automated External Defibrillators
2. Commotio Cordis
3. Communicable and Infectious Diseases in Secondary School Sports
4. Community-Aquired MRSA Infections
5. On-Site Athletic Trainer Coverage for Secondary Schools
6. Steroids and Performance Enhancing Drugs
7. Use of Qualified Athletic Trainers in Secondary Schools
8. Youth Football and Heat Related Illness

Official Statement *NATA*

Statement

The National Athletic Trainers' Association (NATA), as a leader in health care for the physically active, strongly believes that the treatment of sudden cardiac arrest is a priority. An AED program should be part of an athletic trainers emergency action plan. NATA strongly encourages athletic trainers, in every work setting, to have access to an AED.

Athletic trainers are encouraged to make an AED part of their standard emergency equipment. In addition, in conjunction and coordination with local EMS, athletic trainers should take a primary role in implementing a comprehensive AED program within their work setting.

Rationale

According to the American Heart Association (AHA), each year, approximately 250,000 Americans die of sudden cardiac arrest (SCA) outside of the hospital.[1] As many as 7,000 children die of SCA each year.[2] Evidence suggests that the risk of a cardiac event is higher during or immediately following, vigorous exercise. Cardiopulmonary resuscitation (CPR) is critical to maintaining the supply of oxygen to vital organs, but the single most effective treatment for cardiac arrest is defibrillation, a shock delivered to the heart using a small electronic device known as a defibrillator. The AHA recommends defibrillation within 3-5 minutes or sooner.[1]

Most communities cannot meet these guidelines. As a result, nationwide, survival from SCA is only about 5%. In some communities where shocks from an AED and CPR are provided within 3-5 minutes by the first person on the scene, survival rates are as high as 48-74%.[1]

REFERENCES

1. American Heart Association, 2003. Heart Disease and Stroke Statistics – 2003 Update

2. Berger, S.,Dhalia, A.,Freidberg,D.Z.1999. Sudden cardiac arrest death in infants, children and adolescents. *Pediatric Clinics of North America*, 46(2):221-34

Official Statement *NATA*
Commotio Cordis

Statement

According to the U.S. Commotio Cordis Registry, since 1995, 188 athletes have died from blunt force injury to the heart (commotio cordis). Of those 188 fatalities, the mean age was 14.7 years and 96% were male athletes according to the Heart Center at TUFTS New England Medical Center. In an effort to educate the public about the potential risks physically active youth can face, the National Athletic Trainers' Association (NATA) recommends that parents and coaches take proactive steps to protect their athletes against commotio cordis.

Commotio cordis is caused by a blow to the chest (directly over the left ventricle of the heart) that occurs at a certain point of a person's heart beat. The blunt force causes a lethal abnormal heart rhythm called ventricular fibrillation. The force of the blow to the chest is common at speeds of 35-40 mph.

The following suggestions can help prevent commotio cordis and keep young athletes safe:

1. Educate coaches, parents, officials, and players in the recognition of the mechanism and the signs and symptoms of commotio cordis.
2. Encourage all coaches and officials to become trained in cardiopulmonary resuscitation (CPR), automatic external defibrillator (AED) use, and first aid.
3. Proper placement and access of automatic external defibrillator (AED) units at athletic facilities.
4. Educate coaches and officials of the need for immediate CPR and AED care. The longer the delay, the greater likelihood that death may occur.
5. Establish an emergency action plan at all athletic venues. Parents, coaches, and officials should be involved in these plans.
6. Use of sport specific chest protectors during practices and games. At this time the NATA recommends continued research in this area because current information is limited and not proven to prevent commotio cordis. However, use of properly fitted, quality chest protectors is recommended to reduce the risk of traumatic chest injury to the athlete.
7. Ensure all athletic protective equipment fits properly and is used as intended by the manufacturer. Require that all protective equipment meet all appropriate standards of governing bodies such as NOCSAE, ASTM, HECC, and PECC.
8. Teach athletes how to protect themselves and avoid being hit in the chest by projectiles such as baseball, lacrosse balls, and hockey pucks. Do not have athletes step in front of a shot to block it.
9. Encourage youth baseball and ice hockey organizations to utilize softer baseballs and pucks. Support research into modified lacrosse balls for youth play.
10. Maintain an even and clean playing surface (field) for all athletes.

REFERENCES

1. Abrunzo TJ. Commotio cordis. The single, most common cause of traumatic death in youth baseball. Am J Dis Child. 1991 Nov;145(11):1279-82. Review. PMID 1951221

2. Cannon L. Behind armour blunt trauma--an emerging problem. J R Army Med Corps. 2001 Feb;147(1):87-96. Review. PMID 11307682

3. Cooper PJ, Epstein A, Macleod IA, Schaaf ST, Sheldon J, Boulin C, Kohl P. Soft tissue impact characterisation kit (STICK) for ex situ investigation of heart rhythm responses to acute mechanical stimulation. Prog Biophys Mol Biol. 2006 Jan-Apr;90(1-3):444-68. Review. PMID 16125216

4. Geddes LA, Roeder RA. Evolution of our knowledge of sudden death due to commotio cordis. Am J Emerg Med. 2005 Jan; 23(1):67-75. Review. PMID 15672341

5. Kohl P, Nesbitt AD, Cooper PJ, Lei M. Sudden cardiac death by Commotio cordis: role of mechano-electric feedback. *Cardiovasc Res*. 2001 May; 50(2):280-9. Review. PMID 11334832

6. Link MS, Maron BJ, Wang PJ, et al. Reduced risk of sudden death from chest wall blows (commotio cordis) with safety baseballs. Pediatrics. 2002; 109: 873-77

7. Maron BJ, Mitten MJ, Greene Burnett C. Criminal consequences of commotio cordis. *Am J* Cardiol. 2002 Jan 15; 89(2):210-3. Review. PMID 11792344

8. Salib EA, Cyran SE, Cilley RE, Maron BJ, Thomas NJ. Efficacy of bystander cardiopulmonary resuscitation and out-of-hospital automated external defibrillation as life-saving therapy in commotio cordis. J Pediatr. 2005 Dec; 147(6):863-6. Review. PMID 16356450

RESOURCES

Acompora Foundation: www.la12.org

U.S. National Registry for Sudden Death in Athletes: www.suddendeathathletes.org

Tufts – New England Medical Center: www.tufts-nemc.org/medicine/card/commotiocordis.htsm

National Center for Early Defibrillation: www.early-defib.org

Moms Team: www.momsteam.com

Statement

The National Athletic Trainers' Association (NATA) recommends that health care professionals and participants in secondary school athletics take the proper precautions to prevent the spread of communicable and infectious diseases.

Due to the nature of competitive sports at the high school level, there is increased risk for the spread of infectious diseases, such as impetigo, community acquired methicillin-resistant staphylococcus infection (MRSA) and herpes gladiatorum (a form of herpes virus that causes lesions on the head, neck and shoulders). These diseases are spread by skin-to-skin contact and infected equipment shared by athletes, generally causing lesions of the skin.

The following are suggestions from NATA to prevent the spread of infectious and communicable diseases:

1. Immediately shower after practice or competition.
2. Wash all athletic clothing worn during practice or competition daily.
3. Clean and disinfect gym bags and/or travel bags if the athlete is carrying dirty workout gear home to be washed and then bringing clean gear back to school in the same bag. This problem can also be prevented by using disposable bags for practice laundry.
4. Wash athletic gear (such as knee or elbow pads) periodically and hang to dry.
5. Clean and disinfect protective equipment such as helmets, shoulder pads, catcher's equipment and hockey goalie equipment on a regular basis.
6. Do not share towels or personal hygiene products with others.
7. All skin lesions should be covered before practice or competition to prevent risk of infection to the wound and transmission of illness to other participants. Only skin infections that have been properly diagnosed and treated may be covered to allow participation of any kind
8. All new skin lesions occurring during practice or competition should be properly diagnosed and treated immediately.
9. Playing fields should be inspected regularly for animal droppings that could cause bacterial infections of cuts or abrasions.
10. Athletic lockers should be sanitized between seasons.
11. Rather than carpeting, locker or dressing rooms should have tile floors that may be cleaned and sanitized.
12. Weight room equipment, including benches, bars and handles should be cleaned and sanitized daily.

Official Statement *NATA*

Community Acquired Methicillin-Resistant Staphylococcus Infection (MRSA)

Statement

In an effort to educate the public about the potential risks of the emergence of community acquired methicillin-resistant staphylococcus infection (CA-MRSA), the National Athletic Trainers' Association (NATA) recommends that health care personnel and physically active participants take appropriate precautions with suspicious lesions and talk with a physician.

According to the Centers for Disease Control and Prevention (CDC), approximately 25% to 30% of the population is colonized in the nose with Staphylococcus aureus, often referred to as "staph" and approximately 1% of the population is colonized with MRSA[1].

Cases have developed from person-to-person contact, shared towels, soaps, improperly treated whirlpools, and equipment (mats, pads, surfaces, etc). Staph or CA-MRSA infections usually manifest as skin infections, such as pimples, pustules and boils, which present as red, swollen, painful, or have pus or other drainage. Without proper referral and care, more serious infections may cause pneumonia, bloodstream infections, or surgical wound infections.

Maintaining good hygiene and avoiding contact with drainage from skin lesions are the best methods for prevention.

Proper prevention and management recommendations may include, but are not limited to:

1. Keep hands clean by washing thoroughly with soap and warm water or using an alcohol-based hand sanitizer routinely.
2. Encourage immediate showering following activity.
3. Avoid whirlpools or common tubs with open wounds, scrapes or scratches.
4. Avoid sharing towels, razors, and daily athletic gear.
5. Properly wash athletic gear and towels after each use.
6. Maintain clean facilities and equipment.
7. Inform or refer to appropriate health care personnel for all active skin lesions and lesions that do not respond to initial therapy.
8. Administer or seek proper first aid.
9. Encourage health care personnel to seek bacterial cultures to establish a diagnosis.
10. Care and cover skin lesions appropriately before participation.

REFERENCES

1. CA-MRSA Information for the Public. Centers for Disease Control and Prevention.

Official Statement *NATA*

On-Site Athletic Trainer for Secondary Schools

Statement

The National Athletic Trainer's Association (NATA) as a leader in health care for the physically active believes that the prevention and treatment of injuries to student athletes are a priority. The recognition and treatment of injuries to student athletes must be immediate. The medical delivery system for injured student athletes needs a coordinator within the local school community who will facilitate the prevention, recognition, treatment and reconditioning of sports related injuries. Therefore, it is the position of the National Athletic Trainers' Association that all secondary schools should provide the services of a full-time, on-site, certified athletic trainer (ATC) to student athletes.

Official Statement *NATA*

Steroids and Performance Enhancing Drugs

Statement

The National Athletic Trainers' Association (NATA) is concerned with the issue of anabolic steroids and other performance enhancing substances in sports today. NATA recognizes the myriad of problems presented by steroid use - including legal, ethical and sportsmanship boundaries that are jeopardized. NATA's biggest concern, however, is the health and safety of all athletes, which NATA considers compromised by the use of such substances.

NATA supports any and all secondary school, collegiate conference, professional or amateur sports league, international committee or governmental regulations or bans on steroids and other controlled substances not prescribed by a physician for therapeutic purposes. NATA also supports more severe penalties for those who violate imposed regulations or bans. NATA considers this one of the most important issues facing the sports world today. As health care professionals, NATA's members focus primarily on the health and well being of the athletes and patients they serve. Therefore, due to the health risks associated with steroids and other performance enhancing drugs, NATA can never justify their use to improve athletic performance.

NATA's 30,000 members, many of whom work with secondary school or collegiate students, are especially concerned with steroid use among young athletes. The long-term, irreversible, negative effects of banned substances on a young athlete's growing body are a frightening repercussion not worthy of improved athletic performance. While a broad ban on such substances is a start, an equally important weapon in the battle against steroid use is more thorough education of our athletes and parents. Increased research on the dangerous side effects of steroids, combined with more intense dissemination of the facts about the extreme health risks – to athletes of all ages, coaches at all levels and parents of all young athletes – will solidify the message that no on-field victory is worth serious health problems later in life.

Official Statement *NATA*

Use of Qualified Athletic Trainers in Secondary Schools

Statement

The National Athletic Trainers' Association (NATA) is confident the best way to protect the public is to allow only Board of Certification certified athletic trainers and state licensed athletic trainers to practice as athletic trainers. The NATA is not alone in these beliefs. The American Medical Association has stated that certified athletic trainers should be used as part of a high school's medical team.

The American Academy of Family Physicians agrees and states on its web site, "The AAFP encourages high schools to have, whenever possible, a BOC certified or registered/licensed athletic trainer as an integral part of the high school athletic program."

In states with athletic training regulation, allowing other individuals to continue practicing as athletic trainers without a valid state license or BOC certification places the public at risk. Athletic trainers have unique education and skills that allow them to properly assess and treat acute and traumatic injuries in high school athletics. In coordination with the team physician, they routinely make decisions regarding the return-to-play status of student athletes. Other allied health professionals are not qualified to perform these tasks. Finally, most situations encountered by athletic trainers should not be left to a coach or layperson who does not have the necessary education and medical or emergency care training.

Official Statement NATA

Youth Football and Heat Related Illness

Statement

It is important that education about heat illness and hydration occurs at all levels of football. At the youth level, parents and coaches help to prevent heat illness during the warm weather. Most youth football leagues, which include children between the ages of six through thirteen, begin their pre-season practices in the middle of July. The first full-contact activities usually begin in August, when the weather is still hot and humid, a perfect environment to cause heat illnesses.

Both the National Athletic Trainers' Association (NATA) and the Gatorade Sports Science Institute (GSSI) have excellent recommendations on how to prevent heat illness in football during the warm weather. It is important that all youth football leagues review these articles and implement the recommendations into their pre-season and early season systems. These recommended guidelines include:

These recommended guidelines include[1,2]:

1. Proper medical coverage at all practices and games
2. Acclimate the athletes during the pre-season over a two week period
3. Allow proper fluid replacement to maintain hydration
4. Weigh in athletes before and after practices
5. Practice and rest in shaded areas
6. Have proper rest periods during and between practice sessions
7. Minimize the amount of equipment and clothing worn by players in hot and humid conditions.

By minimizing the amount of equipment and clothing worn by players in hot and humid conditions, the NATA - Age Specific Task Force recommends that all players be permitted to remove their helmets during rest breaks of both practices and games. With the football helmet on at all times in hot and humid weather, the body core temperature can increase to a greater extent and that may play a role in the development of an exertional heat illness.[2] The helmet should also be taken off in games between periods and at halftime, during hot weather. By combining proper hydration, rest, and the removal of the helmet for a period of time, this assists in the reduction of core body temperature and reduces the risk of developing a heat illness.

The NATA - Age Specific Task Force recommends that all youth football associations adhere to the guidelines and suggestions researched by the NATA and the GSSI. We hope with the implementations of these guidelines, there will be less chance of a heat related illness in youth football, in the future.

Parents, coaches, and youth football players are advised to adhere to the recommendations made in the 2002 National Athletic Trainers' Association Heat Illness Position Statement and the Gatorade Sports Science Institute Guidelines on Heat Safety in Football.

REFERENCES

1. Binkley HB, Beckett J, Casa DJ, Kleiner DM, Plummer PE. National Athletic Trainers' Association Position Statement: Exertional Heat Illnesses. *Journal of Athletic Training.* 2002;37(3):329-343.

2. Eichner RE. Heat Stroke in Sports: Causes, Prevention, and Treatment. *Sports Science Exchange.* 2002;15:3.

4 *NATA* Support Statements

In This Section: **The following statements give the position of the National Athletic Trainers' Association on issues pertaining to the athletic training profession. This section also contains statements of support for NATA policies from outside health care sources.**

Support Statement *NATA*

The Coalition to Preserve Patient Access to Physical Medicine and Rehabilitation Services

Introduction

The Centers for Medicare and Medicaid Services (CMS) published in the August 5, 2004 Federal Register, pages 47550-47551, a proposal that would limit reimbursement of physicians for "Therapy-Incident To" to a narrow group of providers: physical therapists, occupational therapists and speech and language therapists. Currently CMS regulations allow the physician the freedom to choose any qualified health care professional to perform therapy services at the physician's office or clinic.

We do not support this proposal or similar ones contained in the Medicare Program: Revisions to Payment Policies Under the Physician Fee Schedule for Calendar Year 2005 (CMS docket # 1429-P). We believe the provisions, which will restrict the physician's ability to determine the type of health care provider who administers "Therapy -Incident To" services, are poorly conceived and could have a detrimental effect on the welfare of Medicare patients.

Official Statement

We, the official representatives of the undersigned organizations, wish to formally state our position on Medicare's proposed changes to the "Therapy-Incident To" services.

We believe the health and well being of the Medicare beneficiary should be the primary consideration. To this end, physicians and all other medical professionals authorized to order "Therapy-Incident To" services should have the continued medical authority to determine proper care and treatment for the patient and to select the best available, most appropriate health care professional to provide that care, including "Therapy-Incident To" services. A number of complex factors affect a physician's choice of the most appropriate health care professional to provide "Therapy-Incident To" services in his/her office or clinic. Some examples are type of medical practice; geographic location such as rural or medically underserved areas; availability of qualified allied health care personnel; and patient access to Medicare and secondary health care system providers.

The physician is best equipped to make these medical decisions. We believe any attempt by government entities or other organizations to change this heretofore established right and purview of the physician clearly is not in the best interest of the patient.

We unequivocally request that no changes be made to Medicare or other provisions affecting "Therapy - Incident To" services reimbursement from CMS.

American Academy of Balance Medicine
American Academy of Pediatrics
American Chiropractic Association
American Medical Massage Association
American Optometric Association
American Osteopathic Association of Sports Medicine
California Academy of Family Physicians
Council on Professional Standards for Kinesiotherapy
Florida State Massage Therapy Association, Inc.
Medical Group Management Association
National Athletic Trainers' Association
Society of Teachers of Family Medicine

American Academy of Family Physicians
American Academy of Physical Medicine and Rehabilitation
American Kinesiotherapy Association
American Medical Society for Sports Medicine
American Orthopedic Society for Sports Medicine
American Society of Exercise Physiologists
Connecticut State Medical Society
Florida Orthopedic Surgeons
Lymphedema Stakeholders
Missouri Academy of Family Physicians
National Vision Rehabilitation Association
Texas Medical Association

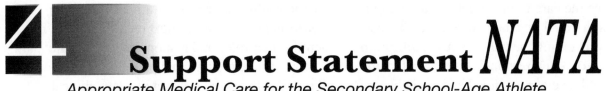

Support Statement *NATA*

Appropriate Medical Care for the Secondary School-Age Athlete

DOCUMENT BACKGROUND

In 2002, the National Athletic Trainers' Association (NATA) developed an inter-association task force to develop recommendations and guidelines for adolescents competing in school and club-level sports. The Appropriate Medical Care for Secondary School–Age Athletes Task Force (AMCSSAA) comprised experts from 17 school, health care, and medical associations who all shared the same goal — ensuring young athletes receive consistent and adequate medical care while participating in practices and games. The group developed a consensus statement stating minimum standards of health care for adolescent athletes. After unanimously approving the document, the task force decided to take the project one step further and put together this scientifically based document that augments the recommendations set forth in the consensus statement.

This communication will help organizations sponsoring athletic programs for this age group justify the importance of providing appropriate medical care and establishing an athletic health care team to identify the resources they should make available to adolescents participating in organized athletic programs. The article can also be used as an evaluation tool to assess current athletic health care delivery programs.

Disclaimer: This communication provides general practice recommendations and guidelines for medical care provided by organizations sponsoring athletic programs for secondary school-age individuals. Actual medical care provided should not be based solely on the information contained in this manuscript, but should be tailored to specific facts and circumstances unique to each entity and location.

PARTICIPATING IN THE DEVELOPMENT AND IMPLEMENTATION OF A COMPREHENSIVE ATHLETIC HEALTH CARE ADMINISTRATIVE SYSTEM

Organizations sponsoring athletic programs for secondary school–age individuals should establish an athletic health care team (AHCT) that functions to ensure appropriate medical care is provided for all participants. To provide appropriate medical care, the AHCT must function in a coherent, coordinated, and efficient manner with coaches and administrators of sponsoring organizations and adhere to commonly accepted standards of good clinical practice.

Medical and allied health professionals representing various disciplines are involved in the provision of athletic health care to adolescents. This communication summarizes the evidence base for points addressed in the consensus statement, which was was prepared and ratified by professional organizations representing numerous disciplines but does not mandate which specific individuals are essential to the AHCT.

Nonetheless, the American Medical Association (AMA), at the request of the American Academy of Pediatrics (AAP), has recommended that athletic medical units (AMUs) include a physician director and an athletic health coordinator, with preference given to NATABOC-certified athletic trainers (ATCs) in this role (AMA Resolution H-470.995 Athletic [Sports] Medicine, 1998).[1] Furthermore, many jurisdictions require that ATCs be supervised by licensed physicians, just as school nurses are supervised by school physicians and emergency medical technicians (EMTs) are supervised by emergency medical services (EMS) physicians.

Therefore, the ATC and team physician form the core of the AHCT, with the ATC being the most appropriate on-site member of the AHCT and the official team physician, if one has been designated, being ultimately responsible for medical decisions made by the AHCT (Figure 1). A designated school official or member of the sponsoring organization should be a liaison to the AHCT when having a member of the AHCT on-site is not possible. Other members of the team, along with the relationships among them, should be dictated by local needs and statutes.

A comprehensive athletic health care system

should enhance the care of the athlete by allowing the strengths of individual members to complement each other and by preventing the unnecessary duplication of efforts. The roles and responsibilities of all team members should be clearly defined and available to all. Regardless of the specifics of a given situation (i.e., local and state qualifications and regulations) or the personnel involved in the AHCT, the extent to which the ATC is responsible for medical decisions must be explicitly understood between the team physician and ATC, with administrative members of the AHCT (e.g., athletic directors) being wholly supportive of the guidelines for decision-making established between the team physician and ATC. At the request of the AAP, in 1998 the AMA passed Resolution H-470.995, which called for the establishment of athletic medical units (AMUs) by all organizations that sponsor athletic programs, school boards, and local boards of health. The scientific rationale for this resolution was thoroughly reviewed and published by the AMA and NATA in 1999.[1]

Expert panels[2] and peer-reviewed journal articles[3] have recommended standardization of sports injury surveillance systems to help improve athletic health care, but little to no primary research has been conducted to demonstrate that AMUs either decrease injury rates or improve athletic health care. The AHCT proposed in this document is similar to the AMU with respect to the allied health care professionals recommended to comprise the team and the roles and responsibilities of the team.

Nonetheless, case law over the past three decades[4,5] has established the precedent that school districts and other agencies sponsoring athletic programs have a legal responsibility to provide medical care for participants. In *O'Brien v. Township High School District* (1979),[6] the court held that a school district has a responsibility to provide proper medical treatment. Care provided by a minor student was not found improper or negligent at the time, but in the interim many states have enacted licensure statutes for athletic training. Therefore, organizations that do not provide appropriate medical care for athletes, defined as that administered by trained and certified professionals, could risk significant liability exposure.

Components of Recommendation

To properly develop and implement a comprehensive athletic health care administrative system, the sponsoring organization must create the AHCT, identify their roles and responsibilities, create the appropriate policies and procedures to ensure all on-site athletic staff adhere to safe clinical practice parameters for adequate medical care, designate appropriate physical space and equipment, document the activities of the AHCT, take part in injury surveillance, and commit to cycles of quality improvement so that appropriate medical care is available for all secondary school–age athletes.

Members of the Athletic Health Care Team

Local availability, needs, and statutes should guide organizations that sponsor athletic programs (e.g., schools, school districts, clubs, youth leagues) to establish desirable team members. Also, organizations should be aware of recommendations made in AMA Resolution H-470.995, the American College of Sports Medicine (ACSM)/American Orthopaedic Society for Sports Medicine (AOSSM) Team Physician Consensus Statement, the National Federation of State High School Associations (NFHS) Sports Medicine Handbook, and the National Collegiate Athletic Association (NCAA) Sports Medicine Handbook. The AHCT should include medical professionals from various organizations, including those listed in Table 1. When appropriate, the AHCT should consult with and develop an on-going coordination of efforts with the athlete, the athlete's parents, coaches, administrators, and other school or organization officials.

Individuals interested in improving the care provided to athletes should generate a needs assessment for their program based on injury risk data collected locally as well as that found in national databases, including the NATA surveillance studies, National Electronic Injury Surveillance System (NEISS), NCAA Injury Surveillance System, and National Center for Catastrophic Sports Injury Research.

Local professionals and groups should be identified and approached to join the AHCT. These may include sports medicine and other physician groups, medical schools, athletic training curriculum programs at local universities, physical therapy groups, physical therapy schools, and nursing schools.

Guidelines such as the NATA Position Proposal

Guide (PPG) for the creation of new programs or the NATA Position Improvement Guide (PIG) for the improvement of existing athletic health care programs are available to the sponsoring organization as resources. Funding issues may need to be addressed by demonstrating savings in liability/health insurance premiums through the establishment of an AHCT and athletic health care delivery program, although such national data are not available.

Roles and Responsibilities

The roles and responsibilities of each team member should be clearly defined and established, especially with each of the areas addressed in the following sections of this document. It is recommended that an "exclusion policy" be instituted whereby any single member of the AHCT, including but not limited to the ATC, team physician, consulting physician, or primary physician, may, based on the member's particular expertise, render an athlete ineligible for participation due to concerns for the health or welfare of the athlete. This exclusion policy should also allow the athlete, his/her parents, coaches, and sponsoring organization to limit participation for reasons justified by their role.

Policies and Procedures

Written policies and procedures for the AHCT should be established and kept in a manual easily referenced by team members as well as outside constituencies (e.g., parent-teacher associations) and governing bodies (e.g., school boards, local boards of health). Specific policies should be established and approved in advance of the athletic season relating to the following:

1) Readiness to participate and return-to-play decisions
2) Facilities inspection and maintenance
3) Proper fit, inspection, and maintenance of athletic equipment
4) Emergency response — the written emergency action plan
5) Environmental conditions protocols
6) Sideline preparedness for practice and competition sessions
7) Nutritional and weight requirements for different activities, such as wrestling
8) Coordination of referrals to consultants
9) Channels of communication
10) Chain of command
11) Documentation and record-keeping
12) Injury surveillance and quality improvement

This communication has been devoted to outlining the recommended roles, responsibilities, policies, and procedures of the AHCT. Several other professional organizations in medicine, sports medicine, and athletic health have also published policies and procedures that may serve as useful templates for local AHCTs.

Physical Space and Equipment

The physical space and equipment necessary for the AHCT must be established and maintained. To obtain and maintain this equipment, the athletic health care annual budgeting process should include input from a member of the AHCT. Recommended standard athletic health care equipment and supplies are detailed later in this communication. In addition, other resources[7] have extensive sections devoted to planning, constructing, equipping, and maintaining facilities for appropriate medical care of the adolescent athlete.

Documentation

Issues relating to the safety of equipment and facilities, as well as athlete injuries, treatment, and reconditioning, should be well documented in accordance with generally accepted standards of their respective state practice acts. To facilitate communication among members of the AHCT as well as with outside consultants and primary treating clinicians, all patient encounters should be documented in adherence with federal, state, and local regulations while keeping within the recommendations set forth by the Health Insurance Portability and Accountability Act of 1996 (HIPAA)[8] and Federal Education Records Protection Act (FERPA)[9] when applicable. Patient records (i.e., personal medical information) should be maintained in such as manner as to ensure privacy and confidentiality in all circumstances.

Injury Surveillance

As detailed later in this document, surveillance is the first step in the cycle of developing effective public health injury control strategies. Anonymous, high-quality injury surveillance and outcomes data should be collected regularly and shared not only with public health officials and other supervisory and regulatory agencies but also with professional health care societies committed to the advancement of their respective fields.

Injury surveillance can be defined on a continuum from action at the local level to the national level. At the local level, injury surveillance can be as simple as a coach removing a field hazard following injury to an athlete so as to not cause additional injuries to other athletes or a coach altering the bullpen throwing schedule if a rash of shoulder injuries occurs to the pitching staff. Injury surveillance at the national level could mean establishing a national secondary school–age sports injury and illness database to begin to collect data regarding the incidence of various injuries and illnesses in this population.

To more easily compare and share such information, it would be ideal to establish uniform sports injury surveillance system standards on the local, state, and national levels. Important elements of sports injury surveillance data may include a clearly defined and standardized definition of injury, type of sports event, position played, and particular activity and moment of injury, level of competition, place where the injury occurred, injury mechanism, level of supervision, nature of the injury, injured body region, severity of the injury (e.g., activity lost, working time lost, need for treatment, cost of treatment, permanent damage, impairment, and disability), characteristics of the injured person, duration and nature of the treatments needed, use of protective equipment, follow-up of game rules, cost of the injury, and well-defined exposure data (population at risk and exposure time), which are critical in determining and comparing incidence rates.[10] However, staffing, time, and cost constraints may limit the feasibility of such extensive injury surveillance.

A cooperative effort between the primary members of the AHCT along with the administrators of sponsoring organizations, coaches, and parents provides the best opportunity to establish an injury surveillance system for each specific group. Analysis of the results of this surveillance system can provide vital information regarding recommendations to improve the overall safety of the athletic activity.

Just as injury surveillance is but the first step in the public health model of prevention, AHCTs and members of the sponsoring organization, including administrators, coaches, and parents, should be committed to ongoing, continuous cycles of quality improvement, whereby local surveillance and outcome data are used to suggest changes in its own members' roles, responsibilities, policies, and procedures. Practices involving quality improvement and injury surveillance need to start locally and move toward a national level.

Ideally, such information would be shared regionally and nationally to contribute to the medical literature and to provide a basis for evidence-based practice of clinical medicine.

Strategies for Implementation

Potential strategies for the prevention of injury and illness as they relate to athletic participation by secondary school–age individuals are described in detail in the following sections of this communication. A brief overview of each consensus statement point is listed.

Consensus Statement Point 1: *Develop and implement a comprehensive athletic healthcare administrative system*

The demands of athletic health care require a team with diverse skills and a comprehensive administrative system. The AHCT should coordinate the various aspects of the athletes' health in a coherent, effective, and professional manner.

Consensus Statement Point 2: *Determine the individual's readiness to participate*

To promote safe participation of the student athlete, the pre-participation physical examination (PPE) is used to identify individuals who may be at risk for the development of injuries related to their activity and those who may be at risk for sudden death due to an underlying medical problem.

Consensus Statement Point 3: *Promote safe and appropriate practice, competition, and treatment facilities*

Sports organizations are expected to provide a safe environment for all athletes, including keeping the premises in safe repair, inspecting the premises for obvious and hidden hazards, removing the hazards if possible or warning of their presence, protecting invitees from foreseeable dangers, and conducting operations on the premises with reasonable care for the invitees. It is recommended that a specific treatment facility be set-up by the organization.

Consensus Statement Point 4: *Advise on the*

selection, fit, function, and maintenance of athletic equipment

Sports organizations should, to the greatest degree possible, ensure that athletes have access to appropriate equipment for the sport and that such equipment is properly fit in accordance with manufacturer recommendations and maintained by qualified personnel.

Consensus Statement Point 5: *Develop and implement a comprehensive emergency action plan*

Based on the activity, skills of participants, and geographic characteristics, various types of emergency incidents are likely to occur. An emergency action plan (EAP) is essential to ensure that all incidents are responded to in an appropriate manner and that the roles of the AHCT members are well defined and communicated in advance.

Consensus Statement Point 6: *Establish protocols regarding environmental conditions*

Environmental conditions pose potential threats to the safety and welfare of athletic participants. It is crucial that organizations responsible for athletic events develop policies and protocols to address the safety of play in hazardous environmental conditions.

Consensus Statement Point 7: *Provide for on-site recognition, evaluation, and immediate treatment of injury and illness, with appropriate referrals*

Injured athletes who do not receive timely evaluation or treatment are at greater risk for improper healing, reinjury, extended time loss from athletic participation and school, and potentially life-threatening consequences. Having a qualified individual on-site and ready to care for the ill or injured person is critical to the safety of the participants and for decision making regarding when an athlete can safely return to play.

Consensus Statement Point 8: *Facilitate rehabilitation and reconditioning*

Although the evaluation and treatment provided immediately after an injury are critical, a rehabilitation and reconditioning program designed to return the individual to their pre-injury level of function is just as important. The process of rehabilitation and reconditioning is fundamental for the safe return of injured athletes to their prior level of competition as quickly as possible and prevention of further injuries.

Consensus Statement Point 9: *Provide for psychosocial consultation and referral*

The AHCT should be able to identify potential psychosocial pathologies (e.g., disordered eating) frequently associated with secondary school–age athletes and refer them for appropriate diagnosis and management. Sponsoring organizations must identify local experts in these medical fields and facilitate the referral of athletes to these consultants.

Consensus Statement Point 10: *Provide scientifically sound nutritional counseling and education*

Nutrition is a key factor for an athlete's health, growth, and performance. It is essential that valid and understandable information regarding nutrition be provided to secondary school–age athletes, parents, and coaches. Even more essential is the ability to refer athletes to appropriate medical personnel for treatment when necessary.

Consensus Statement Point 11: *Develop injury and illness prevention strategies*

Injury and illness can be a heavy burden on the well-being of the secondary school–age athlete. A public health framework can be used to develop effective interventions to reduce the affliction of injuries and illnesses to these young persons.

DETERMINING AN INDIVIDUAL'S READINESS TO PLAY: THE PREPARTICIPATION PHYSICAL EXAMINATION

The number of individuals participating in organized sports has increased dramatically, with various sources estimating close to 6.5 million student participants in high school athletics each year.[11] The National Center for Catastrophic Sports Injury Research (NCCSIR) noted that between fall 1982 and spring 2001, close to 72 million males and 35 million females had participated in high school athletics[12]. These numbers unfortunately do not reflect the number of people participating in non-school-sanctioned programs such as community- or religious group-based leagues and recreational and developmental programs.

The Preparticipation Physical Examination (PPE) is essential to identify athletes at risk for injury and implement corrective actions before injuries occur. Yearly screening of these athletes is imperative because health conditions may change from year to year and the development of subtle problems may be overlooked. The PPE is an important requirement for all participants in any organized program and should be performed by the athlete's primary care physician, school physician, or team physician.

The purpose of the PPE is not to exclude an individual from activity but instead to recognize individuals who may be at risk for developing injuries related to their activity and those who may be at risk for sudden death due to underlying medical problems. The goal is to promote safe participation of the secondary school–age athlete.

There is an inherent risk of injury in secondary school–age athletes through participation in sports and recreational activities. Krowchuk[13] noted that 22% to 39% of high school athletes sustain a significant injury and that as many as 20% of such injuries may be preventable. The value of identifying those at risk therefore is paramount to prevention.

In 1997, Beachy et al[14] noted that over an 8-year time span, 14,318 athletes participating in more than 32 different sports reported a total of 11,184 injuries that required medical help. The male injury rate was 0.90 injury per athlete with 0.33 day-lost injury per athlete; the female injury rate was 0.64 injury per athlete with 0.21 day-lost injury. The overall injury rate for day-lost injuries was 28%. Almost all of the injuries reported in this study were musculoskeletal in nature.

Fortunately, the risk of sudden death is not as common as is that of musculoskeletal injuries. Between 1983 and 1993, 126 non-traumatic deaths among high school athletes were identified by the NCCSIR (overall annual death rate, 4.68:1 million athletes).[13] The impact of an unexpected death in a perceived healthy young person is remarkable and warrants screening measures and education for recognizing those at risk.

Unfortunately, not all injuries and sudden deaths can be prevented, but strategies to minimize the risk are paramount. Periodic assessment of an athlete's medical history and a comprehensive physical examination provide one such prevention strategy.

The AAP noted in a 2001 policy statement that although PPEs are typically not mandated until junior

TABLE 1. MEDICAL PROFESSIONALS WHO SHOULD BE CONSIDERED MEMBERS OF THE ATHLETIC HEALTH CARE TEAM

Certified athletic trainers

Team physicians

Orthopaedic physicians

School physicians

Primary care providers (pediatricians, family practice, nurse practicioners, etc.)

Consulting and other physicians

School nurses and guidance counselors

Physical therapists

EMS Personnel

Physician assistants

Registered dieticians

Public safety personnel

Public health officials

Dentists

Other allied health care professionals

Students and trainees in the above disciplines

high school and high school, annual examinations for younger children afford the opportunity to promote physical activity and to address issues of readiness as they apply to organized sports.[15]

In July 2002, the NFHS released the second edition of their Sports Medicine Handbook, which clearly states that the PPE is "a necessary and desirable pre-condition to participation."[16] It is our objective to have the PPE be required for all participants in all organized programs, including those that are school, community, and religious group based.

Components of Recommendation

In 1992, five organizations (American Academy of Family Physicians, American Academy of Pediatrics, American Medical Society for Sports Medicine, American Orthopaedic Society for Sports Medicine, and American Osteopathic Academy of Sports Medicine) published a consensus report regarding the PPE. This document, herein referred to as the PPE Monograph,[17] clearly outlines the stated goals of the PPE along with guidelines for the organization and administration of the examination. Along with the 1998 American Heart Association guidelines for cardiovascular screening of competitive athletes,[18] these documents set the standard for the PPE.

The PPE should be incorporated to detect conditions that may predispose injury or preclude participation in specific sports; prevent further injuries by identifying and treating musculoskeletal abnormalities; detect medical conditions that may be life threatening or disabling; determine the athlete's general health; assess fitness level for specific sports; advise the athlete in which sports he or she can participate if a condition exists that precludes participation in some sports; develop treatment and rehabilitation plans for problems; counsel the athlete on health-related issues such as nutrition, alcohol, drugs, and other psychosocial issues, and meet legal and insurance requirements. [16-20]

Discovery of limiting or disqualifying conditions
Conditions such as acute, recurrent, chronic, or untreated injuries or illnesses may compromise the performance of the athlete and place him or her at greater risk for the development of other injuries. For example, examination of foot pain in a young gymnast may uncover a chronic stress fracture that may be due in part to an underlying eating disorder and, if left unrecognized, may lead to further disability and injury.

The discovery of a new medical condition during the PPE is very rare. Recently, the Mayo Clinic[21] reported that of 2,739 students screened over a 3-year period, 13.9% were given dispositions other than being cleared for sports. In this group, 1.9% (53 students) were not cleared for sports due to underlying medical concerns. Musculoskeletal abnormalities accounted for the largest proportion of those not cleared (43.4%). Cardiac abnormalities, which included exertional presyncope or syncope and palpitations, were the second leading cause of a "not cleared" disposition.

If medical conditions are identified during the PPE, recommendations for handling these problems should be dealt with on an individual basis and follow guidelines set forth by the AAP[22] and the 26th Bethesda Conference.[23] A summary of these guidelines can be found in various sources, including the PPE Monograph.[17]

Sudden death
The incidence of sudden death in school-age athletes is low compared with the number of musculoskeletal injuries incurred during participation. However, sudden death in a young competitive athlete is usually a devastating and tragic event that affects the community. Most cases of sudden death are related to underlying cardiac abnormalities.

Maron et al[24] evaluated a total of 158 sudden deaths that occurred in trained athletes between 1985 and 1995. A total of 124 deaths were cardiac: 48 (36%) were due to hypertrophic cardiomyopathy and 17 (13%) were due to congenital malformations of the coronary arteries. In 3 individuals (2%), a "normal" heart was found on autopsy with no other apparent cause of death. In the same study, Maron et al[24] noted that PPEs were performed before competition in 115 of the 158 cases reviewed. Of these 115, only 4 (3%) were suspected of having cardiovascular disease and the cardiovascular abnormality responsible for sudden death was correctly identified in only 1 athlete (0.9%).

Given this information, it has been argued that the PPE may not be an adequate tool in assessing risk for sudden death in young athletes. Many articles have been written about using other noninvasive means for screening this population such as the use of echocardiograms, electrocardiograms, and stress tests to identify those at risk. This testing is cost prohibitive and the yield is too low to have a dramatic impact on the overall screening process and therefore is still not required as part of the PPE.[23, 25-28]

However, there remains a critical need for effective, low-cost screening methods. The American Heart Association's[29] history module that consists of five questions has been adopted by some states for use on the PPE and may be a reasonable alternative.

Assessing general health of the athlete

The PPE should be considered as part of an overall health care plan for the secondary school–age athlete and should not be a substitute for the student-athlete's routine medical care. It can be incorporated into a regular examination with the student athlete's primary care physician and should not replace regular scheduled visits and/or checkups. Unfortunately, approximately 80% to 90% of adolescents report that the PPE substitutes for a routine examination.[30]

It is important to recognize that the PPE may be the only contact that some student athletes have with a physician on a regular basis and that attention should be given to issues of routine health maintenance. A standardized form, like that printed in the PPE Monograph,[16, 17] helps address some of these issues and can aid in further screening of potential problems and/or deficiencies.

Assessing fitness level for specific sports

The fitness assessment should include body composition, flexibility, strength, and endurance[16]. Not all of these components can be routinely assessed as part of the PPE, but a review of some of these components and a discussion of the sports in which they want to participate can help establish a baseline for training. For example, an obese male who wants to participate in his high school football program should be counseled on the effects his weight may have on his play. The excess weight may also make him more prone to heat injuries and this should be discussed, by a member of the AHCT, with the athlete, his parents/guardians, and the coaching staff. The athlete should be encouraged to participate because the physical activity is important, but it should also be recommended that he be counseled on proper nutrition, weight training, and aerobic conditioning prior to and during the season to help improve his performance and to avoid injury and illness.

Counseling athletes on health-related topics

The PPE affords an opportunity for the physician to counsel athletes on potentially risky behaviors such as drug, alcohol, and supplement use and nutritional concerns. As previously noted, the PPE may be the only contact a student has with a health care provider during the school year and this opportunity should not be lost.

The use of a standardized PPE form that includes questions about drug, alcohol, and supplement use and concerns about weight can provide a useful screening tool for the physician and coaching staff; any "yes" response should prompt discussions with the athlete at the time of the PPE. Further recommendations for counseling and/or follow-up with the athlete's primary care provider can be made on an individual basis. In female athletes, a review of menstrual history is paramount because many young female athletes have menstrual irregularities that may be related to their training.

Screening for amenorrhea, alterations in body image, and eating disorders can be accomplished by review of the medical history and discussion with the student-athlete at the time of the PPE.

Implement rehabilitation programs

If a chronic condition is uncovered during the PPE or if the athlete has not completely recovered from a prior injury, the examiner should address the potential for reinjury or the risk for other injuries. The medical team should perform a thorough evaluation. Any problems noted during this evaluation should be addressed, treated, or referred to an appropriate medical professional to prevent further injury.

McCoy et al[31] noted that primary care physicians now carry a major responsibility to become familiar with general rehabilitation principles for all types of sports-related injuries and that the reinforcement of a sophisticated plan of applying ice and elevation as treatment for acute injury and range of motion (ROM) exercises followed by strengthening exercises and functional evaluation is critical in the return-to-play decision process. It is no longer acceptable to keep an athlete away from the sport for an indefinite period of time. Short- and long-term goals of treatment need to be established and monitored. In schools or organizations with access to ATCs, this process can usually be accomplished more quickly and efficiently. If ATCs are not available, the responsibility rests with the primary care physician, team physician, school nurse, coaching staff, parents/guardians, and the athlete to ensure proper referrals to appropriate resources for an efficient and safe return to play.

Meeting legal needs

In 1988, Feinstein et al[32] found that 35 states require yearly physical examinations, 3 states require a physical examination every 3 years, 1 state required only 1 physical examination, and 6 states did not specify their requirements. Many local school districts and organizations have their own policies in place with regard to the medical eligibility of secondary school–age athletes, with the PPE, generally the cornerstone of this requirement.

Strategies for Implementation

Implement an optimal time frame for the PPE

While no time frame exists for performing the PPE, it has been suggested that the PPE be performed in advance of the sports season to allow optimum time to address any issues that may arise during the examination – 4 to 6 weeks before the start of a season seems to be most appropriate. In scholastic sports played in the fall season, the PPE should be performed before the end of the preceding school year so that any chronic injuries can be addressed and a treatment plan can be laid out for the student-athlete for the summer months. Many schools and states require yearly evaluations as a prerequisite to participation.

The American Heart Association[18] recommends that both a history and physical examination be performed before participation in organized high school sports, with repeat screening every 2 years. An interim history should be performed in intervening years or sooner if there have been any changes in the student-athlete's health.

The AMA Group on Science and Technology endorses the work of Risser et al[33] and McKeag,[34] who recommend that a PPE be performed at the beginning of any new level of competition with an intercurrent review before the start of each new season.[35] Regardless of the time frames adapted, it is important

to realize the importance of routine screening for injury and illness recognition and prevention.

Methods of performing the PPE

The PPE can be performed in three different ways: (1) by the athlete's private physician in the office setting; (2) by multiple examiners as part of a station examination; or (3) by a physician as part of a mass "assembly-line" examination.[16, 19, 32] Examination by the athlete's private physician would be the most ideal situation because this offers the most continuity of care with the most comprehensive medical history. The physician is likely to have an established relationship with the athlete, and the components of the PPE can be incorporated into a comprehensive health evaluation. Unfortunately, not all physicians are familiar with sports medicine issues, and they may be limited in their ability to detect musculoskeletal abnormalities. Also, many student-athletes do not have a physician whom they see on a regular basis.[13]

Communication issues may arise because the private physician is not usually the school or team physician. Confusion regarding abnormalities, treatment plans and clearance can ensue if concerns are not directly forwarded to the ATC, coaching staff, and/or athletic director by the private physician. Comments from the primary physician should be forwarded to on-site personnel through the AHCT to alleviate any possible problems.

The station method, in which components of the PPE are broken down and delegated to adequately trained support staff, has been more widely accepted as the best model for efficiently performing large numbers of examinations.[16, 18, 19, 33, 17] These stations are often staffed by personnel who are educated in sports medicine and can provide better evaluation of potential problems. The final station is manned by the supervising school or team physician, who reviews each athlete's history and physical examination and makes final recommendations with regard to clearance. This method is very helpful in providing adequate communication with the other members of the AHCT and the coaching staff, as most will be actively involved in the PPE process. A potential drawback to the multistation PPE is lack of sufficient qualified medical personnel to man the stations. In addition, any abnormal findings identified through use of this method should be reported back to the athlete's family physician for follow-up care.

The "assembly line" method or traditional "locker room" examination, in which one physician examines a large number of athletes with little or no support staff, is very inefficient and not recommended.[18]

Identify and use a standard form for all PPEs
The history portion of the PPE is vital in obtaining accurate and up-to-date information regarding the student-athlete's past medical problems, injuries, and current medications. Rifat et al[35] reviewed 2,574 PPEs and showed that the history accounted for 88% of the abnormal findings and 57% of the reasons cited for restriction from a particular sport. Many sources advocate the development of a standardized form to help ensure uniformity; these forms can be given to the student-athlete before the PPE for completion of the history section with their parents/guardians. The history section should include questions that assess for the following[13, 16, 17, 19]:

1) *Past injuries causing the athlete to miss a game or practice.* Specific questions should be posed regarding a prior history of fractures, operations, or use of casts or braces.

2) *A loss of consciousness or memory after a head injury.* Repeated concussions may be criteria for exclusion from contact sports and/or prompt or warrant a comprehensive assessment.

3) *Previous exclusion from sports for any reason*

4) *Syncope, near syncope, chest pains, or palpitations during exercise.* Specific questions regarding passing out, nearly passing out, chest pains, or irregular heartbeats during exercise must be asked because these may be the only clue to an underlying cardiac condition.

5) *Past medical history.* This includes conditions currently being treated, history of asthma or exercise-induced bronchospasm, history of one paired organ, and history of sickle cell disease or trait.

6) *Prior surgical procedures and complications*

7) *Current medications and dosage*

8) *Allergies to medication, stinging insects, foods, and other environmental triggers*

9) *Immunization records, including tetanus*

10) *Family history of sudden death*

11) *Menstrual history with age of menarche and frequency of menses for all female athletes*

12) *History of significant weight gain or loss*

and the athlete's perception of his or her current body weight

13) *History of over-the-counter supplement use.*

The physical examination portion of the PPE form should include the following[13, 16, 17],

1) *Vital signs, including height, weight, blood pressure, and resting and postexercise pulse*

2) *Vision screening with the use of a traditional Snellen chart.* If corrected acuity in either eye is 20/40 or greater, the athlete should be referred to a specialist for follow-up.

3) *Tanner staging*

4) *Assessment of the head, eyes, ears, nose, mouth, and throat for any abnormalities*

5) *Cardiovascular and lung examination*

6) *Abdominal examination with evaluation for hernia in males.* Pelvic examinations in females should be referred to appropriate specialists if the history warrants concerns because these are usually not required as part of the PPE.

7) *Muscle strength testing and brief neurological assessment*

8) *Examination of the skin for any rashes, chronic skin condition, or abnormal moles*

9) *Musculoskeletal evaluation.* This should include ROM testing in the upper and lower extremities; assessment of laxity or instability in the shoulders, elbows, wrists, hips, knees, and ankles; and assessment of the spine for scoliosis and/or abnormalities of the thorax, such as pectus excavatum.

10) *Section to list abnormalities and recommendations for clearance and, if necessary, treatment plans*

11) *Determine Body Mass Index (BMI).*

Preprinted forms that encompass all of the above points can be found in several sources, including the NFHS Sports Medicine Handbook[16] and the PPE Monograph.[17] These forms can be copied and adapted to the needs of the school district or organization.

Communication System
A good communication system should be in place between the medical staff, athlete, parents/guardians, coaches, and athletic director. It is recommended in HIPAA that this communication begin with a formal letter to parents/guardians advising them of the

purpose and nature of the PPE. Consent forms and a copy of the PPE history can be mailed separately or along with the introductory letter with instructions for completion before the PPE. A cover letter should also accompany the PPE to the family physician as a mechanism to avoid any communication problems that could arise. This cover letter should specifically ask for any physician comments on any specific concerns that might affect athletic performance as well as suggested rehabilitation or treatment options for current problems.

Once the data have been collected, it must be kept on file for reference purposes; this should be the responsibility of the school nurse or ATC. If the athlete is participating in a non-school-sponsored program, the sponsoring organization should keep these records up to date. Any abnormalities need to be communicated to the student-athlete, his/her parents/ guardians, the ATC, and the athletic department. If the student opts to have the PPE performed by his or her primary care physician, the use of the standardized PPE form is imperative to maintain uniformity and to ensure that all components of the examination have been addressed.

New regulations instituted by HIPAA may require other specifications with regard to the privacy of these records; this should be part of the organization's overall compliance plan. School-based groups should adhere to FERPA regulations.

PROMOTING SAFE AND APPROPRIATE PRACTICE, COMPETITION, AND TREATMENT FACILITIES

Secondary school–age athletes have a right to play in facilities that are safe and without the potential for unnecessary harm. When injuries do occur, these participants also have a right to be treated in a clean and appropriate environment that is dedicated to this purpose. While the benefits young athletes gain from sports participation are immeasurable, the impact of accidental injuries and deaths to this age group cannot be ignored. Although very few youth sports injuries are fatal, or even catastrophic, their frequency and financial impact warrant our attention. The U.S. Consumer Products Safety Commission has estimated that up to 22% of girls and 39% of boys in organized sports are injured per season.[36] According to the National Youth Sports Safety Council,[37] sports-related

injuries to youths up to 14 years of age cost society more than $49 billion in 1997. These statistics, coupled with a desire to make sports participation a positive experience for children, underscore the need to prevent injuries whenever possible. Making sports facilities safe for young athletes is of paramount importance.

Providing safe facilities is an integral component of effective sports management and is governed by ethical, legal, and other administrative considerations. Safe facilities provide the opportunities for safe participation and a positive experience for the young athlete. The right to participate in safe and healthy environments is contained in The Bill of Rights for Young Athletes.[38] Well-maintained facilities ensure that safety is a priority, and that priority is then carried to the public.

A review of case law shows that sponsoring organizations that do not provide a safe environment expose themselves to unnecessary legal action and the athletes they are supposed to help to undue preventable injury. Facilities that are not maintained routinely also provide opportunity for undue accidental injury.

Countless lawsuits have been filed, and frequently won, by parties who have sustained injuries due to improper inspection and maintenance of facilities,[39-41] hazards in and around facilities,[42-45] unsafe grounds and external walkways,[46-48] and improper facility signage.[49-51] Such litigation depletes the financial resources of sponsoring institutions and reflects a negative image to the public about the specific institution and about sports in general.

Federal, state, local, and professional guidelines regulate certain aspects of most sports facilities. Parties who administer youth sports programs can avoid potential professional censure or criminal proceedings through diligent compliance with regulations pertaining to health and safety.

Components of Recommendation
Athletic facilities can vary greatly in size and complexity. Regardless of the size and purpose of a facility or the resources of its caretakers, entities that sponsor sports opportunities for secondary school– age athletes should ensure that all facilities are safe. The AHCT can play a vital role in sports facility safety issues, specifically maintenance and sanitation, use, and supervision.

Maintenance and Sanitation

A regular maintenance program should be developed for all said facilities and capital equipment. Organizations sponsoring athletic events for the secondary school–age athletes, as well as members of the AHCT, should be aware of maintenance issues in and around the athletic facility. In addition, it is imperative for AHCT members to incorporate proper sanitary procedures when treating the secondary school–age athlete and to provide guidance and recommendations for coaches to comply with proper sanitary, maintenance, and repair procedures.

Maintenance schedules should follow industry or regulatory standards. Individuals who will perform specific maintenance tasks must be familiar with the prerequisite techniques (e.g., pool sanitation, field maintenance) and ensure that these techniques are used. With indoor facilities, appropriate circulation, temperature, and humidity must be maintained. Other health and safety considerations pertaining to sports facilities may include electrical, lighting, signage, and slip control areas of floors.

Locker rooms, bathrooms, and shower areas can present special problems in maintaining a safe environment for young athletes. According to Seidler,[52] "Concrete floors and walls, steel lockers with sharp corners, and standing water, all make locker rooms perhaps the single most dangerous facility in sports and recreation." Because of the potential for injury and infection that these areas pose, they should be checked frequently for hazards, sanitized regularly, and supervised closely to prevent horseplay.

When dealing with outdoor facilities, the sponsoring organization should be concerned with the ground and surface conditions, spacing around fields, and vehicular traffic around the facility. Hazards in any of these areas could pose a risk to participating secondary school–age athletes. Ground hazards requiring immediate attention include holes and depressions in fields, excess moisture, erosion, rocks, broken glass, and playing surfaces or access ways that are abnormally uneven. Prior to athletic competitions, the grounds and/or playing fields should be inspected by the coach or an on-site member of the AHCT as a means of injury prevention. Structures that encroach upon playing areas should be moved. If this is not feasible, then the activity should be repositioned or modified to eliminate potential player impact with the structure. Other hazards include low hanging power lines over playing areas and exposing young athletes to vehicular traffic, either as they play or as they enter and leave the facility.

When a facility hazard is discovered, it is appropriate to either avoid using the facility or modify the sports activity to avoid exposing the young athletes to the hazard. If the problem cannot be corrected on the spot, written reports and requests for repairs should be submitted at the earliest opportunity. Treatment facilities where athletes would be provided injury treatment and rehabilitation should be maintained in a manner consistent with medical facilities.

Use and Supervision

Before activity begins, venue-specific Emergency Action Plans (EAPs) must be formulated, reviewed, and posted within the facility (Section 5 of this document addresses EAPs in detail). Adult sponsors must ensure that first aid/emergency equipment is readily available, that some form of communication is available to contact EMS personnel, and that the facilities are accessible to EMS vehicles. This designation should be clearly marked so all know where help can be obtained. In addition, an area of the facility should be dedicated to sports medicine, with an AHCT member available to provide appropriate treatment and care for injuries sustained through the course of participation in sport.

To minimize injury potential, the activities of young athletes must be supervised. Athletes must also be instructed to use facilities safely. This is particularly true in higher risk venues, such as aquatic facilities. The use of appropriate signage can help instruct the secondary school–age athlete on safe facility use, but should be used in conjunction with appropriate adult supervision. Some signage, such as those marking emergency exit routes, may be required and/or regulated by local fire codes. Signage should comply with the American National Standards Institute (ANSI) and other professional standards for readability, color, and size.

Although specific needs will be unique to a particular facility, safety-oriented signage within sports facilities can include general regulations for facility use, instructions for use of specific equipment (e.g., weight equipment, whirlpools, saunas), the EAP, the location of emergency/first aid equipment, the location of automated external defibrillators (AEDs) if available, warning signs identifying known or potential hazards, and markers to delineate play/activity areas, as well as those used to designate buffer areas around equipment.

Facilities specifically designated for injury treatment and rehabilitation should be used in a manner that promotes a safe environment for all participants and allow direct supervision of all athletes and equipment at all times by a qualified member of the AHCT.

Construction and Design

The opportunities to be involved in the design and construction of sports facilities are limited, but there is little doubt that a well-designed facility can make the job of injury prevention easier. In addressing the significance of design and construction on sports facility safety, it has been noted that poorly planned, designed, or constructed sports and recreation facilities often lead to an increase in the exposure to hazardous conditions for the participants.[52] In addition, these hazardous conditions may make facility maintenance and daily operation more difficult and can increase liability.

Problems commonly encountered in the design and construction of sports facilities include the use of improper building materials, poor access control and security, poorly planned pedestrian traffic flow through activity areas, a lack of proper storage space, inadequate lighting, and inadequate safety zones around courts and fields. It should be noted that once construction on a sports facility has been completed, these problems can be difficult to correct.

Strategies for Implementation

The best implementation strategy begins during the design and construction of new athletic facilities to ensure that all of the safety features listed above are present. However, because most secondary school–age athletes practice and compete in existing facilities, individuals and organizations involved with these athletes should implement strategies to establish procedures, inspect facilities, and record and repair potential hazards.

All parties involved with youth sports activities should regularly and thoroughly inspect their facilities: coaches, administrators, grounds/facilities staff, and members of the AHCT. Some areas, such as fixed building structures, will require less frequent inspections, whereas other areas, such as fields and floors, must be constantly inspected. Young athletes should be encouraged to be a part of this "injury prevention team" by immediately reporting any unsafe conditions to their adult sponsor.

The methods to be used for evaluating the safety of facilities and locations to be inspected should be established and recorded (Table 2). In general, sports safety inspections should include all structures and surfaces used by the athletes. A form or other instrument onto which findings are recorded can be helpful. The individual performing the inspections should sign the tool. As Hossler[53] points out, "It is better to prepare than to repair." This statement underscores the importance of aggressive injury prevention in youth sports. Many strategies for providing safer sports facilities have been previously mentioned in this document. The success of any sports facility safety program depends on the cooperation of many individuals, from players to parents to coaches to administrators. Therefore, it is of paramount importance to involve these persons as the program is planned and then implemented.

In addition, Clover[54] suggests professional staff use the mental cue "S.A.F.E." to ensure safety in the performance of their duties and responsibilities: Supervision from the locker room to the practice field. Aid the athletes when needed. This includes creating and practicing the EAP; keeping proper records of physical examinations, injuries, treatments, insurance, parental releases, and equipment; ensuring first aid kits are available and well stocked; and checking to ensure that water and injury ice are available for the athletes. Facilities must be checked daily for possible hazards. If there is a hazard, the area must be clearly marked or precluded from use. A written work order must be filled out and a time frame for completion of work must be established in writing on the work order. A copy of the work order should be kept on file. Equipment in facilities should be checked daily. From the pitching machine to the modalities used in the athletic training room, all equipment should be well maintained. This ensures the equipment lasts longer and stays in proper working condition.

ADVISING ON THE SELECTION, FIT, FUNCTION, AND MAINTENANCE OF ATHLETIC EQUIPMENT

Participation without proper equipment, or with equipment that is inappropriate or improperly fitted, subjects the participant to an increased risk of injury, illness, and even death. A great number of secondary school–age children want to participate in sports, and most parents allow and encourage their participation. Equipment essential to some sports (helmets, shoulder pads for football, sticks for field hockey) may be supplied by the sponsoring organization or the individual participant. If a sponsoring organization requires the participant to provide such equipment, it is incumbent upon the sponsoring entity to ensure that all equipment worn and used is appropriate and properly fitted. In addition, equipment specific to the purpose of caring for injuries and illnesses of athletes on-site will be addressed.

Proper supervision is also essential when using equipment, including frequent inspections to ensure proper fit and function. Safe, effective, and appropriate equipment should be maintained and provided to the participant. Sponsoring organizations that require the participant to provide their own equipment must ensure that personal equipment complies with requirements outlined by a sports regulatory agency.

Entities that provide guidelines for approval of athletic equipment are the National Operating Committee on Standards in Athletic Equipment (NOCSAE) and the American Society for Testing and Materials (ASTM). Equipment that has not been approved by certifying bodies – that is, inappropriate equipment or appropriate equipment that is improperly fitted or in poor repair or not maintained on a regular schedule – could introduce the athlete to injury that is needless and preventable.

Equipment that is properly fitted and appropriate for the sport or activity is essential for the secondary school–age athlete to be able to enjoy athletic participation in a safe and orderly environment. ATCs and educated coaches of the particular sport are the persons most likely to have the education and qualifications to select, fit, maintain, inspect, and supervise athletic equipment use. An on-site member of the AHCT may be recommended as responsible to perform this activity and a member of the AHCT can be responsible to oversee this in the absence of an on-site AHCT member. A review of case law shows that equipment that is not well maintained or improperly fitted can contribute to, if not cause, injury to participants. In addition, the use of equipment that has not been approved by the appropriate certifying body exposes the athlete to injury as well as liability and negligence to the sponsoring entity.[4-6, 55-65]

Fitting Protective Equipment

Ensuring that all athletes have properly fitting equipment is important to maintaining a safe athletic environment. Sponsoring agencies should ensure that qualified personnel (coach, ATC, equipment manager) fit equipment and that the participant has appropriate equipment for participation. Schutt Inc., a helmet manufacturer, as well as other manufacturers, provide detailed instructions on the fitting of their equipment.[66-68]

Use of these instructions should be followed when fitting participants or the sponsoring agency could be found liable. In the case of Gerritty v. Beatty,[63] the school was found liable when an athlete reported poorly fitting equipment and the school had done nothing about it.

Maintenance and Reconditioning

Once equipment is properly fit to the athlete, sponsoring agencies and members of the AHCT must make sure the equipment is properly maintained and reconditioned. All athletic equipment should be examined periodically during the season and the fit maintained throughout the season (i.e., if an athlete shaves his head, the helmet should be refit).[69] In addition, school and team officials should closely inspect any equipment used by or around participants and know the risks involved in the use of such equipment. Case law has judged in favor of the plaintiffs in cases where a latent defect in a pitching machine caused injury to the face of an athlete while the machine was unplugged[58] and where a vaulting horse was altered and the holes for the pommels were exposed.[65]

Many manufacturers now recommend that equipment be reconditioned on a regular basis, checking for flaws and defects in the product. Most manufacturers state that they will not stand behind the product if the proper reconditioning and checks have not been made.[70] In the case of Gerritty v. Beatty,[63] the school district was found negligent for refusing to furnish well-maintained equipment. Therefore, school districts should ensure that qualified personnel purchase, fit, and maintain appropriate athletic equipment and recondition existing equipment according to manufacturer recommendations. In addition, the sponsoring organization should be cautioned not to accept used equipment passed down from higher level organizations unless the equipment has been properly maintained and reconditioned.

Supervision During Use of Equipment

Finally, all participants in physical education, sports, and recreational teams and events have the right to be supervised by qualified and competent coaches and provided with competent health care.[71] Competent may be defined as being proficient in the skills required by the job description and training. Sponsoring entities and governing bodies should ensure that competent, trained individuals always supervise participants. State or local regulations may influence the parameters of what is required for appropriate supervision. Training should focus on the sport(s) to be supervised, as well as proper fit and use of equipment. In addition, the sponsoring entity or school should provide adequate and appropriate health care as described throughout this monograph.[71, 72]

Lack of appropriate supervision when using equipment in sport can also expose the athlete to undue risk. Two cases, Grant v. Lake Oswego School District Number 759 and Tiemann v. Independent School District #740,[65] provide emphasis that not only should participants be supervised while using equipment but also that the supervisors or coaches should be trained in how to adequately supervise individuals. In both cases, equipment was used that either was set up incorrectly or dangerously (Grant) or was faulty (Tiemann).

Components of Recommendation

The sponsoring organization should identify personnel to educate in the necessary procedures to appropriately select, fit, and maintain all equipment specific to individual sports; protective equipment consistent with specific sports; and protective equipment general to all sports. The person who issues equipment should be trained in the proper fit, function, and use of athletic equipment specific to his/her sport. Members of the AHCT should be educated on the proper selection, fit, and maintenance of athletic equipment and take an active role in reviewing quality and selection of safety equipment provided by a sponsoring organization. Equipment should be chosen based on the appropriateness to the sport, level of competition, age of participants, and overall quality. Maintenance of such equipment should be subject to a predetermined schedule and follow all of the manufacturer's recommendations and rules of the governing sporting association.

Rule changes should be investigated by governing bodies of contact and collision sports and of small ball sports to protect the face and eye from injury. Rules should include requiring the use of eye protection in practice and games.[73, 74] Investigation by a governing body provides the basis for rules changes to be implemented by that governing body. These changes should be based on scientific data. Governing bodies should use such scientific data to amend rules to best protect the participant.

Many times, professional athletes do not wear a complete set of pads, making it enticing for younger athletes to emulate the actions of the professionals. Secondary school leagues and officials should be encouraged to enforce the rules designed to protect these players.

Strategies for Implementation

Coaches, parents, athletes, and members of the AHCT should be aware of the limitations of each piece of equipment and be able to instruct the athlete in its proper use, as well as potential hazards with its misuse. Sponsoring entities should mandate general training as well as sport-specific training for all coaches and individuals dealing with participants, including but not limited to equipment fit, function, and maintenance.[71, 72]

In addition, sponsoring organizations should require appropriately trained personnel to maintain adequate supervision (i.e., within a close proximity as to prevent an inappropriate or dangerous action) of participants at all times.

With respect to equipment, braces should be used to treat or prophylactically prevent injury as directed by, or under the supervision of, a physician.[75] A qualified member of the AHCT should be the designated person to determine and fit appropriate braces, tape, or safety equipment. Shoulder harnesses; braces for the wrist, elbow, ankle, and knee; and custom-made braces should all conform to the rules of the sport and be used under the direction of a physician or other health care provider.[75] No equipment should be modified from manufacturers' standards. Equipment should be used only for the intent it was manufactured. Mouthguard use is recommended for all sports with a risk for mouth and dental injuries. The use of a mouthguard is required by some organizations in football, lacrosse, ice hockey, and boxing for both practices and games.[76-78] Organizations that sponsor sports in which mouthguards are required should provide education to the participants and parents on the appropriate fit and care of mouthguards.[79]

Helmets for all sports should always comply with the appropriate standards. They should be periodically inspected and reconditioned in accordance to the manufacturers' recommendations. Helmets should be used only as directed and should never be used as a weapon or be the point of attack.[16, 69, 80, 81,27] Facial protection or facemasks should be worn in sports where such rules apply or the possibility for injury to the face is high, such as football, ice hockey, men's lacrosse, baseball, and softball. In baseball and softball, it is recommended that children between 5 and 14 years of age wear a batting helmet with a polycarbonate face shield.[82-84] Eyewear is recommended as a wise precaution in limited-contact sports[85] such as racquetball and high school girls' lacrosse.[74] Extra eye protection should be required for any athlete with corrected vision poorer than 20/40 in either eye or with a history of eye injury or surgery.[69, 74] Footwear that fits and is appropriate for the sport and playing surface should be used. The footwear should be replaced when worn out.[69]

Athletic mats, such as those used in wrestling, should be cleaned at least once daily and on a regular schedule with a tuberculocidal cleaner. Further study is recommended to determine the effectiveness of mat-cleaning programs to prevent the spread of skin disorders in wrestling.[86]

Maintenance and reconditioning are essential in providing appropriate safe equipment. A member of the AHCT should document that a designated employee of the sponsoring organization has been trained in the proper fit and care of athletic equipment in the absence of an on-site AHCT member. Sponsoring entities should schedule regular maintenance before equipment is issued to or used by participants. Inspections should be performed on a regular basis throughout the course of the season. In addition, season-end equipment inspections are also recommended to ensure that equipment is repaired or replaced before the start of the next season.

In some sports, forms stating "assumption of risk" for equipment fitting and appropriate use should be used to ensure that there is proper documentation that the participants, and their parents, understand these concepts. If rule changes are to be used to implement improved equipment to protect the participant, care must be used to address public education, the cost of implementation, liability, manpower to implement the rule changes, and the timing of the program.[87]

Additional research has been identified in a number of recommendations. This research is vital in determining how best to protect the participant in any sports program. Every effort or consideration should be made to fund research when it is proposed.

DEVELOPING AND IMPLEMENTING AN EMERGENCY ACTION PLAN

Sports-related injuries and illnesses are common in athletics involving secondary school–age athletes. Members of the AHCT, along with coaches and administrators, need to be prepared for possible emergency situations through the development and implementation of a comprehensive Emergency Action Plan (EAP).

An understood principle within athletics is the possibility that a serious or life-threatening injury and/or illness may occur. There are both intrinsic and extrinsic risks involved with participation in athletics, and it is essential for the sponsoring organization to have a well-developed EAP for such instances to ensure that the appropriate care can be provided in a timely manner. In addition, the EAP should include planning for events that are not athletic related such as natural disasters and crowd control problems that may occur when large groups of people are gathered for athletic events.

In 2002, NATA issued a position statement regarding the need for established emergency plans in all athletic venues and suggested guidelines for developing and implementing the plans.[88] The need for an EAP has been well documented in literature and injury/illness statistics[15,88-94] and supported in case law.[95] In Kleinknecht v. Gettysburg College in

1993,[96] it was decided that an institution owes a duty to each athlete to provide an emergency plan that is adequate for the risks involved in sport participation. This extends beyond the collegiate level and interscholastic athletic events, as seen in Barth by Barth v. Board of Education in 1986,[97] which showed the need for obtaining prompt medical treatment for students injured in physical education activities. In the case of Jarreau v. Orleans Parish School Board in 1992,[98] a school board was found to be vicariously liable for the failure to promptly seek medical attention for an injured athlete. The implementation of an EAP addresses these needs and provides the most efficient opportunity for treatment for injury and/or illness.

Components of Recommendation

The AHCT is an important component of establishing a good EAP. The medical personnel who make up the AHCT often have experience in various areas of emergency athletic care and can contribute to the plan to ensure it is comprehensive and appropriate for school-age athletic events. The development of an EAP requires the input of all members of the AHCT in addition to the administrators of the sponsoring organization, coaches, and facility managers, along with parents and official groups.

This allows for the writing of a comprehensive EAP that fully covers all aspects of emergency situations and environmental conditions and involves the expertise and cooperation of all team members. Examples of individuals to participate in EAP development include the members of the AHCT, coaches, administrators, venue managers, officials, and organizations.

If the event will take place in areas such as city parks, recreation departments, or golf courses, then the governing bodies of these organizations should also be involved or consulted in the development of the EAP. This multiorganization committee would be responsible for developing protocols to manage emergency situations, including establishing the chain of command for emergencies, the specific responsibilities for each team member, emergency situations specific to each sport, emergency situations specific to a particular venue, the necessary emergency equipment and use of said equipment and the training of athletes to help the coach in an isolated situation.

Once the EAP has been developed and implemented, it is essential that all personnel be fully trained in the steps of emergency management, that these training procedures are documented and that there is communication with EMS personnel before the event to ensure cooperation and quicker response to emergency situations. Game and event personnel should also be trained in the necessary skills for emergencies, such as first aid, CPR and AED use, and the prevention of disease transmission.

Minimum athletic emergency equipment should include vacuum splints (or suitable alternative), a long spine board (or scoop stretcher), hard neck (Philadelphia) collars, facemask removal equipment, resuscitation masks, shoulder immobilizers, blankets, crutches, blood pressure cuff, gloves for universal precautions, and a first aid kit.[99]

It is also advisable to have access to an AED during practice and/or competition. This emergency equipment must be readily accessible during all practices and games to all staff responsible for first aid or medical care of the injured athlete.[72]

Steps should also be in place for the documentation of all injury and/or illness situations that occur during the event. A review of the established procedures and all incidences of emergency situations should occur at the conclusion of each event, and a comprehensive review of the entire EAP should occur on an annual basis.

Strategies for Implementation

One of the most important immediate steps is to identify the appropriate personnel to write the EAP. The AHCT should be led by a medical director, preferably the team physician, and include the other members of the team. The members of this team must take into consideration all possible emergency situations that might arise during practice and/or competition. Categories of incidences to consider would be life-threatening injuries, life-threatening illness, and environmental threats.

There should be specific thought given to the types of possible incidents based on the type of activity as well as the specific venue in which it is being held. It is also imperative to ensure that emergency medications, such as an individual athlete's asthma inhaler, EpiPen, Glucagon, or insulin, are available and that the correct protocols for use are followed.

211

Although it is not anticipated that all contingencies will be thought of, a well-developed plan can cover most emergencies and leave a protocol in place to address other issues that arise. The development team should carefully document the emergency treatments and procedures for incidences based on the input and advice of physicians, ATCs, EMS personnel, and other qualified AHCT members. Careful consideration should be given to establishing and documenting specific responsibilities for each member of the AHCT before and during the event.

Written documentation should also include the types and locations of emergency equipment present, methods of communication (e.g., walkie-talkie, cellphone, land line telephone), venue-specific maps, and the location of the hospital or other health care facility for transportation and a list of emergency telephone numbers. Once the EAP has been written, it is essential to review, practice, and revise the EAP so that all duties and responsibilities are clearly outlined and understood. Placing the responsible individuals in mock scenarios is an effective way of testing the EAP for validity. Documentation of all emergency situations during an event is key for liability issues and for revision of the existing EAP. At a minimum, the EAP should be reviewed and practiced on an annual basis and subsequent retraining should take place to refamiliarize the necessary personnel with their duties and responsibilities.

There are several existing documents from supporting organizations that can assist in the development and implementation of an EAP for various venues and athletic settings, including those published by the NATA [88], NFHS[16], NCAA[94, 100], American Academy of Pediatrics [15, 91, 92, 94, 100], AOSSM[101] and The Inter-Association Task Force for Appropriate Care of the Spine-Injured Athlete.[102]

ESTABLISHING PROTOCOLS REGARDING ENVIRONMENTAL CONDITIONS

Secondary school–age individuals participating in athletics are subject to injury due to adverse environmental conditions. Each organization that sponsors an athletics program should establish protocols related to adverse environmental conditions specific to their region. The organizations should identify individuals responsible for ensuring the implementation of the protocols.

Adverse environmental conditions pose varying challenges to athletic events based on geographic regions and the influencing factors specific to those regions. The sponsoring organization's AHCT should be responsible for the development and implementation of policies regarding adverse environmental conditions. Threats can include heat stress, cold stress, lightning, severe weather, air quality, insects, rodents, reptiles, fire, and possible allergic reaction-inducing conditions. Other factors as indicated by geography and climate should be taken into consideration.

It is an understood principle that adverse environmental conditions can pose potential threats to the safety and welfare of athletic participants. Therefore, it is essential that institutions and organizations associated with athletic events have policies and protocols in place to regulate athletic participation.[101] These protocols should be specific to each athletic venue and should take individual geographic effects into consideration.

Some environmental conditions can pose greater threats to athletes in particular regions of the country. There are several environmental considerations and threats that can be included in an individual protocol depending on the venue and geographic region, as given earlier. Several established policies regarding heat stress,[103-107] cold stress,[107, 108] and lightning[109, 110] can be used as models for development. Other environmental condition protocols should be established with the members of the AHCT to ensure that all contingencies have been discussed in detail.

Heat Stress
Exercising in hot temperatures has been shown to have a variety of physiological effects on the human body and can compromise the health of the athlete if not closely monitored.[111, 112] Heat acclimatization is a process through which athletes improve from a physiological standpoint when exposed to exercise in the heat through careful monitoring.[113] Athletes often become acclimatized and adjust to the demands placed on the body by exercise in heat. Throughout this acclimatization period, they should be closely monitored by qualified personnel, most preferably an on-site member of the AHCT.[114] The responsibility of the members of the AHCT should be to allow athletes to acclimatize to heat conditions within certain limits.

There are several position statements and supporting documents that outline safe methods of participation in heat stress conditions and when practice and competition should be suspended.[103, 105, 106, 115] In 2000, the NATA position statement on fluid replacement for athletes outlined the practices that would encourage the optimum fluid replacement for athletes, decreasing the chances for occurrence of heat stress syndromes.[115] In 2002, the NATA position statement on exertional heat illness established recommendations for preventing, recognizing, and treating illnesses that occur from athletic participation.

This position statement,[103] as well as the Inter-Association Task Force on Exertional Heat Illnesses Consensus Statement,[105] contains many details concerning the methods of preventing heat stress syndromes as well as the necessary accommodations that should be made for practices and competitions under given conditions.[103] The NFHS also addresses heat illnesses in detail in their *Sports Medicine Handbook*.[16] The handbook describes the signs and symptoms of heat stress syndromes, as well as treatments and prevention techniques, and provides information on when practices and competitions should be limited based on the ratio of heat to relative humidity.[16] Other organizations that have issued policy statements, position stands, and/or guidelines for heat illnesses include the ACSM,[107] the NCAA,[106] and the AOSSM.[101]

Cold Stress

Cold stress is often an overlooked cause of injury and illness, as heat stress syndromes tend to receive the most attention. However, exposure to cold is obviously more of a concern in certain geographic regions than in others.[116] Extensive research has been done concerning the effects of and possible damage caused by cold on the body during exercise. Exercise and athletic activity in a cold environment can have deleterious effects on performance and human health, which may not be realized by the participant until damage has occurred.[117] Therefore, it is essential to carefully establish a protocol regarding participation in cold environments.

Lightning

Lightning is the second most common environmental cause of death in the United States after floods.[118] It is particularly abundant in early afternoon storms, during which many outside athletic practices and competitions occur.[109] Because there is no absolute protection against the effects of lightning while outside, proper education and a well established protocol can prevent many deaths and injuries.[119, 120]

Table 2. HADDON MATRIX APPLIED TO THE PROBLEM OF ATHLETIC INJURIES

Phases/Factor	Host	Agent	Physical environment	Social environment
Before injury	CS #2 Determine the individual's readiness to participate.	CS #3 Advise on the selection, fit, function and maintenance of athletic equipment.	CS #3 Promote safe and appropriate practice, competition and treatment facilities.	CS #10 Provide scientifically sound nutritional counseling and education
			CS #5 Establish protocols regarding environmental conditions	CS #1. Develop and implement a comprehensive athletic health care administrative system
Injury	Protective responses	Player size and speed	Field condition	Rules enforcement
After injury	CS #8. Facilitate rehabilitation and reconditioning	Exposure to repeat trauma	CS #4. Develop and implement a comprehensive emergency action plan.	CS #9. Provide for pshychosocial consultation and referral
			CS #7. Provide for on-site recognition, evaluation and immediate treatment of injury and illness, with appropriate referrals	

213

The NATA published a position statement on lighting safety for athletics and recreation in 2000 to educate those involved in athletics about the risks involved with participation in a lightning environment and to provide guidelines for safe behaviors during lightning and to advocate appropriate care for lightning strike victims.[109] The NCAA guidelines for lightning safety emphasize many of the same points, including details on an established chain of command and on obtaining weather reports and monitoring of weather systems to provide the most accurate and up-to-date data.[110] The NATA and the NCAA advocate evacuating outside areas as soon as lightning is seen or thunder is heard and seeking shelter in safe buildings. This is the protocol encouraged by the NFHS.[16] The key to lightning injury prevention is to carefully monitor the weather conditions and to allow those individuals in the chain of command to perform their duties in protecting the athletes and participants.

The established environmental protocols should be carefully documented and distributed to all members of the AHCT, coaches and administrators. Opportunities for rehearsing scenarios and revising policies should also be made. It is imperative to ensure that all involved individuals must be aware of the protocols and understand their role in the event of an environmental emergency. An annual revision (similar to that of the EAP) should take place to retrain AHCT members and to address any inaccuracies and inadequacies in the plan.

Components of Recommendation

Before an athletic event or contest takes place, it is essential for the necessary members of the AHCT to meet to develop policies regarding adverse environmental conditions, including lightning, heat stress, and cold stress. The details of this vary as each individual venue and geographic region have concerns that are inherent to that area. The AHCT will begin to develop methods for assessing the site-specific concerns that have been identified. There is a great deal of information available concerning the various environmental conditions and the appropriate planning for prevention and treatment that can be used in identifying the steps to take in each circumstance.[103, 109, 115] Each AHCT will have to decide what is best for each geographic region based on normal environmental conditions for that area.

Taking into account the given possible adverse environmental concerns, written detailed plans that provide for the safety and welfare of all participants will assist the AHCT and event management personnel with decisions regarding participation. In writing these environmental policies, it is also important to carefully delegate responsibility to the appropriate decision makers. Factors to take into consideration include who is responsible for monitoring conditions, what methods will be used to monitor the environment, the time frame parameters for decision making, detailed alternative plans for participants and spectators, and who communicates plans to all relevant individuals.

Strategies for Implementation

There are many members of the AHCT who may be capable of providing input into the development of environmental conditions policies, but it is essential that there is effective communication between the medical director, the ATC, and the administrators of the sponsoring agency. These individuals have the greatest opportunity to effectively design and provide input for the development of these policies. The involvement of all members of the team not only increases the effectiveness of the document but also ensures that all individuals are aware of the policies for safeguarding athletes. It is also essential that communication from the AHCT during contest continues to include the administration and officials.

The use of existing position statements and policies will ease the process of developing individual policies. It is essential that these policies be put into writing so that they may be adequately enforced. Responsibilities for each member of the AHCT should also be put in writing to ensure compliance and to ensure that all members are clear as to what they are to do in given situations. The methods of communication between AHCT members and for the acquisition of necessary environmental information need to be clearly outlined as well (e.g., walkie-talkie, cellphone, CB radio, weather radio).

Heat Stress

Members of the AHCT should be involved with the written guidelines regarding when it is potentially hazardous to participate in athletic events during times of heat and humidity. These guidelines should be implemented by the sponsoring organization and AHCT to determine when it is unsafe for the secondary school–age athlete to participate in sporting events.

Several position statements have been written regarding heat illness, and they recommend that an individual be responsible for evaluating the temperature and humidity. Established local guidelines (limiting personal equipment, increasing fluid replacement breaks, limiting practice intensity and duration, avoiding the heat of the day when possible, etc.) can be followed. Inexpensive sling psychrometers can be used to evaluate wet-bulb and dry-bulb temperatures and humidity, and heat stress.[103, 105, 106,115]

Cold Stress

Sponsoring agencies and the AHCT also need to create guidelines for determining when it is unsafe to participate in athletics due to the cold and/or wind chill. The implementation of these protocols should fall to a designated individual who determines the outdoor temperature with the wind chill and advises whether it is safe for the secondary school–age athlete to participate without the added risk of frostbite or hypothermia. The NCAA has written a guideline for member institutions that reflects the effects of exposure to cold temperature and wind over a period of time and the increased risk for frostbite. These guidelines also include methods of preventing cold illness, such as appropriate clothing, maintenance of energy/hydration levels, and use of a proper warm-up.[108]

The NFHS also addresses cold illness in their Sports Medicine Handbook and includes greater details on the effects of temperature and wind on the body as well as recognition and treatment of frostbite, hypothermia, and related syndromes.[16] Both organizations provide a solid foundation that can be used to develop an individual cold stress protocol to protect athletic populations.

Lightning

A written lightning policy, such as that published by the NATA,[109] should be put into place by the sponsoring agency. It should include the name of a person(s) responsible for monitoring the weather, the criteria for suspension and resumption of activity during lightning, and the safe areas to which the participants and spectators should retreat during inclement weather. Often, the criterion used to determine when activities should cease and resume during lightning is the 30-30 rule, which dictates suspension of activities when the flash-to-bang count nears 30 seconds and resumption of activities after a 30-minute wait following the last lightning flash thunder or after lightning has been seen or heard.[121] In addition, there are other methods of detection, including the weather service radio, lightning detection equipment, and lightning detection services.

There should be a designated person responsible for determining the flash-to-bang count at each outside venue, practice, and competition when severe storms are forecast. It is recommended that this designee be someone other than a game official or coach due to the attention they must pay to the game. This count is determined by beginning to count the seconds from the time the lightning is seen to the time the thunder is heard. The time in seconds between the flash of the lightning and the bang of the thunder is divided by 5 to determine the how far the storm is from the individual who is counting.[119, 121] It is recommended that as the flash-to-bang count nears 30 seconds (means that lightning strike was 6 miles away), all participants and spectators should immediately seek a safe shelter.[109]

Other Environmental Conditions

Special consideration should be given to the incidence of environmental allergens and potential bites from insects, rodents, and reptiles. The on-site member of the AHCT, or the coach when there is no on-site AHCT member, should be aware of those athletes with allergies who might be at increased risk for respiratory ailments or anaphylaxis.
The AHCT should monitor the exposure of those athletes and plan ahead for proper treatment (e.g., have an athlete's EpiPen available) should it occur. Specific information can be gathered from the American Academy of Asthma, Allergy and Immunology (AAAAI) and from organizations such as the National Outdoor Leader School (NOLS) and their Wilderness Medicine School.

PROVIDING ON-SITE RECOGNITION, EVALUATION, AND IMMEDIATE TREATMENT OF INJURIES AND ILLNESSES

Secondary school–age individuals participating

in athletics are subject to injury, including certain injuries and medical conditions unique to this population.[3] Each organization that sponsors an athletics program should develop an EAP that highlights mechanisms for evaluating and treating adolescents sustaining an injury. As part of the EAP, the organization should identify individuals responsible for providing these services and ensure they are educated, trained, and appropriately certified and licensed (if required by state law) to provide these services during every practice and competition.

The ATC offers the best option, offering advanced first aid knowledge, CPR/AED use, and the ability to make return-to-play decisions. The AMA recommends that ATCs provide these services, although the AMA recognizes that EMTs, paramedics, and physicians are viable options in the absence of an ATC.[1, 122] In some cases, the coach is the only person available on-site during practices and games and should be trained in first aid and CPR; however, the coach cannot practice outside of his/her scope of practice, which would include making decisions regarding when it is appropriate for an athlete to return to play following an injury or illness.

Early injury evaluation and treatment encourages proper healing and decreases the risk of reinjury,[1, 3, 123-125] and the initiation of prompt treatment is critical in the management of life- or limb-threatening injuries or conditions. These services should be available to injured athletes at each and every athletic activity.

The amount of epidemiological data concerning the incidence of injury in youth sports participation is increasing.[1, 3, 14, 85, 91, 125-144] The injuries sustained by the participants vary in severity, from relatively minor to catastrophic.[3, 14, 135, 139] It is important to remember that secondary school–age athletes are not miniature adults[124] and are susceptible to injuries that are specific to their age and level of physical maturity, presenting special challenges with respect to their participation in athletic activities.[85]

A thorough, on-site initial evaluation is important in recognizing the nature and severity of the injury, determining if more advanced treatment and care are required, and limiting participation to protect the initial injury and prevent further harm.

One of the primary concerns regarding adolescent injuries is the child's developing musculoskeletal system.[124, 135, 136, 139, 145] The fact that the epiphysis, or growth plates, remain open is the reason physically immature youngsters are at greater risk, especially if they compete against more mature youngsters who have completed puberty and have closed growth plates and more mature muscular support for joints.[124, 145] An adolescent's bones and articular surfaces may not be sufficiently developed to handle the stresses associated with athletic activity. Therefore, adolescents may develop a number of characteristic injuries, including osteochondritis dessicans, spondylolysis, stress fractures, and Salter-Harris fractures, many of which may have long-term consequences.[135, 136, 139, 144, 145]

Adolescents who have sustained an injury should be evaluated immediately to determine the nature and extent of the injury, because its signs and symptoms may change relatively quickly.[1, 3, 123-125] For example, the signs and symptoms of a head injury may resolve soon after the injury, even though a significant, possibly life-threatening, head injury has occurred.[132] This individual may return to play because of resolution of their symptoms; however, Guskiewicz et al[132] report that football players sustaining one concussion were three times more likely to sustain a second concussion during the same season than were athletes who have not had a concussion.

Identifying the head injury through a thorough initial injury evaluation is essential to limiting the "serious sequelae" associated with repeated head injury.[132] An example of this sequelae is second impact syndrome (SIS), which occurs when an individual with a head injury receives a second blow to the head before the brain has recovered from the first injury and can lead

TABLE 3. CHARACTERISTICS OF THE DEVELOPMENTAL STAGES OF ADOLESCENCE

Stage	Characteristics
Early – individuation	During this time, athletes may become confused or question their identity as they encounter the physical and emotional changes of puberty.
Middle – separation/rebellion	This is the phase during which many of the risk-taking behaviors may be initiated or reach their peak
Late – abstract thinking, future/goal orientation	This level of maturity is not often reached during the secondary school years

to death.[127,134] Immediate recognition of the initial concussion by members of the AHCT, as well as team members and coach, is important in the prevention of SIS and can be made through a proper initial evaluation.

An immediate injury evaluation also permits the quick initiation of appropriate medical treatment, which is associated with proper healing and a reduced risk of reinjury.[1,124]

Immediate treatment can mean the difference between life and death. Heat exhaustion, for example, is one condition that can be fatal without prompt recognition and treatment.[103] In addition, improper treatment of a suspected neck or spine injury may lead to secondary injury or a worsening of the original injury.[102]

When identifying the individuals to fulfill these roles, most organizations consider several options: physicians, paramedics or EMTs, coaches, and ATCs. Physicians certainly have the knowledge to complete an injury evaluation. Physicians also possess the medical expertise required to make decisions regarding injury treatment. However, one concern when asking physicians to provide these services is their availability at each practice and competition.

Several studies discuss the medical coverage afforded high schools for athletic activities in a variety of states.[128,143,146] In a survey of 240 California high schools, physicians provided medical coverage at football games over 70% of the time.[146] In contrast, a survey of 119 high schools in Alabama reported physician coverage at less than 25% of school-sponsored sporting events and less than 15% of practices.[128]

Although practice coverage was not addressed specifically, reports from 301 high schools in Wisconsin indicated that only 35.5% of schools had a designated team physician.[143] Hence, although physicians certainly have the skills and training required to provide immediate medical care, they are often not available or able to satisfy the need for immediate injury evaluation and treatment at all practices and games.[1]

Similar results were found when schools were surveyed regarding the presence of an ambulance during practices and competitions. Vangsness et al[146] report that less than 38% of schools had an ambulance with an EMT or a paramedic available at home football games. Culpepper[128] found that at least 80% of schools provided an ambulance during varsity football games, although less than 38% provided an ambulance for junior varsity football games. In a survey of 302 high schools, Rutherford, Niedfeldt, and Young[143] found that almost 79% of schools had an ambulance available or on call for practices or scrimmages. Although this percentage is higher than reports from other states,[146] having an ambulance "on call" does not necessarily mean the ambulance is on-site. In cases where an ambulance is available on-site, that ambulance may be called away at a moment's notice in response to an emergency. An athlete's medical condition can change dramatically in a few minutes, less time than it may take an ambulance to arrive on the scene. Relying on the presence of an ambulance and personnel to provide medical care may not satisfy the need for immediate injury evaluation or treatment.

Coaches are another viable option for providing immediate injury evaluation and treatment. Coaches certainly are available on-site at each practice and competition and are encouraged to become educated about responding to emergencies, including certification in first aid and CPR.[16,85,88,91,123,125,126] In fact, some states require coaches to obtain these certifications.[141,146] However, state laws often prohibit coaches from making return-to-play decisions or care beyond first aid such as taping an injured body part. The U.S. Navy defines first aid as the emergency care and treatment of a sick or injured person before professional medical services are obtained. First aid measures are not meant to replace proper medical diagnosis and treatment – they only provide temporary support until professional medical assistance is available. The purposes of first aid are to save life, prevent further injury, and minimize or prevent infection. Therefore, using coaches as health care providers is not always appropriate.

Moreover, a study by Ransone and Dunn-Bennett[141] questions the ability of coaches to provide these services. They surveyed 104 coaches of boys' and girls' sports at 17 high schools in California. The survey consisted of two separate parts: a test of first aid knowledge and a game situation data sheet that asked coaches to make decisions regarding athletic injuries in nine different athletic scenarios. Of the coaches surveyed, 92% were certified in first aid, yet only 36% passed the first aid assessment. The game situation questionnaire asked coaches to indicate whether they would return a starting player to the game after an injury. The authors note that, in general, coaches tended to return players to the game, especially those coaches who passed the first aid assessment. The authors express concern that coaches may not understand the "ramifications of returning an athlete to competition" and suggest that "additional knowledge on the treatment and rehabilitation of athletic injuries should enable coaches to make more objective decisions."[141] Of additional concern is that standard first aid courses do not teach the specifics regarding athletic-related injuries so many coaches have not been taught how to make these types of decisions. There is also a conflict of interest in allowing coaches to make return-to-play decisions.

Coaches should not be expected to split their attention between evaluating athletes, making return decisions, and their coaching duties. In addition, they do not possess the education to appropriately make the decision to return an athlete to participation following an injury.

In many cases, coaches are asked to fill the role of injury evaluator and treatment provider. However, during the course of an athletic practice or competition, coaches focus their energy on supervising their athletes and instructing them in the skills of the game. In addition, of the coaches responding to Culpepper's survey examining medical coverage in Alabama high schools, "only about half of them said they felt adequately trained to handle a medical emergency."[128] Given the concerns expressed regarding a coach's ability to handle medical emergencies, their expertise in first aid and CPR, and their ability to make objective return-to-play decisions, assigning coaches the additional responsibility of providing immediate injury care may not be the best solution. The CDC will soon release a coach's kit for concussion management that was developed based on input from coaches and an expert task force. The consensus was that coaches should be able to identify a concussion but should make no decisions about return to play based on their preoccupation with all the other players and a limited knowledge.

Providing an individual, such as the ATC, to specifically provide injury evaluation and treatment services at all athletic activities has been recommended.

In summary, while physicians are capable of performing injury evaluations and rendering decisions about injury treatment, they generally are not available to perform these duties at all practices and competitions. And although an ambulance complete with EMTs and paramedics is only a telephone call away, rarely is an ambulance available at each and every athletic activity. Immediate injury evaluation and treatment is a critical component in the successful management of many athletic injuries; however, EMTs are trained in only emergency care and cannot fulfill the role of the comprehensive AHCT. Therefore, organizations that sponsor athletic programs must ensure that an individual or individuals capable of performing these tasks are on-site at each and every athletic event.

The AMA recommends that schools sponsoring athletic programs establish an AMU that consists of a physician and an athletic health coordinator.[1, 122] The AMA suggests that athletic organizations place an ATC in the role of the athletic health coordinator.[1, 122, 147] ATCs are appropriate choices for the athletic health coordinator because they have the skills and knowledge required to perform injury evaluations and to provide immediate treatment.[1]

Components of the Recommendation

Organizations that sponsor athletic programs should establish an AHCT, identify an athletic health coordinator, and develop a comprehensive EAP[1, 122] that includes mechanisms for providing immediate injury evaluation and treatment. Individuals capable of providing these services should be available for all athletic practices and competitions.

Strategies for Implementation

On-site medical professionals such as the team physician or ATC should lead the AHCT. The organization sponsoring the athletics program should identify the individuals responsible for performing injury evaluations and providing injury treatment within applicable state law. The selection of this individual should be based on his/her education and availability to provide these services at each athletic practice and competition. At a minimum, a coach or other individual who is with the team on a regular basis, and is trained in CPR (including AED use) and first aid, should be available to tend to injuries that occur. In addition, protocols should be established, in advance, governing referrals and return-to-play decisions, especially in instances where a sponsoring organization may have multiple events going on at several sites.

Another viable option is the presence of an EMT/paramedic or a registered nurse at practices and games. These individuals would offer a higher level of care than an individual with first aid and CPR training; however, these individuals may be limited in their ability to render return-to-play decisions and apply protective taping and padding following an injury.

FACILITATING REHABILITATION AND RECONDITIONING

Adolescents who participate in athletics are subject to injury. When injuries occur, the injured individual requires proper treatment and rehabilitation to regain full physical function and safely return to athletic participation. This treatment should include not only the care provided immediately after the injury but also the post injury rehabilitation and reconditioning. Rehabilitation and reconditioning programs reduce the likelihood of reinjury and promote a safe return to play. Organizations that sponsor athletic programs should establish an on-site member of the AHCT and identify this individual to manage the postinjury treatment plans of the athletes. Coaches should also be taught to follow the AHCT's recommendations in regard to athlete rehabilitation.

Injuries are a common occurrence in all levels of athletics. For most athletes, a return to activity after the injury is expected. However, when the individual returns to competition, the likelihood of reinjury is directly dependent on the care this individual receives after the injury. Although the evaluation and treatment provided immediately after the injury are critical, a rehabilitation and reconditioning program designed to safely return the individual to play is just as important.

Trauma to the body causes tissue damage and cell death, resulting in swelling, pain, and decreased ROM.[148] Prolonged periods of disuse can further limit ROM and lead to decreases in strength, cardiovascular conditioning, and muscular endurance.[148]

Effective postinjury care can limit the long-term consequences of the initial injury by decreasing pain and increasing ROM, muscular strength, and overall function.[149-151] Programs designed to return an injured individual to a preinjury level of function can be described using a variety of terms, including injury treatment, rehabilitation programs, and therapy. In general, these programs consist of exercise, therapeutic modalities, and functional activities specific to the individual and his/her injury.[148, 152, 153] The goals of rehabilitation and reconditioning programs include preventing further injury and promoting a safe return to play.[148] Adolescents who are injured during athletic performance should complete a rehabilitation and reconditioning program to promote a safe return to play.

Adolescents who sustain an athletic injury should receive treatment. This, as a whole, consists of two distinct parts or phases. The first component is the treatment received immediate after the injury; the second component is the postinjury rehabilitation and reconditioning. The rehabilitation and reconditioning component should be viewed as a process that lasts days, weeks, or months, with the length dependent on the severity of the injury.

Programs designed to return an injured individual to a preinjury level of function can be described using a variety of terms, including injury treatment, rehabilitation and reconditioning programs, therapy, and physical therapy. Although these terms are familiar to most, the concepts behind them are less well known. Understanding these concepts is best achieved by describing the characteristics and goals of rehabilitation and reconditioning programs. The first primary goal of every rehabilitation and reconditioning program is injury prevention.[3, 148] The second goal is a safe and timely return of injured athletes to their preinjury level of competition.[148] Rehabilitation and reconditioning programs consist of individualized therapeutic exercise that is performed in orderly, progressive steps until return to play.[148]

One of the hallmarks of rehabilitation and reconditioning programs is the progression of therapeutic exercise. This is enhanced through the setting of both short- and long-term goals. Short-term goals tend to focus on increasing ROM, strength, and flexibility and on restoring proprioception.[130, 148] Long-term goals tend to focus on optimizing the individual's functional status.[148, 154] Achieving these goals depends on many factors, of which perhaps the most important is frequent reevaluation of the athlete to modify the goals and treatments as needed.[148] Therefore, qualified personnel capable of re-evaluating and modifying the rehabilitation and reconditioning program as needed should be available.

The benefits of completing rehabilitation and reconditioning programs are also well known. Stylianos[155] notes that individuals participating in "effective rehabilitation programs will often surpass expectations for functional recovery." Entering into a rehabilitation and reconditioning program after injury permits injured athletes to return to play sooner with fewer long-term disabilities.[136] Individuals have noted decreased pain and disability and increased ROM and functional activity following the completion of rehabilitation programs for patellofemoral pain and neck pain, respectively.[149, 151] Gilbey et al[150] found that individuals who completed an exercise program before total hip arthroplasty and continued with the program after surgery exhibited an earlier return to functional activity.[150] In a study of injury patterns in select high school sports, Powell and Barber-Foss[3] noted that, as part of an overall injury prevention program, rehabilitation after the initial injury minimized the risk of reinjury.

Adolescents who return to participation before completing a rehabilitation and reconditioning program are risking reinjury and other long-term consequences. There are a number of reasons why an adolescent may not successfully complete a rehabilitation and reconditioning program. An adolescent may lack access to such a program or choose not to participate in the program. Compliance with rehabilitation and reconditioning programs and the length of time an individual receives these services correlates strongly with better treatment outcomes.[156, 157]

The rehabilitation and reconditioning of athletic injuries represents a major component of a comprehensive injury prevention program and should be undertaken by a selected member of the AHCT. The NATABOC-certified athletic trainer (ATC) is the choice of the AMA because they have the appropriate training and educational background to provide appropriate care for injured athletes and to make sound decisions regarding when an athlete can return to play.[1, 122] Although it has been noted that not all organizations have the resources to hire an ATC or implement a sophisticated sports medicine program, they can designate a qualified member of the coaching staff to work with a member of the

AHCT to prevent injuries, provide medical care, and rehabilitate injured athletes.[1]

Components of Recommendation

Organizations that sponsor athletic programs should identify an individual who is responsible for coordinating rehabilitation and reconditioning programs with physicians and other health care professionals. This individual should also be responsible for determining return-to-play following rehabilitation.

Strategies for Implementation

Organizations that sponsor athletic programs should establish an AHCT consisting of a team physician and an athletic health coordinator.[1, 122] The organization may choose to provide an athletic health coordinator such as an ATC who is qualified to evaluate injured individuals and develop appropriate rehabilitation and reconditioning programs.

If the organization cannot provide an ATC, it should identify both (1) an athletic health coordinator to provide rehabilitative care and (2) an athletic health coordinator to work with health care providers outside the organization to ensure their recommendations regarding treatment and participation are being followed.

The on-site member of the AHCT can ensure injured athletes receive appropriate rehabilitation and reconditioning services in several ways. An ATC possesses the education and credentials to design the rehabilitation and reconditioning program, supervising and reevaluating individuals as they progress through it. In cases where the athletic health coordinator does not have the training to provide these services, s/he can coordinate with outside health care providers to ensure that the recommendations of the treating physician, physical therapist, and others are followed. Regardless of the athletic health coordinator's qualifications, this individual plays an important role in injury rehabilitation and reconditioning.

PROVIDING FOR PSYCHOSOCIAL CONSULTATION AND REFERRAL

Members of the AHCT may be the health care professionals who most often interact with adolescent athletes. In some cases, a PPE or injury management may be an adolescent's only interaction with any health care system. Members of the team must therefore be capable of identifying potential psychosocial pathologies and referring the athlete for appropriate diagnosis and management. Organizations that sponsor athletic programs must identify local experts who specialize in these areas.

Adolescents are at significant risk for morbidities associated with substance abuse, sexual activity, depression, eating disorders, suicidal tendencies, weapon use, violence, and vehicular recklessness. Adolescent athletes in particular may have an increased risk of depression associated with injury or athletic "burn-out." Furthermore, although adolescent athletes may have a decreased risk of cigarette smoking, some studies have suggested an increased use of smokeless tobacco, unsafe sexual activity, alcohol abuse, vehicular recklessness, and other risk-taking behaviors among certain adolescent athletes.

The AMA has estimated that the athletic PPE serves as the only routine health maintenance for 80% to 90% of adolescents.[30] Even though the consensus PPE monograph recommends counseling and screening for psychosocial problems,[17] some have called the PPE a "missed opportunity"[158] to adequately evaluate the physical, emotional, and psychological well-being of secondary school–age athletes.

Studies have shown that not only do secondary school–age athletes engage in numerous health risk behaviors,[159] they may also have a higher rate of certain behaviors than their non-athletic peers. Due to the requirement for parental consent, conducting research to estimate the prevalence of health-risk behaviors is difficult in secondary school–age athletes. However, if one extrapolates conclusions from data in the collegiate population, to which many secondary school–age athletes aspire and will graduate, some conclusions can be made regarding athletes and risky health habits.

Nattiv and Puffer[160] found that collegiate athletes have higher proportions of risky behaviors than do their non-athletic peers, including a higher quantity of alcohol consumed, lower use of contraception, higher number of sexual partners and sexually transmitted diseases, greater rates of driving while intoxicated with alcohol or other drugs and riding with an intoxicated driver, and lower use of seatbelts and of helmets when riding a motorcycle or moped.

In addition, high school athletes have been found to have a higher rate of accidental non-athletic injuries[161] and to demonstrate earlier sexual contact[162] compared to non-athletes.

The risk-taking behaviors seem to vary by gender, with male athletes disproportionately more likely to engage in them than female athletes.[163] Nattiv et al[164] confirmed this finding in a follow-up study to their prior work and further identified participants in contact sports as at the highest risk. They also showed that athletes who engage in one high-risk behavior are more likely to engage in multiple high-risk behaviors. There are suggestions that addictive disorders, such as gambling, may often be seen as a comorbid factor with depression among athletes.[165] An excellent review of certain risk-taking behaviors of athletes and the studies comparing health risk behaviors in athletes and nonathletes was published by Patel and Luckstead.[166]

Of importance is that the same studies also demonstrated important benefits of athletic participation, including lower likelihood to smoke cigarettes or marijuana, greater likelihood to engage in healthy dietary behaviors, and lower likelihood to feel bored or hopeless[161]; a significant decrease in drug and alcohol use and abuse over all 4 years of high school[162]; and less depression, less suicidal ideation, and fewer suicide attempts.[167] Looking more critically at the Nattiv and Puffer[160] data, if certain male contact sports were removed from the sample, the remaining athletes may have demonstrated no greater risk-taking behaviors than the general student body.

In general, then, athletic participation seems to correlate with improved emotional wellbeing in adolescents.[168] Injured patients in sports medicine clinics may therefore experience significant psychological distress associated with the loss of this participation.[169] Interestingly, among injured adolescent athletes who reported higher athletic self-identity, higher depressive symptom scores were measured.[170]

The health professionals best positioned and suited to address these psychosocial concerns in the athletic setting may be ATCs, because the necessary skills and knowledge are standard to their professional practice and because they are more likely to be consistently available on-site.[171]

Components of Recommendation

Members of the AHCT team and coaches often develop close and/or long-term relationships with adolescent athletes and may be well positioned to identify subtle early warning signs of common psychosocial problems. Coaches should work with members of the AHCT to provide for psychosocial consultation and referral of adolescent athletes with the following guidelines:

• Coaches and AHCT members should be aware of the psychosocial problems of adolescence, including disordered eating, substance abuse, sexual activity, athletic "burn-out," depression, suicidal tendencies, weapon use, violence, and vehicular recklessness.

• At least one AHCT member should review the PPE to look for specific warning signs.

• Coaches and AHCT members should be aware that psychosocial problems of adolescent athletes might manifest themselves as overtly as dropping out of participation or as subtly as small decreases in performance.

• AHCT team members should be able to easily refer athletes to identified consultants who can further evaluate and treat these suspected conditions.

• The organizations that sponsor athletic programs must establish systems to facilitate these referrals by identifying local mental health providers, ensuring prompt access to them, and minimizing barriers such as insurability and payment.

• At least one, if not all, of the AHCT members should be aware of the specialized developmental needs and stages of growing adolescents.

• At a minimum, one on-site AHCT or coach should be well versed in the recognition of psychosocial issues and the referral system established by the sponsoring organization

Strategies for Implementation

Members of the AHCT may be well positioned but, because of their training, not well suited to identify emerging psychosocial problems. Implementation of this recommendation would therefore require some, if not all, of the following elements: As detailed in the PPE monograph,[17] thorough psychosocial screening should be an important component of the PPE and should be conducted, ideally, by the athlete's primary care provider. If not conducted by the primary care provider, a thorough psychosocial screening could be conducted by another health care professional who is comfortable with adolescents and familiar with the basic tenets of confidential and sensitive interviewing. The issues that can be addressed in a thorough psychosocial screening can include questions regarding home life and family dynamics, education (school performance and relationships), activities (sports, jobs, and leisure enjoyment), diet, drug use, safety issues (violence, weapon use vehicular recklessness), sexuality (contraception, type, number and frequency of partners), depression, and suicidal tendencies.

Texts such as Neinstein's Adolescent Health Care[172] provide more detailed examples of the content of and techniques for adolescent psychosocial screening. Other tools for screening specific conditions include a screening instrument that can reliably and validly identify disordered eating behaviors in the secondary school–age population and ones that evaluate depressive symptoms such as sleep disturbances, irritability, guilt, low energy levels, inability to concentrate, changes in appetite, and suicidal tendencies.

Team members should be provided education and training by local experts in adolescent health such as the multidisciplinary members of the Society for Adolescent Medicine (SAM) (http://www.adolescenthealth.org). Curricular goals could include understanding of the basic cognitive, emotional, physical, and psychosocial developmental stages of adolescence (Table 3) and identifying signs and symptoms of common psychosocial problems, such as disordered eating, substance abuse, sexual activity, athletic "burn-out," depression, suicidality, weapon use, violence, and vehicular recklessness.

While a sports psychologist may be a valuable member of or consultant to the AHCT, ATCs are specifically trained in the components listed and often practice on-site with adolescent athletes and therefore would be extremely valuable members of the AHCT.

In addition, the ATC should refer any athletes with identified problems to the school counselors and, if comfortable, discuss the issue with the athlete and/or his or her parents.

PROVIDING SCIENTIFICALLY SOUND NUTRITIONAL COUNSELING AND EDUCATION

Sports nutrition is a key factor in an athlete's growth, development, and performance. It is well known that adolescents have unique nutritional requirements that are further complicated by sport participation. The massive industry of supplements marketed to enhance sports performance and the lack of regulation as to the effectiveness and safety of such products pose an additional risk to secondary school–age athletes. Athletes need guidance to make sound nutritional decisions in an age where fad diets and performance enhancement products are prevalent.

Sponsoring organizations of athletic programs have a responsibility to provide a safe environment including sound, scientifically based information regarding nutrition and supplements. A solid knowledge of nutritional concepts is crucial to any AHCT; especially those caring for secondary school–age athletes. In addition to basic growth and development, competition puts an increased demand on daily nutritional requirements. Factors such as ethnicity, social and economic status, family history and environment, peer pressure, and inaccurate diet information can complicate the prescription for good nutrition. In addition, adolescents' tendencies to skip meals, snack on junk food, and feast at fast food restaurants can add to poor eating habits.

A system for reviewing an athlete's nutritional status is the basis of providing appropriate information to athletes and parents regarding long-term nutritional health.

Childhood obesity is on the rise in United States and puts children at risk for heart disease, illness, and injury.[173] A review of an athlete's nutritional status could alert the child and parents to a problem. If a child is found to have poor nutritional habits, an allied health care professional should help combat the problem by creating a plan to address the issues identified in the nutritional review.

Included within the topic of nutrition is proper hydration, especially during activities conducted in high heat stress environments. The availability of hydration fluids in a clean, noninfectious environment at all sport settings should be ensured. It has been well documented in the NATA's Heat Illnesses Position Statement[103] that one major preventative measure is to maintain proper hydration. Not only should the athlete be given the opportunity to consume the appropriate amount of fluid, but s/he should also be educated as to how much to consume and why it is important. Athletic performance may decrease due to hypohydration.[115] Education of

athletes, coaches, and parents in regard to hydration is crucial in the prevention of unwanted injuries and illness and should be a consideration of any group working with adolescent athletes. In addition, coaches or other personnel should never restrict fluids for exercising athletes.

Pre-event and post-event nutritional needs are important considerations for the secondary school–age athlete. For optimal performance, an athlete needs to know what to eat and when to stop eating before a competition. Eating the wrong foods at the wrong time will not give an athlete the appropriate energy for competition and may cause bloating and discomfort.[174]

After exercise, it is important to replenish the nutrients used. Athletes, parents, and coaches should have an avenue to find out the necessary information. Resources reflecting sound scientific material should be used; examples are provided in the Identification of Additional Resources section of this document.

Body weight has a direct influence on some sports such as wrestling and crew and is associated with performance in many other sports such as gymnastics and dance. It has an aesthetic impact in sports such as cheerleading. The pressure to achieve or maintain a low body weight during the secondary school years can lead some to develop disordered eating. There should be a system in place to identify athletes at risk for eating disorders and to treat those who have been identified. It is important that someone close to the athlete knows what to look for. People with eating disorders are very manipulative; so once they have been identified, it is very important to have a plan set in place to provide referral to an appropriate allied health care professional who specializes in this field.

Use of sports supplements and performance-enhancing drugs is fairly common among secondary school students.[175] Young people are taking them to perform better or to build muscle, as well as to look better. The main sources of knowledge regarding supplements and performance-enhancing drugs are friends and advertising. Most athletic governing bodies prohibit the use of supplements and drugs that are designed to enhance performance.[16] Supplements marketed to enhance athletic performance often are touted as "herbal" or "natural," which implies an element of safety. This, coupled with the massive marketing campaigns and use by professional athletes, provides for the "easy path to success" for the secondary school–age athlete. Society's emphasis on winning and a child's desire to please parents and coaches make for a potentially deadly combination. While young people may realize that supplements and performance-enhancing drugs are dangerous, few are reported to know the potential side effects.[175]

Dietary supplements are not required to be standardized in the United States. In fact, no legal or regulatory definition exists in the United States for standardization as it applies to dietary supplements.[176] Studies conducted on sports supplements rarely include subjects of adolescent population. Adverse potential side effects of sports supplements may include, but are not limited to, heart failure/cardiac anomalies, organ malfunction, personality disorders, reproductive disorders, headache, and acne.

Members of the AHCT should be well versed in proper sports nutrition for the adolescent and have a basic knowledge of proper nutrition and eating habits. They should also have access to a professional nutritionist or dietician.

Components of Recommendation
Sponsoring organizations should establish components of a comprehensive sports nutritional support system, based on current scientific facts, and should include, 1) A system for reviewing an athlete's nutritional status, 2) Policies to ensure the availability of hydration fluids in a clean, noninfectious environment at all sport settings, 3) Encouragement of appropriate pre-exercise and post-exercise food, 4) A system to identify athletes at risk for disordered eating and a system to treat those who have been identified, and 5) The use of scientifically supported literature when developing rules that restrict the use of performance-enhancing supplements, drugs and substances, or educational programs to inform coaches, athletes, and parents of the dangers of ergogenic aids.

Strategies for Implementation
Reviewing the athlete's nutritional status
Information sheets with general nutrition goals for an active secondary school–age athlete can be provided by the sponsoring organization. Each athlete should have a basic understanding of what nutritional requirements s/he needs to have for normal growth and activities of daily living as well as the additional

needs that exist because of the energy expenditure caused by his/her sport. Reference to appropriate print and Web media can also be provided; sources are available later in this document. Coaches, as well as members of the AHCT, should be alert to the athletes' nutritional well-being and provide additional information and interaction when circumstances warrant.

Maintaining adequate hydration
The sponsoring organization, via the coaches and members of the AHCT, has a responsibility to provide an environment and information to facilitate or help athletes maintain adequate hydration during physical activity. Several documents are available to assist with the development of a fluid replacement program such as NATA's Position Statement on Fluid Replacement,[115] as well as educational materials that can be provided to athletes, coaches, and parents, such as NATA's Exertional Heat Illness Consensus Statement.[105] Encouraging fluid replacement adequate to replace fluids lost due to sweating before, during, and after intense physical activity is essential to maintain performance levels and general health.

Pre-exercise and post-exercise nutrition
There should be an encouragement of appropriate pre-exercise and post-exercise food. For optimal performance, an athlete needs to know what to eat and when to stop eating before a competition. Informational handouts with recommendations based on accurate scientifically proven information can be provided to athletes and parents. Sponsoring organizations that provide opportunities for athletes to travel (e.g., youth travel soccer) can lead by example and provide the teams with nutritionally sound eating opportunities, both before and after exercise. Members of the AHCT should investigate available resources such as community-based wellness centers and hospitals that have registered dietitians and nutritionists on staff to provide appropriate information to the team, coaches, and parents.

Identify athletes at risk for disordered eating
Disordered eating can have a variety of signs and symptoms. Providing information to coaches about the signs and symptoms of disordered eating can encourage early recognition. The complexity of

dealing with disordered eating necessitates referral of athletes who exhibit signs and symptoms to an appropriate professional. Appropriate professionals include physicians, psychologists, school nurses, and nutritional counselors. Establishing, in advance, a systematic protocol to follow when an athlete is suspected of disordered eating is essential to ensure athletes receive the appropriate support.

Performance-enhancing supplements

Supplements marketed to enhance athletic performance come in many different forms. Most athletic governing bodies prohibit the use of supplements and drugs that are designed to enhance performance. Sponsoring organizations should support rules prohibiting supplement use and provide education addressing the potential health risks associated with them. Caution should be taken when researching information on specific supplements and drugs to ensure it is from a reputable source.

DEVELOPING INJURY AND ILLNESS PREVENTION STRATEGIES

Injuries and illnesses are a heavy burden on the well-being of secondary school–age athletes and a leading reason why people stop participating in physical activities. There are many interventions that have proved to be effective in reducing the severity of athletic injuries.[177-180] Still, many opportunities for prevention remain. This document establishes recommendations for the prevention, care, and appropriate management of athletic-related injury and illness specific to the secondary school–age individual. This overview presents a public health framework for developing effective interventions to reduce the burden of injuries to secondary school–age athletes.

Participation by secondary school–age children in sports, recreation, and exercise is widespread, with nearly 6.5 million high school students participating in organized athletics.[11] However, many of these activities involve elevated risks of injury. As a result, approximately 715,000 sports- and recreation-related injuries occur in the school setting each year.[181] These injuries may lead to a number of costs, some of which are financial and some of which affect a person's quality of life.[182] In the short term, costs include medical care expenses and time lost from classes and athletic play. Of U.S. schoolchildren

who received medical attention for a sport/recreation injury, 20% had one or more days of lost time from school.[183] Long-term costs may include medical and rehabilitation expenses, restriction of future athletic activities, loss of some amount of physical function, and increases in insurance premiums.

A wide variety of injury control interventions have been accepted in the athletic community over the years, including changes to the environment (e.g., break-away bases),[184] use of protective equipment in contact sports (e.g., helmets),[185] and rule changes (e.g., football's prohibition of spearing).[186] Scientific progress has demonstrated that certain sports, certain positions, and certain competitive situations have greater risks of injury than others. By recognizing the greatest risks, we can develop ideas that reduce the chances of a serious injury to a young athlete.

Developing a comprehensive approach to injury control strategies for athletics is difficult. To begin to establish this direction, NATA sponsored the development of recommendations for appropriate medical care of secondary school–age athletes. This effort addresses more than basic emergency care during sports participation; it involves virtually all aspects of prevention, and activities of ongoing daily athletic health care.

The recommendations are intended for use by the sponsoring organizations of athletic programs, and the AHCT they establish, in consultation with administrators, coaches, parents, and participants. Establishing an AHCT should be one of the sponsoring organization's first priorities and should include medical professionals such as ATCs, allopathic or osteopathic physicians, school nurses, and other allied health care providers.[1] By approaching the issue of athletic injuries in a comprehensive way, we develop a better sense of where the problems lie and what can be done to eliminate or reduce them.

This holistic approach involves considering characteristics of the athlete (host), the environment associated with athletic performance (both physical and social-cultural), and the energy that is transferred to the body that causes damage. These elements and their relationships are represented as a public health framework. This framework has long been used in the study of disease and has recently been applied to the topic of athletic injury. As described by Weaver et al,[125] "The public health framework suggests that multiple types of social environments…operate within a physical environment, and provide the context in which an energy vector acts on an athlete to cause an injury. Each of these components and their multiple interactions can be further investigated as a potential target for injury prevention efforts."

Athletics includes a long history of interventions designed to protect players from specific injuries. However, not all of these efforts have been scientifically evaluated to demonstrate their effectiveness. Also, not all interventions have been found to be acceptable to players, and enforcement of protective rules may be rejected by the athletic community, who view the rule change as an offense to the sport's tradition.[182]

Nevertheless, games are constantly evolving with safety concerns often driving the changes. The following outline presents some examples of the best practices for injury control in modern sport using elements of the implementation hierarchy previously described.

Engineering controls

Although safety balls have long been assumed to cause fewer injuries, no epidemiological study had examined their effectiveness before the study of Marshall et al[84]. In a 3-year nationwide study involving more than 6.7 million player-seasons, the use of safety balls was associated with a 23% reduced risk of ball-related injury in Little League Baseball. The effect was more dramatic among younger divisions than among older divisions. The authors also suggest that concerns of poorer performance by the reduced-impact ball, the greatest barrier to wider acceptance, are based on misperception "of the ball's play, rather than the actual performance of the ball."[84]

Administrative controls

Based on surveillance data of head and neck injuries occurring in tackle football, axial loading was identified in 1975 as the primary cause of serious cervical spine injuries.[187] The incidence of catastrophic head and neck injuries increased in 1976 as a result of the new helmets, which led some athletes to consider themselves indestructible.

Subsequent rule changes in high school and college play banned "spearing" and using the top of the helmet as the initial point of contact in striking an opponent during a tackle or block. Once the actual mechanism of injury was understood, modification of the rules to affect a change in playing technique was very effective. From 1976 to 1984, cervical spine injury rates sharply decreased and injuries that resulted in quadriplegia decreased 85% from 34 to 5 incidences.[186]

Educational intervention

In a prospective controlled intervention study, a prevention program that focused on education and supervision of soccer coaches and players demonstrated 21% fewer injuries in the intervention group among male youth amateur players.[178] The effects were more dramatic for injuries that were mild, resulted from overuse, or occurred during training. Also, the program was more successful with low-skill teams, demonstrating the potential of education strategies for a great number of youth teams.

Personal protective equipment

A good case study of the need for personal protective equipment involves the long-running debate over whether protective eyewear should be required in women's lacrosse. Proponents of protective equipment cite a fast-moving sport, the use of sticks and a hard rubber ball, and documented eye injuries as evidence of the need for protective eyewear. Opponents suggest that by requiring protective equipment, players will feel secure enough to increase their aggression and ultimately change the nature of the game from one of incidental contact to one of full contact, similar to the men's game. Further, it is argued that this increase in aggression will eventually cause more injuries than the original intervention (protective eyewear) prevents.

To assess the true effect of protective eyewear, Webster et al[188] collected field data from 700 varsity and junior varsity players in central New York over a 2-year transition from sparse to almost complete eyewear use. The findings indicated a 16% reduction in overall head/face injuries among goggle wearers, with an even greater effect in game situations (51% reduction). This and similar studies[189] demonstrated a beneficial use of eyewear and provided the basis for strategic decisions on how best to prevent head and facial injuries in young athletes. One such change is the recent decision by the U.S.

Lacrosse Women's Division Board of Governors

to amend the rules of women's lacrosse to highly recommend the use of protective eyewear meeting current ASTM lacrosse standards for 2004 and to mandate use beginning in 2005.[190]

Components of Recommendation

There is a well-accepted scientific process for addressing a public health injury problem, and in this case, athletic injury among secondary school–age athletes. This public health approach[191-194] includes the following five components, which are then described in greater detail: 1) Determine the existence and size of the problem, 2) identify what may cause the problem, 3) determine strategies and interventions that may prevent the problem, 4) implement prevention strategies, and 5) monitor and evaluate the effectiveness of prevention efforts.

Determine the existence and size of the problem
The success of the first step relies on a complete and accurate collection of relevant data. This includes a good description of the circumstances surrounding the injury, including person, place, and time. Surveillance describes such characteristics as the magnitude of the problem ("How many players have been injured?"), the physical location of the problem ("Where on the field do injuries occur?"), what body parts are at greatest risk of injury ("Are there more head injuries than shoulder injuries?"), and who is affected ("Are more boys injured than girls?").[195] Along with the descriptive injury data, it is imperative that injury surveillance also takes into consideration exposure data (athlete-exposures). Additional information should be collected to allow for comparisons to be made within and between positions, sports, and those with and without a previous injury history. Only with a strong surveillance effort can we be sure that the biggest problems are being addressed and our efforts to reduce them are successful.

Identify what may cause the problem
This information suggests why certain people may be at greater risk of injury while others are protected. This type of data requires long-term, expensive longitudinal studies. However, some risk factors have already been identified in high school athletes and interventions can be developed from these known risk factors (e.g., landing biomechanics and anterior cruciate ligament [ACL] injury in females has led to jump training programs). Understanding which risk factors are involved is often overlooked, yet is crucial to developing effective interventions.

Determine strategies and interventions that may prevent the problem
Developing strategies for injury prevention is usually based on the approach introduced by William Haddon, known as the Haddon Matrix.[196] It is based on Haddon's observation that all injury events come from the uncontrolled release of physical energy.[197] Efforts focused on prevention can occur at one of three times: before the injury (when the energy becomes uncontrolled), during the injury (when the energy transferred to the body is more than can be safely absorbed), or after the injury (when the body attempts to heal the damage). In addition to the time axis, the Haddon Matrix includes an axis of risk factors also found in the public health framework; the host (potentially injured person), the agent (the energy and the way in which it is transferred), and the environment (both physical and social). The resulting 12-cell matrix can be used as a brainstorming tool to devise interventions according to a specific time phase and a specific risk factor. An example of the use of the Haddon Matrix applied to the problem of athletic injuries is found in Table 4. A strong prevention program incorporates interventions that address the different risk factors and span the time axis.

Implement prevention strategies
Once potential strategies are identified, the next step is to assess which strategies should be implemented and how to put them into action. Recently, Runyon[198] added another dimension to the Haddon Matrix to help with this decision. A set of value criteria is included as a starting point for planners to consider. Depending on the nature of the injury problem, some criteria will be weighted more heavily than others; these criteria include

- Effectiveness: How well does the intervention work when applied?
- Cost: What are the costs of implementing and enforcing the program?
- Freedom: Do the freedoms of some groups have to be sacrificed to achieve the goal?
- Equity: Are people treated equally or in a universal

fashion?
- Stigmatization: Does a program result in a person/team being stigmatized?
- Preferences: Are preferences recognized to encourage compliance?
- Feasibility: Can the intervention actually be produced?

Another strategy for developing effective interventions for athletic injuries is to consider whether players are protected from injury without having to take additional precautions.[125, 199] A passive strategy, such as adding padding to an outfield wall, provides automatic protection without requiring the cooperation of the athlete to be effective. An active strategy, such as a rule change to ban slaps to the side of the helmet, requires an athlete to modify his or her play or cooperate in some other way.

Passive strategies are generally considered to be more effective because they do not rely on player compliance each and every time a potential injury situation presents itself. Different types of interventions can be classified according to the degree of compliance required of athletes. This principle is presented in an intervention implementation hierarchy that includes engineering modification to the athletic environment, administrative changes to a rule, educational efforts to introduce a safer technique or less risky behavior during play, and the use of personal protective equipment.[200] Engineering controls are typically considered to be most effective because they require the least amount of effort/cooperation from the athlete to provide safety, although they also require a greater commitment and resources from the organization with overall responsibility for player safety. Educational controls and personal protective equipment are more active interventions because they require the players to consider the risk of a situation and to act in a safe manner every time the situation presents itself during play.

Monitor and evaluate the effectiveness of prevention efforts
The evaluation step provides answers to the ultimate questions, "Does our intervention work?" or "Have injuries been reduced?"[195] We return to our first step of surveillance for data that support or deny the effectiveness of the interventions that have been implemented. Although we are most interested in this primary question, we also must consider whether there may be other reasons, unrelated to the intervention, which might explain why injuries were reduced. Another key issue is whether there are any unintended consequences (good or bad) that are a direct result of the intervention. A bad unintended consequence may ruin any positive effect of the intervention, so it must be determined not only whether fewer injuries occurred, but also whether the intervention had a positive effect on the athletes' overall well-being. Evaluation requires the conduct of well-designed randomized controlled effectiveness studies.

Strategies for Implementation
The potential strategies for the prevention of injury and illness in the secondary school– age athlete have been presented in the previous 10 sections of this monograph. These interventions address various aspects of the framework previously described, including the athlete, energy transfer, and environment. They also relate to efforts that affect the safety and welfare of athletes before, during, and after the injury or illness.

CONCLUSIONS
Appropriate medical care of the secondary school–age individual involves more than basic emergency care during sports participation. It encompasses the provision of many other health care services. While emergency medical care and event coverage are critical, appropriate medical care also includes activities of ongoing daily athletic health care. The athletic health care team (AHCT) comprises appropriate health care professionals in consultation with administrators, coaches, parents, and participants.

Appropriate health care professionals could be certified athletic trainers, team physicians, consulting physicians, school nurses, physical therapists, emergency medical services (EMS) personnel, dentists, and other allied health care professionals.

Organizations sponsoring athletic programs for secondary school–age individuals should establish an AHCT that functions to ensure appropriate medical care is provided for all participants.

REFERENCES

1. Lyznicki JM, Riggs JA, H.C. C. Certified athletic trainers in secondary schools: report of the council on scientific affairs, American Medical Association. *J Athl Train*. 1999;34:272-276.
2. Shulman LE. *Preface*. Conference on Sports Injuries in Youth: Surveillance Strategies. Bethesda, MD;1992.
3. Powell JW, Barber-Foss KD. Injury patterns in selected high school sports: a review of the 1995-1997 seasons. *J Athl Train*. 1999;34:277-284.
4. *Mogabgab v. Orleans Parish School Board*, La. App. 239 (S. 2d).
5. *Stineman v. Fontbonne College*, 664 (F.2d).
6. *O'Brien v. Township High School District*, 392 (N.E.).
7. Ray R. *Management strategies in athletic training*. Champaign, IL:Human Kinetics; 2000.
8. Health Insurance Portability and Accountability Act,. Public Law 104-191, 104th Congress. 1996.
9. Family Educational Rights and Privacy Act. (20 U.S.C. § 1232g; 34 CFR Part 99).
10. Parkkari J, Kujala UM, Kannus P. Is it possible to prevent sports injuries? Review of controlled clinical trials and recommendations for future work. *Sports Medicine*. 2001;31:985-95.
11. National Federation of State High School Associations. *2000-01 Handbook*. Indianapolis:NRSHSA; 2000.
12. National Center for Catastrophic Sports Injury Research. *Nineteenth Annual Report*. July 10 2002.
13. Krowchuk D. The preparticipation athletic examination: a closer look. *Pediatr Ann*. 1997;26:1.
14. Beachy G, Akau C, Martinson M, Older T. High school sports injuries: a longitudinal study an Punahou School: 1988 to 1996. *Am J Sports Med*. 1997;25:674-681.
15. American Academy of Pediatrics (AAP). Organized sports for children and preadolescents: policy statement. *Pediatrics*. 2001;107:1459-1462.
16. Shultz SJ, Valovich TC, Zinder SM. *Sports Medicine Handbook*. Indianapolis:National Federation of State High School Associations; 2002.
17. Smith DM, Kovan JR, Rich BSE, Tanner SM. *Preparticipation Physical Evaluation, 3rd Edition*. New York:McGraw-Hill; 2004.
18. Maron BJ. American Heart Association: cardiovascular preparticipation screening of competitive athletes. *Med Sci Sports Exerc*. 1996;28:1445-1452.
19. Bratton RL. Preparticipation screening of children in sports. *Sports Med*. 1997;24:300-307.
20. Hergendroder AC. The preparticipation sports examination. *Pediatr Clin North Am*. 1997;44:1525-1539.
21. Smith J, Laskowski E. The preparticipation physical exam: Mayo Clinic experience with 2,739 examinations. *Mayo Clinic Proc*. 1998;73:419-429.
22. American Academy of Pediatrics (AAP). Recommendations for participating in competitive sports. *Pediatrics*. 1988;81:737-739.
23. 26th Bethesda Conference. Recommendations for determining eligibility for competition in athletes with cardiovascular abnormalities. *Med Sci Sports Exerc*. 1994;26:S223-S283.
24. Maron BJ. Sudden death in competitive athletes. *JAMA*. 1996;276:199-204.
25. Epstein SE, Maron BJ. Sudden death and the competitive athlete: perspectives on preparticipation screening studies. *J Am Coll Cardiol*. 1986;7:220-230.
26. Fuller C. Cost effectiveness analysis of screening of high school athletes for risk of sudden cardiac death. *Med Sci Sports Exerc*. 2000;32:887-890.
27. Faharenbach M, Thompson P. The preparticipation sports exanination: cardiovascular considerations for screening. *Cardiol Clin*. 1992;10:319-328.
28. Weidenbener EJ, Krauss MD. Incorporation of screening echocardiography in the preparticipation examination. *Clin J Sport Med*. 1995;5:86-89.
29. American Heart Association. Accessed April 6, 2004 www.americanheart.org
30. Technology GoSa. Athletic preparticipation examinations for adolescents: report of the board of trustees. *Arch Pediatr Adolesc Med*. 1994;148:93-98.
31. McCoy R, Dec K, McKeag D. Caring for the school-aged athlete. *Primary Care*. 1994;21:781-799.
32. Feinstein RA, Soileau EJ, Daniel WA. A national survey of preparticipation physical examiniation requirements. *Phys Sportsmed*. 1988;16:51-59.
33. Risser WL, Hoffman HM, Bellah GG. Frequency of preparticipation sports examinations in secondary school athletes: are the University Interscholastic League guidelines appropriate? *Tex Med*. 1985;81:35-39.
34. McKeag DB. Preseason physical examination for the prevention of sports injuries. *Sports Med*. 1985;2:413-431.
35. Rifat SF, Ruffin MT, Gorenflo DW. Disqualifying criteria in preparticipation sports evaluations. *J Fam Pract*. 1995;41:42-50.
36. U.S. Consumer Product Safety Commission. Estimates for Sports Injuries: National Electronic Injury Surveillance System. *National Youth Sports Injury Foundation*. 1994;
37. National Youth Sports Injury Foundation. Information on standards for safety equipment in sports.
38. National Association for Sport and Physical Education (NASPE). The bill of rights of young athletes. In: *Guidelines in Children's Sports*. R Martens and V Sefeldt (Eds.) Reston: NASPE, 1979.
39. *Bush v. Parents Without Partners*, 21 CR2d 178 (1993).
40. *Short v. Griffiths*, 255 S.E. 2d 479 (VA 1979).
41. *Ardoin v. Evangeline Parish School Board*, 376 So. 2d 372 (LA 1979).
42. *Domino v. Murcurio*, 193 N.E. 2d 893 (NY 1963).
43. *Dawson v. Rhode Island Auditorium, Inc*, 242 A. 2d 407 (RI 1968).
44. *Pedersen v. Joilet Park District*, 483 N.E. 2d 21 (IL 1983).
45. *Singer v. School District of Philadelphia*, 513 A. 2d 1108 (PA 1986).
46. *Flournoy v. McCoumas*, 488 P. 2d 1104 (1971).
47. *Taylor v. Oakland Scavenger Company*, 17 C. 2d 594 (1941).
48. *Horynak v. The Pomfret School*, 783 F. 2d 284 (1st Cir. 1986).
49. *First Overseas Investment Corporation v. Cotton*, 491 So. 2d 293 (Fla. Dist. Ct. of App. 1986).
50. *Markowitz v. Arizona Park Board*, 706 P. 2d. 364 (146 Ariz. 352 1985).

51. *Jacobs v. Commonwealth Highland Theatres, Inc,* 738 P2d 6 (Col. Ct. of App. 1986).

52. Seidler TL. Planning facilities for safety and risk management. In: *Facilities Planning for Health, Fitness, Physical Activity, Recreation and Sports: Concepts and Applications.* TH Sawyer (Ed.): Sagmore Publishing, 2002.

53. Hossler P. *The High School Athletic Training Program: An Organizational Guide.* Dubuque, IA:Kendall/Hunt Publishing Co.; 1983.

54. Clover J. *Sports Medicine Essentials: Core Concepts in Athletic Training.* Clifton Park, N.Y.:Delmar Learning, Inc.; 2001.

55. *Locilento v. John A. Coleman Catholic High,* 523 N.Y.S. (2d).

56. *McKeever v. Phoenix Jewish Community Center,* 374 P. (2d 875 (AZ 1962)).

57. *Kungle v. Austin,* 330 S.W. (2d).

58. *Dudley Sports Co., Inc. v. Lawrence Robert Schmitt b/n/f/ Joseph Schmitt,* 151 Ind. App. 217 (279 N.E.2d).

59. *Grant v. Lake Oswego School District Number 7,* 515 P. (2d).

60. *Byrns v. Riddell, Inc,* 113 Ariz. 264 (550 P.2d).

61. *Kobylanski v. Chicago Board of Education,,* 63 Ill. 2d 165; 347 N.E.2d 705; 1976 Ill (Supreme Court of Illinois).

62. *Everett v. Bucky Warren, Inc.,* 380 N.E. (2d).

63. *Gerritty v. Beatty,* 71 Ill. 2d 47 (373 N.E.2d 1323).

64. *Berman v. Philadelphia Board of Education,* 456A (2d).

65. *Tiemann v. Independent School District #740,* 331 (N.W.2d).

66. Schutt Sports. *Sizing, Fitting, & Maintaining the Schutt Helmet & Shoulder Pad Systems.* Schutt Sports; 2002. [Videotape].

67. Schutt Sports. *Proper Helmet Fitting.* Schutt Sports,; 2003.

68. Schutt Sports. *Recommended Shoulder Pad Fitting Procedure.* 2003.

69. Michigan Governor's Council on Physical Fitness HaS. *Position Statement: The Prevention of Injuries in Amateur Football.* January http://www.mdch.state. mi.us/pha/vipf2/football.htm.

70. Schutt Sports. *Schutt Football FAQ.* May 31, 2003 http:// www.schuttsports.com/faq_fb.html.

71. Hergoenroeder AC. Prevention of Sports Injuries. *Pediatrics.* 1998;101:1057-1063.

72. AAHPERD. *Certified Athletic Trainers in U.S. High School.* Jan 2003 http://www.aahperd.org/NASPE/pdf_files/ pos_papers/resource-trainer.pdf.

73. Nelson LB, Wilson, T.W., Jeffers, J.B. Eye Injuries in Childhood: Demography, Etiology, and Prevention. *Pediatrics.* 1989;84:438-441.

74. Risser WL, Anderson, S.J., Bolduc, S.P., Coryllos, E., Greisemer, B., McLain, L., Tanner, S. Protective Eyewear for Young Athletes (RE9630). *Pediatrics.* 1996;98:311-313.

75. Martin TJ. Technical Report: Knee Brace Use in the Young Athlete (RE9844). *Pediatrics.* 2001;108:503-507.

76. American Dental Association. ADA Says Mouthguard Important Piece of Children's Athletic Gear. *ADA News Releases.* 2002;

77. American Dental Association. Do you need a mouthguard? *Journal of American Dental Association.* 2001;132:

78. American Dental Association. *Policy on Orofacial Protectors.* American Dental Association; 1995.

79. Nowjack-Raymer RE, Gift, H.C. Use of Mouthguards and Headgear in Organized Sports by School-aged Children. *Public Health Report.* 1996;111:82-86.

80. NOCSAE. *Shared Responsibilities in Reducing Sports Related Injuries.* January http://www.nocsae.org/ nocsae/STANDARDS/SharedResponse.htm.

81. Heck JF, Clarke KS, Peterson TR, Torg JS, Weis MP. National Athletic Trainers' Association Position Statement: Head-Down Contact and Spearing in Tackle Football. *J Athl Train.* 2004;39:101-111.

82. American Society for Testing and Materials. Standard Specifications for Face Guards for Youth Baseball. 1986;

83. International Federation of Sports Medicine. *Eye Injuries and Eye Protection in Sports: A Position Statement.* July 19, 2003 http://www.fims.org/fims/frames.asp.

84. Marshall SW, Mueller FO, Kirby DP, Yang J. Evaluation of Safety Balls and Faceguards for Prevention of Injuries in Youth Baseball. *JAMA.* 2003;289:568-574.

85. American Academy of Pediatrics Committee on Sports Medicine and Fitness. Medical Conditions Affecting Sports Participation. *Pediatrics.* 1994;95:757-760.

86. Kohl T, Giesen D, Moyer JJ, Lisney M. Tinea Gladiatorum: Pennsylvania's Experience. *Clinical Journal of Sports Medicine.* 2002;12:165-171.

87. International Academy of Sports Dentistry. Position Statement on Athletic Mouthguard Mandates. *IASD Newsletter.* 1999;14:7-8.

88. Anderson JC, Courson, R.W., Kleiner, D.M., McLodas, T.A. National Athletic Trainers' Association Position Statement: Emergency Planning in Athletics. *Journal of Athletic Training.* 2002;37:99-104.

89. Centers for Disease Control and Prevention. Nonfatal sports and recreation related injuries treated in emergency departments-United States, July 2000-June 2001. *MMWR.* 2002;51:736-740.

90. Walsh K. Thinking proactively: the emergency action plan. *Athl Ther Today.* 2001;6:57-62.

91. American Academy of Pediatrics (AAP). Guidelines for emergency medical care in school: policy statement. *Pediatrics.* 2001;107:435-436.

92. American Academy of Pediatrics (AAP). Physical fitness and activity in schools: policy statement. *Pediatrics.* 2002;105:1156-1157.

93. National Association for Sport and Physical Education (NASPE). Guidelines for after-school physical activity and intramural sports programs: postion paper. 2001;

94. National Collegiate Athletic Association. NCAA Guideline 1f, emergency care and coverage. In: *NCAA Sports Medicine Handbook, 15th Edition* Indianapolis: NCAA, 2002.

95. Cotton D, Wilde TJ. *Sports Law.* Iowa:Kendall Hunt; 1997.

96. *Kleinknecht v. Gettysburg College,* 786 F. Supp 449 (3rd Cir. 1993).

97. *Barth by Barth v. Board of Education,* 490 N.E. 2d 77 (Ill. App. 1 Dist. 1986).

98. *Jarreau v. Orleans Parrish School Board,* 600 So.2d 1389 (La. 1992).

99. Almquist JL, et. al.,. The Position Improvement Guide for the Secondary School Athletic Trainer. *National Athletic Trainers' Association*. 2003;

100. Courson R. Example template: sports medicine emergency plan. *www1.ncaa.org/membership/ed_outreach/health-safety/care-coverage/emergency_plan*.

101. American Orthopaedic Society for Sports Medicine (AOSSM). *Sideline Preparedness for the Team Physician: A Consensus Statement*. 2002.

102. Kleiner DM, Almquist JL, Bailes J, Burruss P, Feuer H, Griffin, L.Y., Herring S, McAdam C, Miller D, Thorson D, Watkins RG, Weinstein S. *Prehospital Care of the Spine-Injured Athlete: A document from the Inter-Association Task Force for Appropriate Care of the Spine-Injured Athlete*. Dallas:2001.

103. Binkley H, Beckett J, Casa D, Kleiner D, Plummer P. National Athletic Trainers' Association Position Statement: Exertional Heat Illness. *J Athl Train*. 2002;37:329-343.

104. Convertino V, Armstrong L, Coyle E, Mack G, Sawka M, Senay L, Sherman WM. *Exercise and Fluid Replacement*. American College of Sports Medicine Position Stand. 1996

105. Inter-Association Task Force. *Inter-Association Task Force on Exertional Heat Illness Consensus Statement*. 2003;

106. National Collegiate Athletic Association. NCAA Guideline 2c Prevention of Heat Illness. In: *NCAA Sports Medicine Handbook* Indianapolis: NCAA, 2002.

107. Armstrong L, Epstein Y, J. G, Haymes E, Hubbard R, Roberts W, Thompson P. Heat and Cold Illnesses During Distance Running. *American College of Sports Medicine Position Stand*. 1996

108. National Collegiate Athletic Association. NCAA Guideline 2m, Cold Stress. In: *NCAA Sports Medicine Handbook* Indianapolis: NCAA, 2002.

109. Walsh K, Bennett B, Cooper M, Holle R, Kithil MBA, Lopez R. National Athletic Trainers' Association Position Statement: Lightning Safety for Athletics and Recreation. *J Athl Train*.2000;35:471-477.

110. National Collegiate Athletic Association. NCAA Guideline 1d, Lightning Safety. In: *NCAA Sports Medicine Handbook* Indianapolis: NCAA, 2002.

111. Casa D. Exercise in the heat. I. Fundamentals of thermal physiology, performance implications, and dehydration. J Athl Train. 1999;34:246-252. .

112. Casa D. Exercise in the heat II. Fundamentals of thermal physiology, performace implications, and dehydration. *J Athl Train*. 1999;34:253-262.

113. Armstrong L. Heat acclimatization. In: Encyclopedia of Sports Medicine and Science. TD Fahey (Ed.): *Internet Society for Sports Medicine*, 1998.

114. Sparling P, Millard-Stafford M. Keeping sports participants safe in hot weather. *Phys Sportsmed*. 1999;27:27-35.

115. Casa D, Armstrong L, Hillman S, Montain S, Reiff R, Rich B, Roberts W, Stone J. National Athletic Trainers' Associaiton Position Statement: Flluid Replacement for Athletes. *J Athl Train*.2000;35:212-224.

116. Kanzenbach T, Dexter W. Cold injuries. *Postgrad Med*. 1999;105:43-50.

117. Noakes T. Exercise in the cold. *Ergonomics*. 2002;43:1461-1479.

118. Zimmerman C, Cooper MA, Holle RL. Ligtning safety guidelines. *Ann Emerg Med*. 2002;39:665- 670.

119. Holle R, Lopez R, Zimmerman C. Updated recommendations for lightning safety. *Bull Am Meteor Soc*. 1999;2034-2041.

120. Cherington M. Lightning injuries in sports: situations to avoid. *Sports Med*. 2001;31:301-308.

121. Vavrek JR, Holle RL, Lopez RE. Updated lightning safety recommendations. In: *Preprints of the American Meteorological Society 8th Symposium on Education* Dallas, TX, 1999.

122. American Medical Association. Report 5 of the council on scientific affairs (A-98): Certified athletic trainers in secondary schools. Retrieved May 25, 2003, from http://www.amaassn.org/ama/pub/article/2036-2373.html.

123. National Athletic Trainers' Association. Minimizing the risk of injury in high school athletics. Accessed February 19, 2003, from www.nata.org/publications/brochures/minimizingtherisks.htm.

124. Shimon JM. Youth sports injury: prevention is key. *Strategies*. 2002;15:27-30.

125. Weaver NL, Marshall SW, Miller MD. Preventing sports injuries: opportunities for intervention in youth athletics. *Patient Educ Counseling*. 2002;46:199-204.

126. American Academy of Pediatrics (AAP). Injuries in youth soccer: a subject review. Accessed November 3, 2002, from www.aap.org/policy/re9934.html.

127. Cantu RC. Head and spine injuries in youth sports. *Clin Sports Med*. 1995;14:517-532.

128. Culpepper MI. The availability and delivery of health care to high school athletes in Alabama. *Phys Sportsmed*. 1986;14:131-137.

129. DeLee JC, Farney WC. Incidence of injury in Texas high school football. *Am J Sports Med*. 1992;20:575-580.

130. DiFiori JP. Overuse injuries in children and adolescents. *Phys Sportsmed*. 1999;27:75-80.

131. Gomez JE. Upper extremity injuries in youth sports. *Pediatr Clin North Am*. 2002;49:593-626.

132. Guskiewicz KM, Weaver NL, Padua DL, Garrett WE. Epidemiology of concussion in collegiate and high school football players. *Am J Sports Med*. 2000;28:643-650.

133. Kocher MS, Waters PM, Micheli LJ. Upper extremity injuries in the pediatric athlete. *Sports Med*. 2000;30:117-135.

134. Luckstead EF, Patel DR. Catastrophic pediatric sports injuries. *Pediatr Clin North Am*. 2002;49:581-591.

135. Maffulli N, Baxter-Jones ADG. Common skeletal injuries in young athletes. *Sports Med*. 1995;19:137-149.

136. Martin TJ, Martin JS. Special issues and concerns for the high school- and college-aged athletes. *Ped Clin North Am*. 2002;49:533-552.

137. Messina DF, Farney WC, DeLee JC. The incidence of injury in Texas high school basketball. *Am J Sports Med*. 1999;37:294-299.

138. Pasque CB, Hewett TE. A prospective study of high school wrestling injuries. *Am J Sports Med*. 2000;28:509-515.

139. Patel DR, Nelson TL. Sports injuries in adolescents. Med

Clin North Am. 2000;84:983-1007.

140. Powell JW, Barber-Foss KD. Sex-related injury patterns among selected high school sports. *Am J Sports Med*. 2000;28:385-391.

141. Ransone J, Dunn-Bennett LR. Assessment of first-aid knowledge and decision making of high school athletic coaches. *J Athl Train*. 1999;34:267-271.

142. Rauh MJ, Margherita AJ, Rice SG, Koepsell TD, Rivara FP. High school cross country running injuries: a longitudinal study. *Clin J Sport Med*. 2000;10:110-116.

143. Rutherford DS, Niedfeldt MW, Young CC. Medical coverage of high school football in Wisconsin in 1997. *Clin J Sport Med*. 1999;9:209-215.

144. Ryu RKN, Fan RSP. Adolescent and pediatric sports injuries. Pediatr Clin North Am. 1998;45:1601-1635.

145. Marsh JS, Daigneault JP. The young athlete. *Curr Opin Pediatr*. 1999;11:84-88.

146. Vangsness TC, Hunt T, Uram M, Kerlam RK. Survey of health care coverage of high school football in Southern California. *Am J Sports Med*. 1994;22:719-722.

147. Fandel D. Athletic Trainer Credentialing. Dallas:National Athletic Trainers' Association Board of Certification; 2002.

148. Prentice WE. Rehabilitation Techniques in Sports Medicine (2nd ed.). St. Louis:Mosby; 1994.

149. Crossley K, Bennell K, Green S, Cowan S, McConnell J. Physical therapy for patellofemoral pain: a randomized, double-blinded, placebo controlled trial. *Am J Sports Med*. 2002;30:857-865.

150. Gilbey HJ, Wang AW, Trouchet T. Exercise improves early functional recovery after total hip arthroplasty. *Clin Orthop*. 2003;408:193-200.

151. Wang TJ, Olson SL, Campbell AH, Hanten WP, Gleeson PB. Effectiveness of physical therapy for patients with neck pain: an individualized approach using a clinical decision-making algorithm. *Am J Phys Med Rehabil*. 2003;82:203-218.

152. Harris GR, Susman JL. Managing musculoskeletal complaints with rehabilitation therapy: summary of the Philadelphia panel evidence-based clinical practice guidelines on musculoskeletal rehabilitation interventions. *J Fam Pract*. 2002;15:1042-1046.

153. Hurwitz EL, Mogenstern H, Harber P, Kominski GF, Belin TR, Adams AH. A randomized trial of medical care with and without physical therapy and chiropractic care with and without physical modalities for patients with low back pain: 6-month follow up outcomes from the UCLA low back pain study. *Spine*. 2002;27:2193-2204.

154. Griffin KM. Rehabilitation of the hip. Clin Sports Med. 2001;20:837-845. 155. Stylianos S. Late sequelae of major trauma in children. *Ped Clin North Am*. 1998;45:853-859.

156. Chen C, Neufeld PS, Feely CA, Skinner CS. Factors influencing compliance with home exercise programs among patients with upper-extremity impairment. *Am J Occ Ther*. 1999;53:171-179.

157. Kirk-Sanchez NJ, K.E. R. Relationship between duration of therapy services is a comprehensive rehabilitation program and mobility at discharge in patients with orthopedic problems. *Phys Ther*. 2001;81:888-895.

158. Cavanaugh RMJ, Miller ML, Henneberger PK. The preparticipation athletic examination of adolescents: a missed opportunity? *Curr Probl Pediatric* 1997;27:109-120.

159. Patrick K, Colvin JR, Fulop M, Calfas K, Lovato C. Health risk behaviors among California college students. *J Am Coll Health*. 1997;45:265-272.

160. Nattiv A, Puffer JC. Lifestyles and health risks of collegiate ahtletes. *J Fam Pract*. 1991;33:585-590.

161. Baumert PW, Henderson JM, Thompson NJ. Health risk behaviors of adolescent participants in organized sports. *J Adolesc Health*. 1998;22:460-465.

162. Forman ES, Dekker AH, Javors JR, Favison DT. High-risk behaviors in teenage male athletes. *Clin J Sport Med*. 1995;5:36-42.

163. Kokotailo PK, Henry BC, Koscik RE, Fleming MF, Landry GL. Substance abuse and other health risk behaviors in collegiate athletics. *Clin J Sport Med*. 1996;6:183-189.

164. Nattiv A, Puffer JC, Green GA. Lifestyles and health risks of collegiate athletes: a mulit-center study. *Clin J Sport Med*. 1997;7:262-272.

165. Miller TW, Adams JM, Kraus RF, Clayton R, Miller JM, Anderson J. Gambling as an addictive disorder among athletes: clinical issues in sports medicine. *Sports Med*. 2001;31:145-152.

166. Patel DR, Luckstead EF. Sport participation, risk taking, and health risk behaviors. *Adolesc Med State Art Rev*. 2000;11:141-155.

167. Oler MJ, Mainous AG, Martin CA, Richardson E, Haney A, WIlson D. Depression, suicidal ideation, and substance use among adolescents. Are athletes at risk? *Arch Fam Med*. 1994;3:781- 785.

168. Steptoe A, Butler N. Sports participation and emotional well-being in adolescents. Lancet.1996;347:1789-1792.

169. Brewer BW, Linder DE, Phelps CM. Situational correlates of emotional adjustment to athletic injury. *Clin J Sport Med*. 1995;5:241-245.

170. Manuel JC, Shilt JS, Curl WW, Smith JA, Durant DH, Lester L. Coping with sports injuries: an examination of the adolescent athlete. *J Adolesc Health*. 2002;31:391-393.

171. Joint Review Commission for Athletic Training. Standards and Guidelines.

172. Neinstein LS. Adolescent Health Care: A Practical Guide. Philadelphia:Lippincott, Williams, & Wilkins; 2002.

173. Ogden CL, Flegal KM, Carroll MD, Johnson CL. Prevalence and trends in overweight among US children and adolescents. *JAMA*. 1999-2000;288:1728-1732.

174. Perriello V. Aiming for healthy weight in wrestlers and other athletes. Contemporary Pediatrics. 2001;9:55.

175. BlueCross BlueShield. *National Performance-Enhancing Drug Study*. 2001;

176. Office of Dietary Supplements. http://ods.od.nih.gov.

177. Caraffa A, Cerulli G, Projetti M, Aisa G, Rizzo A. Prevention of anterior cruciate ligament injuries in

soccer. A propsective controlled study of proprioceptive training. *Knee Surg Sports Traumatol*. 1996;4:19-21.

178. Junge A, Rosch D, Peterson L, Graf-Baumann T, Dvorak J. Prevention of soccer injuries: a prospective intervention study in youth amateur players. 2002;30:652-659.

179. Perna FM, Antoni MH, Baum A, Gordon P, Schneiderman N. Cognitive behavioral stress management effects on injury and illness among competitive athletes: a randomized clinical trial. *Ann Behav Med*. 2003;25:66-73.

180. Tyler TF, Nicholas SJ, Campbell RJ, Donellan S, McHugh MP. The effectiveness of a preseason exercise program to prevent adductor muscle strains in professional ice ockey players. *Am J Sports Med*. 2002;30:680-683.

181. National Center for Injury Prevention and Control. CDC Injury Research Agenda. Atlanta:Centers for Disease Control and Prevention; 2002.

182. Janda DH. The prevention of baseball and softball injuries. *Clin Orthop*. 2003;409:20-28.

183. Conn JM, Annest JL, Gilchrist J. Sports and recreation related injury episodes in the US population, 1997-1999. *Injury Prev*. 2003;9:117-123.

184. Janda DH, Wojtys EM, Hankin FM, Benedict ME. Softball sliding injuries: a prospective study comparing standard and modified bases. *JAMA*. 1988;259:1848-1850.

185. Marshall SW, Waller AE, Dick RW, Pugh CB, Loomis DP, Chalmers DJ. An epidemiologic study of protective equipment and injury in two contact sports. *Int J Epidemiol*. 2002;31:587-592.

186. Torg JS, Vegso JJ, Sennett B, Das M. The national football head and neck injury registry. 14- year report on cervical quadraplegia, 1971 through 1984. *JAMA*. 1985;254:3439-3443.

187. Torg JS, Vegso JJ, O'Neill MJ, Sennett B. The epidemiologic, pathologic, biomechanical, and cinematographic analysis of football-induced cervical spine trauma. *Am J Sports Med*. 1990;18:50-57.

188. Webster DA, Bayliss GV, Spadaro JA. Head and face injuries in scholastic women's lacrosse with and without eyewear. *Med Sci Sports Exerc*. 1999;31:938-941.

189. Waicus KM, Smith BW. Eye injuries in women's lacrosse players. *Clin J Sport Med*. 2002;12:24-29.

190. US Lacrosse. Women's division, Umpiring: eyewear update. Accessed August 2, 2003, from www.uslacrosse/org/wdoc/Rule%20Info/Eyewear.htm.

191. Jones BH, Hansen BC. An Armed Forces epidemiological board evaluation of injuries in the military. *Am J Prev Med*. 2000;18:14-18.

192. Jones BH, Knapik JJ. Physical training and exercise-related injuries: surveillance, research and injury prevention in military populations. *Sports Med*. 1999;27:111-125.

193. Mercy JA, Rosenburg ML, Powell KE, Broome CV, Roper WL. Public health policy for preventing violence. *Health Affairs*. 1993;Winter:7-29.

194. Robertson LS. Injury Epidemiology. New York:Oxford Press; 1992.

195. Sleet D, Bonzo S, Branche C. An overview of the National Center for Injury PRevention and Control and the Centers for Disease Control and Prevention. *Injury Prev*. 1998;4:308-312.

196. Haddon W. Options for the prevention of motor vehicle crash injury. *Isr J Med Sci*. 1980;16:45-65.

197. Bonnie RJ, Fulco CE, Liverman CT. Reducing the Burden of Injury: Advancing Prevention and Treatment. Washington, D.C.: *National Academy Press;* 1999.

198. Runyon CW. Using the Haddon Matrix: introducing the third dimension. *Injury Prev*. 1998;4:306-307.

199. Bell NS, Amoroso PJ, Baker SP, Senir L. Injury control, part II: strategies for prevention. In: *U.S. Army Research Institute for Environmental Medicine Technical Report* TN 00-4 Natick, MA: U.S. Army, 2000.

200. Levy BS, Wegman DH. Preventing occupational disease. In: Occupational Health: Recognizing and Preventing Work-Related Disease, 2nd ed Boston: Little, Brown, and Company, 1988.

Support Statement *NATA*

Appropriate Medical Coverage for Intercollegiate Athletics

INTRODUCTION

In February 1998, the National Athletic Trainers' Association (NATA) created the Task Force to Establish Appropriate Medical Coverage for Intercollegiate Athletics (AMCIA) to address concerns regarding the increased exposure of student-athletes to injury from the expansion of traditional seasons, non-traditional season practices and competitions, skill instruction sessions, and year-round strength and conditioning.

Of additional concern were the elevated number of injuries, serious injuries and deaths of student-athletes at the collegiate level. The mission of the task force was to establish recommendations for appropriate medical coverage to assist institutions in providing the best possible health care for all intercollegiate student-athletes without discrimination. The AMCIA Recommendations and Guidelines (originally created in 2000) were based on accepted medical criteria (e.g., injury rates and severity), not on gender, sport or level of competition. The sole intent of the recommendations was to address student-athlete welfare issues with regard to the amount and quality of medical coverage provided them.

To systematically determine the appropriate level of medical coverage for each sport at an institution, the task force devised a rating system utilizing injury rates, the potential for catastrophic injury, and treatment/rehabilitation demands for both time loss and non-time loss injuries per sport. In addition to these indices, other relative factors, such as prolonged season exposure, squad size, travel requirements, and health care administrative duties, were used to determine health care loads and medical staffing needs. To form the basis for the recommendations and indices, the task force relied on existing literature, and where data were inadequate or unavailable, relied on the professional consensus and expertise of task force members.

Since the publication of this document in 2000, the NATA commissioned a two-year research study (conducted by John W. Powell, PhD, ATC, Michigan State University) with the goal of obtaining treatment and injury data for both time loss and non-time loss injuries for sports and all competitive divisions levels. The purpose of the study was to substantiate the AMCIA Recommendations and Guidelines with scientific data where previously the task force had to rely on expert consensus alone.

Injury rate and treatment data were tracked on all sport teams at 50 colleges and universities over two seasons. In addition to providing information on sports not previously reported on, these data confirmed that a considerable amount of time is spent in care of injuries not resulting in time loss, which suggests that both time loss and non-time loss injury rates should be considered when determining the health care needs of a particular sport. Based on the results of the Powell study, as well as up-to-date time loss injury rate data provided by the Big 10 Athletic Association and the NCAA's Injury Surveillance System, the AMCIA Recommendation and Guidelines were revised.

Since the 2003 revision there again has been an increase in exposure to injury because of rules changes. It should be noted that the document can account for this by increasing the yearly percentage (# of days) that a sport needs coverage. If football needs year around coverage then adjust the percentage accordingly.

All updated data were instrumental in improving the accuracy and applicability of the system for determining health care loads. We are confident the Revised AMCIA Recommendations and Guidelines reflect a more scientifically defensible document that relies heavily on actual data, and less on expert consensus alone.

Institutions are encouraged to view these recommendations as guidelines, not mandates, taking into consideration their unique individual needs. We encourage institutions to consider these recommendations a "living document" because further revisions may be required as more data become available, or as preventative techniques, rules and policies change.

DEFINITION FOR APPROPRIATE MEDICAL COVERAGE

Appropriate medical coverage involves more than basic emergency care during sports participation. It encompasses the provision of many other health care services for the student-athlete. While emergency medical care and event coverage are critical, appropriate medical coverage also includes activities of ongoing daily health care of the student-athlete, such as:

- Determination of athletes' readiness to participate, in conjunction with the team physician (e.g., pre-participation evaluation and post-injury/ illness return)
- Risk management and injury prevention
- Recognition, evaluation and immediate treatment of athletic injuries/illnesses
- Rehabilitation and reconditioning of athletic injuries
- Psychosocial intervention and referral
- Nutritional aspects of injuries/illnesses
- Health care administration
- Professional development to maintain and improve knowledge and skills

SYSTEM FOR DETERMINING HEALTH CARE LOADS FOR EACH SPORT AND INSTITUTION

Each student-athlete, without consideration for sport, gender or level of competition, shall have equitable access to appropriate medical care, which should be directed by a college- or university-appointed team physician working in conjunction with a certified athletic trainer. After comprehensive study and analysis, the National Athletic Trainers' Association has issued the following recommendations for appropriate medical coverage.

In addition to those services provided by a qualified team physician, a system has been devised to assist in determining each collegiate setting's medical coverage needs. Items considered when creating this system were injury rates for both time-loss and non-time loss injury, time required for treatment and rehabilitation of these injuries, potential for injury based on number of exposures over the length of season, travel requirements, onsite coverage needs and administrative demands placed on the athletic health care staff. To that end, the ensuing model has its foundation in health care units (HCU). As described in the sections to follow, each sport is assigned a base Health Care Index (HCI). The base HCI for each sport falls in the range of 1-4 units. While these values are based on available injury risk and treatment data, institutions can adjust these numbers as their own injury risk and treatment data dictate.

It is reasonable that one certified athletic trainer can only manage so much in a given academic year (i.e.,~ one sport/season). Therefore, one full-time certified athletic trainer may be responsible for ~12 health care units, which should be considered a starting point for each institution. For example, if after applying the system a college or university has 48 total health care units, then that institution should

---

Certified Athletic Trainer: An allied health professional who, upon graduation from an accredited college or university, and after successfully passing the NATABOC certification exam, is qualified and appropriately credentialed according to state regulations to work with individuals engaged in physical activity in the prevention of injuries and illnesses, the recognition, evaluation and immediate care of injuries and illnesses, the rehabilitation and reconditioning of injuries and illnesses and the administration of this health care system. This individual must have current certification in CPR and be qualified in first aid and blood borne pathogens. Other health care professionals with equivalent certification and/or licensure would also meet this standard.

Team Physician: The team physician must have an unrestricted medical license and be an MD or a DO who is responsible for treating and coordinating the medical care of athletic team members. The principal responsibility of the team physician is to provide for the well-being of individual athletes, enabling each to realize his or her full potential. The team physician should possess special proficiency in the care of musculoskeletal injuries and medical conditions encountered in sports. The team physician also must actively integrate medical expertise with other health care providers, including medical specialists, athletic trainers and allied health professionals. The team physician must ultimately assume responsibility within the team structure for making medical decisions that affect the athlete's safe participation.

have the equivalent of 4 (48 divided by 12) full-time certified athletic trainers, unless some of the units fall in the category of minimally qualified personnel. (Please see item "B," under Recommendations and Guidelines for Health Care Providers.) If an institution finds it equitable to increase or decrease the HCU load for its athletic trainers, it may do so with consideration to the health and welfare of the student-athlete.

Base Health Care Index (Table 1)

The base health care index is founded on the injury risk (IR), and treatment demands associated with those injuries (Tx/I), as the means to determine the base health care needs for each sport. Aggregate injury rate and treatment data reflecting both time loss and non-time loss injuries (across all competitive divisions) comprised the IR and Tx/I, with values representing rates per 1,000 athletic exposures (or opportunity for injury). (See Table 7 for Actual Data Sources.) Institutions may use specific competition level injury rates by referencing the AMCIA Injury Surveillance Study.

IR = Injury Rate: The IR reported for each sport is based on available multi-year sport injury surveillance data. Injury rate is defined as the number of athletic injuries per 1,000 exposures resulting from both time loss and non-time loss (at least one day of missed practice/competition) injuries. Table 7 has been revised to provide the most up to date time loss injury risk data.

Tx/I = Treatments/Injury: The Tx/I is intended to characterize each sport on the basis of time devoted to the ongoing treatment and rehabilitation of the injured student-athlete. This value provides as estimate of the volume of care that is required to manage injuries on an ongoing basis and to restore an athlete to full activity after time loss injury. Hence, the Tx/I reflects the average number of reported treatments provided per injury for that particular sport. Tx/I represents the aggregate care provided for both time loss and non-time loss injuries (Powell & Dompier, 2003).

Base HCI: To determine an index of total health care load, IR and Tx/I indices were multiplied to provide an estimate of the relative workload for that

236

sport. Each value was then normalized to a relative 4-point scale, with 0 representing no risk/demand and 4 representing the highest risk/demand. To determine the maximum risk (value of 4), the IR*Tx/I recorded for each sport was divided by the highest IR*Tx/I recorded for any one sport where sufficient representative data was available (i.e. women's basketball).

$$\frac{\text{Aggregate IR*Tx/I}}{528 (= \text{max IR*Tx/I recorded})} \ (\text{x } 4) = \text{Base Health Care Index/ Sport}$$

Adjustments to Base Health Care Index Based on Actual Athlete Exposures (Table 2)

The base HCI is calculated on injury and treatment rates per 1,000 exposures. However, the actual number of athlete exposures (thus injuries encountered) can vary considerably between sports, depending on squad size (# of athletes) and the actual number of days engaged in activity (length of season). In order to accurately reflect the potential injury risk and treatment demands for a particular sport, an estimate of the total athlete exposures for that sport should be calculated.

1. Calculating Total Athlete Exposures (Column E): An exposure is one athlete participating in one coach-directed session involving physical activity. Hence, the base HCI must be adjusted for the actual number of athletes and days of activity anticipated for each sport season.

Total Days Engaged in Physical Activity (Table 2, Column C): Depending on competitive division and sport, the number of days athletes are actually engaged in practice and/or competition may differ (e.g. safety exception sports, non-traditional seasons, etc). In order to accurately determine injury risk exposure, an estimate of actual days each sport will be engaged during an average season is needed. This value should reflect both traditional, and where applicable, non-traditional seasons. Skill instruction sessions or other out of season activities requiring the presence of an athletic trainer or other health care professional should also be considered, depending on the perceived risk and the number of athletes associated with those activities. It should be noted that even if an athletic trainer is not present but there is a risk exposure (as allowed by recent rules changes) then the exposure must be counted.

Total Athletes per Sport Team (Table 2, Column D): Injury risk exposure is also based on total number of athletes engaged in any one activity (i.e. team size). While two sports may have similar season lengths, actual athlete exposures will be substantially lower for teams with small squad sizes compared to teams with larger squad sizes.

2. Adjusting Base HCI for Total Exposures (Table 2, Column G): The actual number of athlete exposures is divided by 1,000 (Column F) to determine the factor by which the base HCI should be multiplied.

Since the base HCI is founded on injuries per 1,000 exposure, dividing the actual # of exposures in Column E allows one to calculate the actual "anticipated risk" for that sport. The adjusted HCI (Column G) therefore provides an estimate of health care load for each sport based on the number and severity of injuries one would expect to encounter in a given season.

3. Adjusting HCI for Active Time of Sport Per Year (Column I): Based on the number of allowable days of activity for each sport, no sport is exposed to the risk of injury represented in the adjusted HCI year

---

Examples:

Division 1 football, which allows 105 regular season practice days and 15 days for spring practice, is active a total of 120 days per academic year. If the team roster includes 100 athletes, the total number of athlete exposures is:

$$120 \text{ days X } 100 \text{ athletes} = 12,000 \text{ TAE}$$

Example only. If football team requires more coverage based on exposure, increase the number of days, eg. summer conditioning.

Women's gymnastics, a safety exception sport, is allowed to participate year round and will have more practice days (144) per academic year. However, given the smaller squad size (eg. 10 athletes), women's gymnastics will have far fewer total athletes exposures per year:

$$144 \text{ days X } 10 \text{ athletes} = 1,440 \text{ TAE}$$

Formula:
Base HCI (Column B) X TAE/1,000 (Colmun F) = Adjusted HCI (Column G)

Examples:

If men's football has 12,000 exposures per season that means the number of exposures is 12 times greater than what is reflected in the base HCI. Thus, potential for injury (and associated medical care for those injuries) is 12 times greater. To account for the anticipated volume of injury and treatment for that sport, the following adjustments are made to the base HCI:

$$3.0 \text{ (Base HCI) X } 12 \text{ (Exposure Modifier)} = 36 \text{ Adjusted HCI}$$

If women's golf fields 10 athletes, only minor adjustments are needed to base HCI to account for the actual exposures associated with that sport:

$$1.0 \text{ (Base HCI) X } 1.3 \text{ (Exposure Modifier)} = 1.3 \text{ Adjusted HCI}$$

round. The health care demands calculated for that sport must primarily reflect what can be expected while the sport is actively engaged in traditional and non-traditional season activities. To appropriately adjust for inactive periods, the HCI is divided by the proportion of the year that the sport is active. For simplicity, this adjustment has been standardized at 50% for the academic year. This standard proportion is based on: (1) a conservative estimate of the number of allowable active days for each sport (~120-144 days) in a 10-month athletic calendar (10 months @ 4 weeks x 6 work days/week = 240 days), and (2) the assumption that full-time health care staff are able to care for two high risk sport teams in a given year (providing no significant overlap in seasons exists). Although it can be argued that the treatment of injuries continues throughout the year, the potential for an athlete to sustain an injury is limited to the actual days of activity.

Other Adjustments Based on Ancillary Staff Responsibilities

Formula:
Adjusted HCI (Column G) X % of Year (Column H)= Adjusted HCI/Year (Column I)

1. Travel: Traveling with an individual team removes a health care provider from the institution, which reduces the health care resources available to other student-athletes during that time period. This must be accounted for when determining the overall health care provider load. To more accurately reflect the impact of travel on athlete health care, this adjustment has been revised to represent the proportion of anticipated travel days for each staff member in a given academic year. Based on a 12 HCU load per staff member and a 10-month athletic calendar (240 work days), one HCU is assigned for every 20 days of anticipated staff travel per academic year:

2. Administrative Duties: A variety of administrative duties and responsibilities can remove the health care provider from direct athlete care during part of the workday. This time must be accounted for when determining the total health care load of the institution (see Table 2, final totals), as well as the total health care load for each full-time health care provider (i.e., 12 units). Theoretically, if an administrative duty is assigned a value of 3, that duty

Formula:

Administrative Duties	*Health Care Units*
25% of total work time	3 units
16% of total work time	2 units
8% of total work time	1 unit
<8% of total work time	.5 unit

should consume approximately 25% of one's time (e.g., 1½ days per week, 1 week per month, etc). As a guideline, the following table is provided:

The following list, although not comprehensive, identifies examples of administrative duties to be considered:

- *Budget*
- *Pre-participation Physical*
- *Insurance*
- *Medical Records and Injury Reporting*
- *Coordination of Student Workers*
- *OSHA*
- *Staff Education*
- *Special Assistance Fund*
- *Computer Systems*
- *Classroom Instruction*
- *Facility Maintenance*
- *Drug Testing*
- *Scheduling*
- *Head Athletic Trainer*
- *Purchasing*
- *Clinical Supervision and Instruction of Athletic Training Students*
- *Team Travel Arrangements*
- *Athlete Education*

Formula:
240 work days per year/12 HCU per staff member = 1 HCU per 20 travel days

5 travel days = .25 HCU
10 travel days = .50 HCU
15 travel days = .75 HCU

Example (Table 3):
If an athletic trainer travels with women's basketball an estimated 30 days per season, 1.5 HCUs are added to the total health care index for that sport.

4.0 HCI/Year (Column 1)+ 1.5 HCU for travel (Column F) = 5.5 HCU (Column H)

3. Other factors: Additional factors such as the number and location of full-service athletic training facilities, location of practice and competition venues (relative to each other, distance from the athletic treatment facilities), and geographic locale (i.e., distance from emergency medical services/hospital care) may either reduce or increase health care demands. Institutions should consider these factors and make appropriate adjustments in the total health care load, based on sound decisions of how to best handle their individual medical care coverage needs.

Recommendations and Guidelines for Health Care Providers

The following recommendations and guidelines are provided to assist institutions in making appropriate decisions for onsite medical coverage of sport activities. These decisions should be based on the potential for serious or catastrophic injury, not on gender, sport profile or level of competition. Hence, primary factors for determining onsite practice or game coverage, and the level of qualifications of the health care member providing that coverage, are overall injury rate and the potential for catastrophic injury for that sport.

Example:
If two venues are within 3-5 minutes* of each other, one qualified provider (based on the qualifications required for the sport with the highest base unit/risk as defined in the next section) could cover both venues. Individual factors may necessitate adjjustments in the sport health care unit derived from the system worksheet.
*A 3-5 minute response time is recommended based on current emergency standards

---

IR = Injury Rate Index: The IR Index classifies each sport on the potential for injury, based on the aggregate injury rate values presented in Table 1. The relative risk of each sport (4-point scale rating) is then combined with the risk for catastrophic injury.

CI = Catastrophic Index: The CI classifies each sport on the basis of its potential for life-threatening situations, spinal cord injury, major head injury or permanent disability. The catastrophic injury index provides a separate measure for determining the level of qualified medical personnel required at practice and/or competition. Catastrophic injury rates were obtained from the most recent report from the National Center for Catastrophic Sports Injury Research. The relative risk of CI for each sport was then determined by converting these risk values to a 4-point scale using 10 injuries per 100,000 participants (i.e. football) as the highest IR recorded (4) for any one sport (Table 3).

It is recommended that personnel providing medical coverage of institutionally sponsored athletic activities and treatment facilities possess the following qualifications:

A. NATA recommends all personnel who are associated with medical coverage for intercollegiate sports participation shall be at least minimally qualified as stated in Guideline 1 c-7 of the *NCAA Sports Medicine Handbook*.

"Certification in cardiopulmonary resuscitation techniques (CPR), first aid, and prevention of disease transmission (as outlined by OSHA guidelines) should be required for all athletics personnel associated with practices, competitions, skills instruction and strength and conditioning. New staff engaged in these activities should comply with these rules within six months of employment." Additionally this training shall include certification in AED usage. Athletic activities where an institution decides a certified athletic trainer need not be in attendance then one individual with the qualifications above must be present.

B. Sports that are considered lower risk (combined IR and CI less than 4.0) and sports-related activities that include strength/conditioning, individual skill sessions and voluntary summer workouts must have an individual physically present who possesses the minimum qualifications as specified in A above. Based on the values in Table 3, the following sports are considered to be of low risk:

> Baseball
> Crew (M&W)
> Cross Country (M&W)
> Fencing (M&W)
> Golf (M&W)
> Outdoor Track (M&W)
> Softball
> Swimming (M&W)
> Tennis (M&W)
> Water Polo (M&W)

C. Sports with moderate risk (combined IR and CI of 4.0 - 5.0 or CI of 3.0) should have a certified athletic trainer, or other designated person with the designated minimal qualifications (Recommendation A), physically present. If no athletic trainer is present, a certified athletic trainer must be able to respond within 3-5 minutes. Based on the values in Table 3, the following sports are considered to be of moderate risk:

> Basketball (W)
> Diving (M&W)
> Field Hockey
> Indoor Track (M&W)
> Lacrosse (M&W)
> Soccer (M&W)
> Volleyball (M&W)

D. Sports with increased risk (combined IRE and CI of 6.0 or greater or CI of 4.0) should have a certified athletic trainer physically present for all practices. Based on the values in Table 3, the following sports are considered to be of increased risk:

> Basketball (M)
> Football
> Gymnastics (M&W)
> Ice Hockey (M&W)
> Skiing
> Wrestling

E. Any sport with a combined IR and CI of 3.0 or greater should have a certified athletic trainer physically present during all home competitions. While the task force encourages the physical presence of certified athletic trainers at all home competitions, competition coverage of sports with lower unit values (e.g., golf, outdoor track) will be left to institutional discretion.

F. A certified athletic trainer must directly supervise all full-service athletic training facilities during institution declared hours of service.

G. Visiting teams and athletes shall be provided with equitable access to health care.

H. NATA supports the implementation of NATA guideline that states each institution shall have a venue-specific emergency care plan in place that includes:

1) Each institution or organization that sponsors athletic activities must have a written emergency plan. The emergency plan should be comprehensive and practical, yet flexible enough to adapt to any emergency situation.

2) Emergency plans must be written documents and should be distributed to certified athletic trainers, team and attending physicians, athletic
240

training students, institutional and organizational safety personnel, institutional and organizational administrators, and coaches. The emergency plan should be developed in consultation with local emergency medical services personnel.

3) An emergency plan for athletics identifies the personnel involved in carrying out the emergency plan and outlines the qualifications of those executing the plan. Sports medicine professionals, officials, and coaches should be trained in automatic external defibrillation, cardiopulmonary resuscitation, first aid, and prevention of disease transmission.

4) The emergency plan should specify the equipment needed to carry out the tasks required in the event of an emergency. In addition, the emergency plan should outline the location of the emergency equipment. Further, the equipment available should be appropriate to the level of training of the personnel involved.

5) Establishment of a clear mechanism for communication to appropriate emergency care service providers and identification of the mode of transportation for the injured participant are critical elements of an emergency plan.

6) The emergency plan should be specific to the activity venue. That is, each activity site should have a defined emergency plan that is derived from the overall institutional or organizational policies on emergency planning.

7) Emergency plans should incorporate the emergency care facilities to which the injured individual will be taken. Emergency receiving facilities should be notified in advance of scheduled events and contests. Personnel from the emergency receiving facilities should be included in the development of the emergency plan for the institution or organization.

8) The emergency plan specifies the necessary documentation supporting the implementation and evaluation of the emergency plan. This documentation should identify responsibility for documenting actions taken during the emergency, evaluation of the emergency response, and

institutional personnel training.

9) The emergency plan should be reviewed and rehearsed annually, although more frequent review and rehearsal may be necessary. The results of these reviews and rehearsals should be documented and should indicate whether the emergency plan was modified, with further documentation reflecting how the plan was changed.

10) All personnel involved with the organization and sponsorship of athletic activities share a professional responsibility to provide for the emergency care of an injured person, including the development and implementation of an emergency plan.

11) All personnel involved with the organization and sponsorship of athletic activities share a legal duty to develop, implement, and evaluate an emergency plan for all sponsored athletic activities.

12) The emergency plan should be reviewed by the administration and legal counsel of the sponsoring organization or institution.

CONCLUSION

The health and safety of the student-athlete should be paramount to all involved in sports at the collegiate level. In an effort to safeguard the student-athlete, the National Athletic Trainers' Association has issued these recommendations as guidelines to provide appropriate medical coverage. While these recommendations represent an appropriate level of care, institutions of all sizes and/or divisions are encouraged to provide enhanced care as consistent with the stated philosophy of their institution.

APPENDIX A

System Worksheet and Narrative

Application of the Health Care Unit System

NATA's Recommendations and Guidelines for Appropriate Medical Coverage of Intercollegiate Athletics (Revised) offer college and university health care providers a system by which they can evaluate their current level of coverage for student-athletes. These recommendations have been created for the safety of student-athletes competing at the collegiate level. To that end, certified athletic trainers in these settings must have a thorough understanding of the recommendations before implementing the system.

Constants: The following remain constant throughout the system regardless of the size of your program or the level of competition:

➢ The estimated health care load for one athletic trainer is 12 health care units (HCU). The concept is constant however, the institution may adjust the load as they see fit.

➢ Each sport has an assigned base Health Care Index (HCI) value derived from injury rates (IR) for both time loss and non-time loss injuries, and the treatments associated with those injuries (Table 1).

➢ Each sport has an assigned base HCI value to represent the risk of catastrophic injury (Table 3).

➢ Full-service athletic training rooms should have a certified athletic trainer present during institution-declared hours of operation.

Variables: Variable items affecting HCU totals that can be added (or omitted) at the discretion of the institution are:

➢ Travel

➢ Administrative Duties

Consider using these variables as negotiation points. For instance, after having applied the system at your institution, you determine that two additional certified athletic trainers (24 health care units) are needed in order to deliver appropriate medical coverage. Your administrator states that, at this time, you will only receive one additional staff member. You can suggest reducing the length/vigor of non-traditional seasons, reducing squad size, eliminating travel requirements or reassigning time-consuming administrative duties to other areas. This would reduce total health care units, thus ensuring appropriate medical coverage.

Application of the System

1. The Health Care Index for each sport is listed on the System Worksheet (Table 4), which will be used to calculate the total health care needs of your institution. Disregard those sports not offered at your institution. (Refer to Table 2 for the examples provided.)

2. The load for an institution is not only based on the sports offered and their respective HCI, but on the actual athlete exposures, which is a function of squad size and the number of practice/competitions. In Column C place the number of days (practices/competitions) for a given team. This number should reflect the number of days team members are active, both during the traditional and non-traditional seasons. (Depending on the perceived risk of injury, institutions may also wish to account for skill instruction sessions). In Column D place the number of athletes on the roster for that team. Column E represents the total number of athlete exposures for a sport, which is derived by multiplying exposures (Column C) by the number of athletes (Column D).

> *Example:*
>
> *Women's soccer practices/competes for 132 days (based on allowable traditional + non-traditional practice days for NCAA Division I soccer) and has 30 athletes. Therefore, women's soccer has 3,960 total exposures*

3. Next, divide the total exposures (Column E) by 1,000 to obtain the exposure modifier and then place this value in Column F.

> *Example:*
>
> *From above, women's soccer has 3,960 total exposures, so the modifier is 3.96 when divided by 1,000 (rounded to 4.0 in the Sample Worksheet).*

4. The value in Column E now represents the HCI modifier for that sport at that institution. The value in Column F is then multiplied by the HCI in Column B to calculate the actual health care load for that sport. The institution adjusted HCI value is then placed in Column G.

> *Example:*
>
> *The exposure modifier for women's soccer from Column F is 4.0. This means that 4 times the number of exposures will actually occur in this sport than what is calculated in the base HCI. The base HCI for women's soccer (Column B) is therefore multiplied by this value (Column F), to obtain the adjusted HCI for that sport (2.6 x 4.0 =13.9). This value is then placed in Column G.*

5. Because the number of allowable participation days prevents sports from being actively engaged throughout the entire year, the unit values in Column G are too high to reflect the true health care demands of that sport. The assumption is made that the health care professional is providing care for that sport's athletes for half of the year. Therefore, the value in Column G is divided by 50% (Column H) resulting in a new adjusted HCI/year (Column I). (The proportion in Column G should be adjusted by individual institutions if they anticipate that the sport will be activity engaged more or less than 50% of the year.)

> *Example:*
>
> *Continuing with our example, women's soccer has an adjusted HCI of 13.9. Half of 13.9 is 6.9 HCI/year.*

6. The last adjustment for each sport is to add in anticipated travel responsibilities. One (1) unit is assigned for every 20 days of travel or a portion thereof.

> *The adjusted HCI/year for women's soccer is 6.9. The team travels 20 days, so the new value for women's soccer is 7.9*

7. Add all adjusted health care units (Column K) to determine a SUBTOTAL of health care units for the institution.

8. Next list administrative duties carried out by the health care staff and assign each a value based on the time requirement for that duty. Remember, for an administrative duty to receive 3 units, it must account for 25% of the athletic trainer's total work time in a given year. (1 unit = 8.33%)

9. Add all administrative units together.

10. Add the administrative units to the to health care unit subtotal. This number represents the TOTAL health care units expended by the institution.

11. Divide the total health care units by 12 (the recommended allowable load for one athletic trainer). This value represents the number of full-time AT equivalents needed to provide appropriate medical coverage for student-athletes at the institution.

Table 1: Base Health Care Index by Sport

Sport	IR	TX/I	IR*TX/I	HCI
Baseball	19.3	11.5	222	1.7
Basketball-M	29.3	11.0	322	2.4
Basketball-W	32.4	16.3	528	4.0
Crew-M	7.2	12.9	93	0.7
Crew-W	22.0	13.0	286	2.2
Cross Country-M	21.7	8.6	187	1.4
Cross Country-W	23.7	9.4	223	1.7
Fencing-M	15.7	16.2	254	1.9
Fencing-W	24.1	12.6	304	2.3
Field Hockey	34.8	10.8	376	2.8
Football	42.5	9.7	412	3.1
Golf-M	6.5	9.8	64	0.5
Golf-W	13.8	11.0	152	1.2
Gymnastics-M	29.0	16.8	487	3.7
Gymnastics-W†	48.1	27.9	1342	4.0
Ice Hockey-M	33.9	7.2	244	1.8
Ice Hockey-W	12.3	10.7	132	1.0
Indoor Track-M	31.9	11.4	364	2.8
Indoor Track-W	32.3	11.8	381	2.9
Lacrosse-M	23.9	10.0	239	1.8
Lacrosse-W	27.9	11.8	329	2.5
Outdoor Track-M	18.3	8.0	146	1.1
Outdoor Track-W	21.1	7.1	150	1.1
Soccer-M	35.0	10.7	375	2.8
Soccer-W	42.3	11.2	474	3.6
Softball	28.1	10.7	301	2.3
Swim & Diving -M	12.8	7.6	97	0.7
Swim & Diving-W	15.5	9.5	147	1.1
Tennis-M	21.7	9.3	202	1.5
Tennis-W	24.5	10.7	262	2.0
Volleyball-M†	35.0	22.7	795	4.0
Volleyball-W	36.8	12.6	464	3.5
Water Polo-M	12.0	18.3	220	1.7
Water Polo-W	22.2	7.9	175	1.3
Wrestling	41.8	9.1	380	2.9

†To determine the maximum risk (value of 4), the IR*Tx/I recorded for each sport was divided by the highest IR*Tx/I recorded for any one sport where sufficient representative data was available (i.e., women's basketball). Sports indicated by an (†) recorded higher IR*Tx/I, but were based on limited data.

Table 2: Sample Worksheet – Adjustments to Base Health Care Index

A	B	C	D	E	F	G	H	I	J	K
Sport	Base HCI (Table 1)	#Days/ Season†	#Athletes/ Team	Total Athlete Exposures (C*D)	Exposure Modifier (E/1,000)	Adjusted HCI (B*F)	% of Year	Adjusted HCI/Yr	Travel (20 days = 1 HCU)	Admin Duties
Baseball	1.7	132	30	3960	4.0	6.7	50%	3.3	1.5	
Basketball – M	2.4	132	15	1980	2.0	4.8	50%	2.4	1.5	
Basketball – W	4.0	132	15	1980	2.0	7.9	50%	4.0	1.5	
X-Country – M	1.4	144	10	1440	1.4	2.0	50%	1.0		
X-Country – W	1.7	144	10	1440	1.4	2.4	50%	1.2		
Field Hockey	2.8	132	25	3300	3.3	9.4	50%	4.7	0.5	
Football	3.1	120	100	12000	12.0	37.5	50%	18.7	0.5	
Gymnastics – W	4.0	144	10	1440	1.4	5.8	50%	2.9	0.5	
Lacrosse – M	1.8	132	30	3960	4.0	7.2	50%	3.6		
Outdoor Track – M	1.1	132	40	5280	5.3	5.9	50%	2.9		
Outdoor Track – W	1.1	132	40	5280	5.3	6.0	50%	3.0		
Rowing – M	0.7	132	50	6600	6.6	4.6	50%	2.3		
Soccer – M	3.6	132	30	3960	4.0	11.2	50%	5.6	1.0	
Soccer – W	2.8	132	30	3960	4.0	14.2	50%	7.1	1.0	
Softball	2.3	132	25	3300	3.3	7.5	50%	3.8	1.5	
Volleyball – W	3.5	132	15	1980	2.0	7.0	50%	3.5	1.0	
Wrestling	2.9	132	30	3960	4.0	11.4	50%	5.7	0.5	
TOTALS								75.8	11.0	

TOTAL HEALTH CARE UNITS   87
(Add all units in Column I-K)

TOTAL FULL TIME ATs   7.25
(Total Heath Care Units)
            12

†Figures represent total number of allowable practice days for both in and out of season for NCAA Division I. Individual institutional values should be adjusted based on competitive level and the extent of both traditional and non-traditional season activities.

Table 3. Injury and Catastrophic Risk Indices for Medical Coverage

Sport	CI Index (Table 11)	IR Index (Table 1&7)	CI + IR	Coverage Category
Baseball	1	2	3	B
Basketball-M	4	3	7	D
Basketball-W	1	4	5	C
Crew-M	1	1	2	B
Crew-W	1	2	3	B
Cross Country-M	1	2	3	B
Cross Country-W	1	2	3	B
Fencing-M	1	2	3	B
Fencing-W	1	2	3	B
Field Hockey	1	3	4	C
Football	4	4	8	D
Golf-M	1	1	2	B
Golf-W	1	1	2	B
Gymnastics-M	4	4	8	D
Gymnastics-W	4	4	8	D
Ice Hockey-M	4	2	6	D
Ice Hockey-W	4	1	5	C
Indoor Track-M	1	3	4	C
Indoor Track-W	1	3	4	C
Lacrosse-M	3	2	5	C
Lacrosse-W	1	3	4	C
Outdoor Track-M	1	1	2	B
Outdoor Track-W	1	1	2	B
Soccer-M	1	3	4	C
Soccer-W	1	4	5	C
Softball	1	2	3	B
Swimming-M	2	1	3	B
Swimming-W	1	2	3	B
Tennis-M	1	2	3	B
Tennis-W	1	2	3	B
Volleyball-M	1	4	5	C
Volleyball-W	1	4	5	C
Water Polo-M	2	1	3	B
Water Polo-W	1	2	3	B
Wrestling	2	4	6	D

Table 4: System Worksheet - Adjustments to Base Health Care Units

A	B	C	D	E	F	G	H	I	J	K
Sport	Base HCI (Table 1)	# Days/ Season	# Athletes/ Team	Total Athlete Exposures (C*D)	Exposure Modifier (E/1,000)	Adjusted HCI (B*F)	% of Year	Adjusted HCI/Yr	Travel (20 days = 1 HCU)	Final Adjusted HCU (I + J)
Baseball	1.6									
Basketball-M	2.4									
Basketball-W	4.0									
Cheerleading										
Crew-M	0.7									
Crew-W	2.1									
Cross Country-M	1.4									
Cross Country-W	1.6									
Fencing-M	1.9									
Fencing-W	1.2									
Field Hockey	2.8									
Football	3.0									
Golf-M	0.5									
Golf-W	1.1									
Gymnastics-M	3.8									
Gymnastics-W	4.0									
Ice Hockey-M	1.9									
Ice Hockey-W	0.9									
Indoor Track-M	2.7									
Indoor Track-W	2.8									
Lacrosse-M	1.8									
Lacrosse-W	2.5									
Novice Crew	1.9									
Outdoor Track-M	1.1									
Outdoor Track-W	1.1									
Soccer-M	2.6									
Soccer-W	3.5									
Softball	2.2									
Swimming-M	0.7									
Swimming-W	1.1									
Tennis-M	1.5									
Tennis-W	1.9									
Volleyball-M	4.0									
Volleyball-W	3.4									
Water Polo-M	1.6									
Water Polo-W	1.3									
Wrestling	2.8									
					Total Health Care Units (Add Column K)					
					Add Administrative Units					
					Total Units					
					Total ATs (Total Units ÷ 12)					

Table 7 (Revised 3/03). Comparative Multi-Sport Injury Rate Data (indicates the number of time loss injuries per 1,000 athlete exposures)

Sport	NCAA ISS (~1985-2002) Practice	NCAA ISS (~1985-2002) Game	NCAA ISS Aggregate Injury Rate†	Big Ten Conference (1995-2000)	AMCIA 2 Year Study (2000-2002)	Time Loss Injury Rate (Combined)
Baseball	2.1	6.1	3.2	4.9	3.5	3.9
Basketball - M	4.6	9.2	5.5	5.0	6.0	5.5
Basketball - W	4.4	10.0	5.6	3.7	6.1	5.1
Crew - M					1.4	1.4
Crew - W					4.7	4.7
Cross Country - M					3.8	3.8
Cross Country - W					3.3	3.3
Cheerleading						
Diving						
Fencing - M					4.8	4.8
Fencing - W					6.2	6.2
Field Hockey	4.1	8.5	5.0	4.4		4.7
Football	4.1	36.0	6.7	9.5	9.8	8.7
Football (Spring)	9.5	19.3	10.5			10.5
Golf – M					1.9	1.9
Golf – W					2.5	2.5
Gymnastics - M	5.5	5.5	5.5	5.9	8.9	6.8
Gymnastics - W	7.5	18.5	8.4	6.4	8.5	7.8
Ice Hockey - M	2.2	17.6	5.9		8.6	7.3
Ice Hockey - W	2.8	13.6	5.6		4.1	4.9
Indoor Track – M					5.2	5.2
Indoor Track – W					4.1	4.1
Lacrosse - M	3.7	14.6	5.5		7.6	6.6
Lacrosse - W	3.6	7.5	4.3		5.1	4.7
Outdoor Track – M					3.7	3.7
Outdoor Track – W					3.1	3.1
Skiing - M						
Skiing - W						
Soccer - M	4.7	20.2	7.8	4.8	7.7	7.8
Soccer - W	5.7	17.6	8.3	5.4	6.4	7.4
Softball	3.2	4.9	3.9	3.3	4.1	3.8
Swimming - M					1.6	1.6
Swimming - W					2.1	2.1
Tennis - M					2.6	2.6
Tennis - W					4.2	4.3
Volleyball - M					7.5	7.5
Volleyball - W	4.5	4.8	4.6	2.9	4.2	4.4
Water Polo - M					2.3	2.3
Water Polo - W					1.5	1.5
Wrestling	6.9	29.7	9.4	9.3	9.0	9.3

NCAA ISS data based on injuries recorded from the start of individual sport surveillance through the 2001-02 seasons (http://www1.ncaa.org/membership/ed_outreach/health-safety/iss/index.html). Big Ten data based on time loss injuries recorded from 1995-96 through 1999-2000 seasons (Big Ten Conference, Sports Medicine Committee). AMCIA data based on the time loss and non-time loss injuries recorded for the 2000-01 through 2001-02 seasons (Powell & Dompier, In Review). †Aggregate NCAA injury rate for combined practice and games represent the weighted average (percentage of total exposures) of injuries attributed to practice vs. game. Proportions were calculated based on a representative season for that sport.

Table 11 (Revised 1/07). Catastrophic Index Based on Catastrophic Injury Rate Data by Gender and Sport. The CI Rate was converted to a 4-point scale by dividing each CI Rate by 10, then multiplying by a factor of 4 and rounding up to nearest full digit.

Sport	Injury Rate/ 100,000 Participants†	(IR/10)*4	AMCIA CI Index
Baseball	2.49	1.0	1
Basketball - M	8.94	3.6	4
Basketball - W	.35	0.1	1
Cross Country - M	.42	0.19	1
Cross Country - W	.00	0.0	1
Cheerleading‡	N/A	<4.0	4
Diving‡	3.23	1.3	2
Fencing	N/A		1
Field Hockey	1.56	0.6	1
Football	9.48	3.8	4
Golf – M	N/A		1
Golf – W	N/A		1
Gymnastics - M	27.98	<4.0	4
Gymnastics - W	8.7	<4.0	4
Ice Hockey - M	14.82	<4.0	4
Ice Hockey - W	8.43	<4.0	4
Lacrosse – M	7.14	2.87	3
Lacrosse – W	2.3	.92	1
Rifle	N/A		1
Rowing – M	N/A		1
Rowing – W	N/A		1
Skiing – M	6.54	2.6	3
Skiing – W	7.43	2.97	3
Soccer – M	1.35	.54	1
Soccer – W	1.56	.62	1
Softball	.00	0	1
Swimming - M	3.35	1.3	2
Swimming - W	.00	0	1
Tennis – M	.57	.23	1
Tennis – W	.56	.22	1
Track – M (Indoor/Outdoor)	1.23	.49	1
Track – W (Indoor/Outdoor)	.17	.07	1
Volleyball - M	.00	.00	1
Volleyball - W	.72	.29	1
Water Polo - M	4.39	1.76	3
Water Polo - W	.00	.00	1
Wrestling	2.55	1.02	2

†Data obtained from the most recent study of Mueller and Cantu[24] on athletes participating in college sports. Number of participants reflects the cumulative total number of participants since tracking began respective for each sport. ‡Cheerleading numbers are based on like sport (gymnastics) and diving ratings were derived from the pooled data of men's swimming.

Support Statement *NATA*

Support and Endorsement From Outside Groups

From the:

American Academy of Family Physicians

The AAFP encourages high schools to have, whenever possible, a National Athletic Trainers Association (NATA)-certified or registered/licensed athletic trainer as an integral part of the high school athletic program. (1989) (2007)

Copyright © 2008 American Academy of Family Physicians http://www.aafp.org/online/en/home/policy/policies/s/athletictrainhsathletes.html.

From the:

American Medical Association

Policy H-470.995
July 1998
H-470.995 Athletic (Sports) Medicine

The AMA believes that:

(1) the Board of Education and the Department of Health of the individual states should encourage that an adequate Athletic Medicine Unit be established in every school that mounts a sports program;

(2) the Athletic Medicine Unit should be composed of an allopathic or osteopathic physician director with unlimited license to practice medicine, an athletic health coordinator (preferably a NATABOC certified athletic trainer), and other necessary personnel;

(3) the duties of the Athletic Medicine Unit should be prevention of injury, the provision of medical care with the cooperation of the family's physician and others of the health care team of the community, and the rehabilitation of the injured;

(4) except in extreme emergencies, the selection of the treating physician is the choice of the parent or guardian and any directed referral therefore requires their consent;

(5) the Athletic Medicine Units should be required to submit complete reports of all injuries to a designated authority;

(6) medical schools, colleges, and universities should be urged to cooperate in establishing education programs for athletic health coordinators (NATABOC certified athletic trainers) as well as continuing medical education and graduate programs in Sports Medicine;

(7) high school administrators, athletic directors, and coaches to work with local physicians, medical societies, and medical specialty societies, as well as government officials and community groups to undertake appropriate measures to ensure funding to provide the services of a certified athletic trainer to all high school athletes; and

(8) not all high schools have the resources to procure the services of a certified athletic trainer and further recognizing that athletic trainers cannot be present at all practices and competitions, that the AMA encourage high school administrators and athletic directors to ensure that all coaches are appropriately trained in emergency first aid and basic life support.

(Res. 112, A-69; Reaffirmed: CLRPD Rep. C, A-89; Modified and Reaffirmed by Ref. Cmt. D, I-96; Amended and Appended by CSA Rep. 5, A-98)
References: Report of the Coucil on Scientific Affairs
CSA Report 5-A-98 Subject: Certified Athletic Trainers in Secondary Schools (Resolution 431, A-97)

From the:

American Academy of Pediatrics

The American Academy of Pediatrics endorses and accepts as its policy the National Athletic Trainers' Association guideline, *Lightning Safety for Athletics and Recreation*.

From the:

National Collegiate Athletic Association

The health and safety principle of the NCAA's constitution provides that it is the responsibility of each member institution to protect the health of, and provide a safe environment for, each of its participating student athletes.

In light of the lengthened playing seasons (regular, non-traditional seasons, vacation periods, summer months) and increased expectations on athletes regarding participation in practice times (weight lifting, conditioning, skill instruction), the NCAA Committee on Competitive Safeguards and Medical Aspects of Sports (CSMAS) recommends that NCAA institutions examine the adequateness of their sports medicine coverage. In particular, whether the increased time demands placed on certified athletic trainers reduces their ability to effectively provide high quality care to all student athletes.

At its June meeting, the CSMAS reviewed the National Athletic Trainers' Association (NATA) revised document "Recommendations and Guidelines for Appropriate Medical Coverage of Intercollegiate Athletics." The CSMAS encourages NCAA institutions to reference the NATA AMCIA in their assessment of the adequateness of their sports medicine coverage.

The addition of sports teams, non-traditional seasons, scrimmages outside of the regular season, skill instruction sessions, junior varsity teams and host coverage for championship events have added significant hours that are driving professionals away from athletic training. In addition, the highly competitive nature of today's athletics in all divisions require athletes to spend more time in treatment and rehabilitation of injuries rather than merely event coverage. Consequently, additional administrative duties are required in conjunction to these tasks, including educational programming, drug testing, medical record keeping and filing insurance claims.

The latest trends imply that certified athletic trainers are leaving the college setting or the profession as a whole due to the stress of the job from long hours, low pay, consecutive days without time off and high travel demands. Stress within the job setting can lead to fatigue, short tempers and impatience and is linked to depression, anxiety, weight gain and cardiovascular disease, all of which can adversely effect the adequacy and quality of sports medicine provided to NCAA student athletes.

All persons participating in, or associated with, NCAA intercollegiate athletics share the responsibility to protect student athlete health and safety through appropriate medical coverage of its sports and supporting activities.

About the
National Athletic Trainers' Association

Athletic trainers are unique health care professionals who specialize in the prevention, diagnosis, treatment and rehabilitation of injuries and illnesses. The National Athletic Trainers' Association represents and supports over 30,000 members of the athletic training profession. NATA advocates for equal access to athletic trainers for patients and clients of all ages and supports H.R. 1846. NATA members adhere to a code of ethics. *www. nata.org*

Attention Students!

Kick start your athletic training career by joining the NATA now and receive **$20 off** your first full year of dues*.

Fill out the form below, send it to the national office and we'll e-mail you a special code good for a $20 discount on your membership dues…It's that easy! Once you join the association, you'll have access to all of the great services and programs NATA has to offer. What are you waiting for?

Name: _____   E-mail: _____

Address: _____   Phone: _____

City: _____ State: _____ Zip code: _____

Date of birth: _____   Last four digits of SSN: _____

Undergraduate institution: _____

Mail completed coupon to:
NATA Membership Department
2952 Stemmons Freeway, Ste. 200
Dallas, TX 75247
800.879.6282

* Discount applies to new members only.